A LOVING TESTIMONY

Other Books by Lesléa Newman

Novels

Fat Chance
Good Enough to Eat
In Every Laugh a Tear

Short Story Collections

Every Woman's Dream
A Letter to Harvey Milk
Secrets

Poetry Collections

Just Looking for My Shoes
Love Me Like You Mean It
Sweet Dark Places

Nonfiction

SomeBODY To Love: A Guide to Loving the Body You Have
Writing from the Heart: Inspiration and Exercises for Women Who Want to Write

Anthologies

The Femme Mystique
Eating Our Hearts Out: Personal Accounts of Women's Relationship to Food
*Bubbe Meisehs By Shayneh Maidelehs: An Anthology of Poetry by
Jewish Granddaughters about Our Grandmothers*

Children's Books

Belinda's Bouquet
Felicia's Favorite Story
Gloria Goes to Gay Pride
Heather Has Two Mommies
Saturday Is Pattyday
Too Far Away to Touch

A LOVING TESTIMONY

REMEMBERING LOVED ONES
LOST TO AIDS

AN ANTHOLOGY EDITED BY LESLÉA NEWMAN

The Crossing Press
Freedom, CA 95019

Copyright © 1995 by Lesléa Newman
Cover design by Amy Sibiga
Book design by Victoria May
Printed in the U.S.A.

Library of Congress Cataloging-in-Publication Data

A loving testimony : remembering loved ones lost to AIDS / edited by
   Lesléa Newman.
      p. cm.
   Includes bibliographical references (p.).
   ISBN 0-89594-752-8
      1. AIDS (Disease)—Patients—United States—Literary collections.
   2. AIDS (Disease)—Patients—United States—Biography.
   3. Friendship—United States—Literary collections. 4. Family—
   United States—Literary collections. 5. American literature—20th cen-
   tury. 6. Grief—Literary collections. I. Newman, Lesléa.
   PS509.A43L68 1995
   810.8'0356--dc20   95-2627
                                                       CIP

Credits

"Lovers" by Maureen Brady was first published under the title "The Calling" in the anthology *Lovers*, edited by Amber Coverdale Sumrall, Crossing Press, 1992.

"Wool" by C.A. Carmel first appeared in *Christopher Street*, March 1994.

"Barry and Me and the Angels" by Louie Crew first appeared in *Christianity & Crisis*, March 2, 1992.

"David Lemieux" by Denise Duhamel is reprinted from *Smile!* (Warm Spring Press, 1993).

"Author, Brother, Hero, Barosaurus" by Marny Hall originally appeared in *Lambda Book Report*, Vol. 3, No. 9, March/April 1993.

"AIDS: Notes of a Survivor" by David Israels first appeared in *The San Francisco Bay Guardian*, Vol. 23, No. 29, April 26, 1989.

"AIDS Death #54,911" by Robert Kaplan was originally published in *Beyond Definition: New Gay and Lesbian Writing from San Francisco* (Manic d Press, August 1994).

"When My Friend Died of AIDS" by Margaret McMullan originally appeared in *Glamour*, March 1991.

"No More Poems For The Dead" by Victor Mingovits originally appeared in *The Missoula Independent*, Volume 3, No. 2, August 28, 1992.

"Birds" by J. Fraser Nelson first appeared in *PW Alive* (Minneapolis, MN).

"Charisma" by Marcy Sheiner appeared in *Five Fingers Review*, 8/9, San Francisco, CA, 1990.

"In the Room the Women Come and Go" by Deborah Shouse first appeared in *Art & Understanding*, Volume 1, No. 4, July-August 1992.

Photo Credits

Scott Caldwell and Kathryn Udevitz Hulings by James R. Hulings, "Incomplete"

Kenneth Dawson by Wendy Jane Workman, "Ken"

Blare Feulner & Nels Highberg by Deborah Garza, "What I Did on My Summer Vacation"

Keith Gann by Michael Kiesaw Moore, "To Pluto's House: An AIDS Odyssey"

Bart Hammond by William McBride, "Angels on Your Pillow"

Rachel Ellyn Hertzberg-Thurman by Marcia Rose, "Dearest Rachel"

Dennis Janis by Nina Haritos, "Dennis"

Raymond Navarro by Marilyn Humphries, "To Ray Ray, Little Raymond, Mijo"

Duane Puryear by Scott Lokitz, "Passover Wish"

Marco Vassi by Annie Sprinkle, "Tested"

TABLE OF CONTENTS

For Keith Gardner

INTRODUCTION

As I sit down to write the introduction to *A Loving Testimony*, I find myself restlessly wandering about my study, distracted by my neighbor packing her car outside my window, the pile of mail waiting to be answered, the bookshelves that need dusting. I force myself to sit down at my writing table where I am faced with what I don't want to see, never wanted to see, and must see every day for the rest of my life: a photo of my friend, Gerard Rizza, taken shortly before he died of AIDS at thirty-two years of age. No wonder I don't want to write this introduction. When it is over, Gerard will still be dead. And I will have finished another book that Gerard will never read.

Gerard and I met in Boulder, Colorado, in 1979, two out-of-place New Yorkers amid the mountains and the cowboys. His Staten Island accent was like a breath of fresh air out there among all those positive ions. We became roommates and quickly developed the instant intimacy that forms when two people share toothpaste and secret dreams. Both of us wanted to be famous writers someday; we even had hopes of winning the Yale Series of Younger Poets award. Well, both of us can scratch that ambition off our lists: Gerard is no longer writing poetry and I am no longer "younger." That summer we did give our first poetry reading together, though, which was a step in the right direction.

That summer Gerard also fell in love. It was inevitable, as he was the most beautiful man I'd ever seen. Heads, both male and female turned 180 degrees whenever we walked down the street, and I knew they weren't turning for me. Gerard knew it, too, and didn't help matters any by wearing shorts so short they should have been illegal, or jeans so tight they left nothing to the imagination.

Gerard fell in love and he fell hard. Soon he and his beau moved back to New York, and after a year I followed. New York City became our playground and we took in poetry readings, experimental theatre, and other entertainment listed on the "Cheap Thrills" page of the *Village Voice*. I lived in the city for a year and then moved to New England. Gerard and I stayed in touch with birthday and holiday cards and the occasional midnight phone chat. He'd call to tell me he'd just had a poem accepted for publication in *The World*, or that he was giving a reading at the St. Marks Poetry Project. Always pursuing his dream.

Time passed and our contact became spotty. We were both very busy, and who knew we didn't have forever? I called Gerard whenever I went to New York, but he was never in, and he never returned my calls. I figured he was busy. I didn't know he was busy fighting for his life.

And then one day when I was in New York, I called Gerard and he answered the phone. His voice sounded woozy, like he was on drugs (he was, but not the kind I was thinking of). He told me he'd love to see me, "but," he said, "mobility's a big problem right now." Instantly I knew what he was talking about and I rushed right over. And though I knew Gerard had AIDS, nothing prepared me for what I was about to see.

Gerard, whose long-legged stride was impossible to keep up with, whose hands moved a mile a minute when he talked, which was all the time, whose eyes widened and smile deepened whenever he saw anyone or anything of interest, lay in bed motionless except for the tears that began to stream out of his left eye when I walked into the room. I had to move his legs over to make room to sit next to him on the bed. There are no words to describe what he looked like (thin and gaunt don't even come close). There is no language to describe what remained of his beautiful face. And there is no way to describe how I felt that day, knowing that even though we made a date to go to the St. Mark's Bookstore next time I was in town, I knew there would be no next time. Next time I was in town my friend would be dead. And there was nothing I could do.

When I went to Gerard's memorial service months later, I was surprised that except for his mother, his sister and one friend, I was the person there who knew him the longest. People spoke about how brave he was and what a fighter he was, and while that was all true, I wanted someone to speak about how funny he was, how vain he was, even how obnoxious he could be. I wanted someone to speak about what he was like before he became a PWA (Person with AIDS). I wanted someone to speak about his life as well as his death. I realized that someone was me.

I developed an incessant need to write about Gerard: stories, poems, even a children's book. It was never enough though, because every time I put my pen down, Gerard was still dead. And again I felt helpless. There was nothing I could do.

And then I decided there was something I could do. I couldn't bring Gerard back, but I could help other people who had lost loved ones by putting together a book that gives voice to our experiences. I know, from being a writer and a reader, the healing power of sharing stories. Knowing that other people have gone through the same thing, at the very least, makes one feel less alone, and that somewhere, someone understands. I have also experienced the profound impact of seeing the NAMES project, each six-foot by three-foot panel a loving testimony made for someone who has died. I wanted the words that went along with the images. I wanted to hear people's *stories*.

In September of 1993, I sent out a call for manuscripts that spoke about what it was like to lose a loved one to AIDS. Six months later, the pile in my study was a force to be reckoned with. I handled each essay, story and poem carefully, as if it was a broken heart. I read each manuscript more than once, and though I knew the inevitable outcome of each one, I hoped against hope that it would not be so. At times my grief overwhelmed me, and I had to go outside and take a break. Each time I did so, I was very aware that I had that choice while many other people did not. I would also become especially upset when I read about someone who had died who was my age or younger, or when I read about someone who had died on my birthday or anniversary. Once I read a poem about a person who had died a year ago that very day. Reading the manuscripts reminded me that whenever I am doing anything—eating a piece of birthday cake, drinking champagne with my lover, running out to the store for a loaf of bread, or writing this introduction—someone, somewhere is suffering from AIDS.

I received stories from all types of people about all types of people: parents, children, siblings, spouses, lovers, friends, neighbors, and coworkers wrote about those they've lost: men, women and children from all races, religions, professions, nationalities, economic backgrounds and sexual preferences. I'm sure none of these people ever expected to see themselves and their loved ones in such a book, but here they are: housewives, radical lesbians, political prisoners, drag queens, businessmen, Republicans, ACT UP members and others, all thrown together because we share a common bond: we are all susceptible to a disease that we know too much and too little about. Editing this book reminded me that anyone can contract HIV and develop AIDS, and anyone who does is not guilty of anything, except perhaps one thing: being a human being.

I felt my friend Gerard's presence all during the year I worked on this project. One night I had a dream in which he said to me, "You forgot about the tape, *mameleh*. It's in your closet." Sure enough, when I woke up I went to my closet and there was a tape recording of the first poetry reading we did together that summer so long ago. I hadn't listened to that tape for ten years, but I played it many, many times while I worked on *A Loving Testimony*. Many other people wrote of similar experiences, reminding me that while our loved ones are gone, they are always near at hand.

Here are our stories. They are filled with sorrow and grief, anger and rage, compassion and courage. Most of all, they are filled with love. I'd like to thank my agent, Charlotte Raymond, and my editors, John Gill and Elaine Goldman Gill, for their commitment to this project. I'd also like to thank Mary Grace Vazquez for her love, patience and support. Most of all, I'd like to thank everyone who sent me their stories, poems, essays, photos, memorial programs, prayers, warm wishes and encouragement. As a way to give something back, a portion of the proceeds of this book will be donated to AIDS organizations that give direct care to people living with AIDS. How I wish that Gerard Anthony Rizza was still one of them.

Lesléa Newman

August 1994

Prologue

What To Do When Someone You Love Is Dying

Brooke Wiese

1. Take your finger,
   stick it in your eye.
   Deny the sight of dying:
   the tubes, fat and thin
   going out, going into
   every orifice,
   bringing liquid food or
   backing up with blood;
   the always curtained sky;
   the constant wash of bright
   light over the face,
   mouth a wooden 'O' around
   a plastic tube taped in place;
   another in a withered thigh.

2. Press your palms
   over your ears
   to muffle the moans
   filling the room,
   queer, and grim;
   climbing over the metal bars of the bed,
   under the rims of metal trays;
   in your bones,

in your head;
moving every molecule of air:
always there.

3. Hold your nose.
   With your fingers
   squeeze it closed
   against the cloying smells
   of disinfectant, disease, hospital,
   repellant breaths expelled.
   Death has a special smell.

4. To stifle the fright
   fiercely feared,
   as your heart, or other part
   rises in your throat;
   to fight the urge to retch;
   to still the quickening queasiness,
   the choking hold of
   your own cowardice
   that catches you off guard—
   bite down hard.

5. As instructed,
   wear gloves
   against the ooze
   and leak of death.
   First, turn them inside out,
   shake, then blow
   the fingers out
   so talcumed inside
   now is outside,
   blocked from touch:
   even baby powder
   hurts too much.

For John Carl O'Brien
Sept. 27, 1953–Sept. 3, 1989

THE STORIES

A HALO AROUND OUR WORLD

DANIEL J. BARONE

O41565658...041565658...on and on as if a mantra... reassuring yet jarring. Trying to hang on to something, anything familiar, while all else is spiraling. 041565658... I must remember. It is the key to help. My saying those numbers reminds me that Paul is helpless and I'm scared. However, announcing that magical number with no hesitation establishes my position as someone important in Paul's life. This is paramount. I am not the "next of kin," just the "partner," "friend," "lover," "significant other." Emphasis on "other," not significant when it comes to decision-making. Saying his social security number over and over again while awaiting The Outcome is remotely reminiscent of the soothing monotony and familiarity of the Hail Mary. It represents a desperate attempt to remain in this world; all the while being hurled into The Unknown. 041565658...forwards, backwards, in different rhythms and possible configurations, this number provided tiny, hairlike roots, tenuously anchoring me in the here and now, while blurring the omnipresent pain of the moment. The pain of not knowing The Outcome. Always unable to shake The Fear. Will this be The End? Confidence Shattered. I had managed to be important to Paul but only for those who checked Paul into the Emergency Room. Still, the Virus remained unscathed by the Power of the Social Security Number Mantra. This mantra had met its match and was found wanting. My mantra was not strong enough to ward off disease progression. A bittersweet quality pervades this number.

041565658... Remembering this collection of numbers helps fight back tears by keeping me numbly focused on the act of remembering while the quick recall of these numbers provides calming consolation. Ironically, as strength was usurped from Paul's body, it was methodically transferred to his social security number. It provided an entree to medical care: one of the first questions asked. Also, while triggering memories of illness and Emergency Room questioning, it evokes a happier time in Paul's life. After all, this is the number that followed him throughout his work life and his computer career was an important identification for him.

I didn't know Paul as a sailor, but, in many ways it seemed a happy time for him. He was so bright and the Navy gave him an opportunity to shine. He was very proud of the fact that he got to navigate his ship during the 1976 bicentennial. Since I am not even remotely Navy, I never remember the important distinction between ship and boat, and "navigate" is probably the incorrect term. But Paul's endless patience in describing these terms and distinctions was unwavering. This was also a scary time for Paul: the beginning of his struggle with his sexuality. Paul described his first passion for a man's physique in his journal. Paul's early queries into his sexuality were not purely lust-filled campaigns. He was exploring the depth of his emotional attachments to men. A sea of depression and confusion followed. Paul had an endearing public side that I marvelled in watching. Paul on stage! Paul was an eloquent speaker when relating his experiences as a person living with HIV. He seemed energized by the impact of his words. He wanted to keep people from becoming infected and to let them know that having AIDS was not a death sentence for him or for them. He also would talk about the obstacles he saw to the provision of quality medical and home care services. This was the public version of Paul on stage. His more private "on stage" side included silly posing for the camera while soaking in the tub. Also, he did animated re-enactments of the parrot on the Whiskas commercials. This was always effortlessly offered with barely any prompting or encouragement. Paul was a better Rita Moreno in *The Ritz* than the star herself. Anticipating each line with an indiscernible drum roll that prepared you for the caricature to follow. Paul's being on stage was unpretentious, unpredictable and totally disarming.

Paul's most striking virtue was his patience. It was both boundless and far-reaching. Paul was treated at a "teaching hospital," which, when translated, means *a place where one goes to be continually prodded and probed.* One time, a doctor stuck Paul twenty-seven times trying to do a spinal tap and never got any spinal fluid. Paul was so patient and kind. He waited until the twentieth time before asking him to stop, which, of course, only limited the remaining tries to seven! Paul somehow always found the strength to be patient. Paul could sit quietly while they took pictures of his eyes at the National Institutes of Health. He was so thrilled to be helping, to hopefully be part of THE CURE, that he sat calmly, intently, for hours. Paul was not passively removed from this research. He actively engaged doctors, nurses and techs to understand the impact of the research. He was patient to a fault. I would always have to ask him if he were in pain; he rarely admitted to any.

Despite his unfathomable optimism and patience, Paul experienced frustration with THE DISEASE. He poignantly described his despair in this poem, written on October 10th, 1990.

> No way to live!
> No way to live!
> That cough,
> is it pneumonia?
> That infected cut,
> will it heal?
> That fever,
> some major virus?
> Others have died.
> That waxy skin.
> That lack of breath.
> These things to look forward to?
> To take your life would be a blessing.
> To take your life would be understandable.
> To take your life would be peace.
> No way to live!
> No desire to make life plans.
> No reason to.
> No way.

Paul's creative side also evidenced great patience. Paul poured much detail into the creation of our wedding cake. He lovingly constructed a three tier-cake that was as delicious to look at as it was to taste. He fashioned an eggshell-colored delight, resplendent with rose petals, leaves, florid trim and silver candies, overseen by two dashingly elegant men frozen atop a mound of cream cheese luxury.

The true epiphany of Paul's patience showed in his training of our pup, Beauchamp. One of Paul's regrets in life was not having children. However, we did parent The Monster. I was "the dad" and he was "the other dad." "The other dad" was home with Beauchamp all day and responsible for his training. I should preface all this with the more than minor detail that Beauchamp is a Jack Russell Terrier (pronounced Terror; (the "i" in his case is silent).

Paul also demonstrated infinite patience when it came to preparing me for his death. He rarely showed his fear of The Unknown. He tenderly reminded me of his love for me, his reluctance to leave but the inevitability of his impending journey. Paul was neither morbid nor defeatist about his disease. Each new assault was met with courage and strength. Tantrums and self-pity were not part of his repertoire. Despite his resiliency, the toxicity of the KS drugs began to take its toll. As the KS progressed and the frequency of administering cancer-fighting drugs increased, Paul's patience began to wear thin. His time became divided between alternating periods of comfort and misery. After being infused with the blood-red drug, vomiting, depression and constant unsteadiness of gait inevitably ensued. The Chemoclock was unrelenting. One quarter of each month was spent coping with side effects, while another quarter was spent gearing up for them. In addition, ten days out of each month included self-injections of Neupogen to bolster his white blood counts. Finding flesh to inject became a painful pursuit for Paul. This is also when Paul developed a burning hatred for the color Red. Red food was religiously avoided.

Despite this drug regimen, the purple dots began to win. They multiplied, combining to form bigger dots. The dots became islands which turned into peninsulas which led to continents, until finally it seemed that these land masses would swallow up all else. Hope became a scarcer commodity. Paul took a vacation from this madness to prepare for our wedding. He wanted to have some hair and no nausea for our nuptials. Paul got his wish.

Amazingly, Paul still found the resolve to help me through this time. Not only did he endlessly explain procedures to me and constantly console me, he managed to nurture normalcy in our day-to-day relationship. As Paul got sicker, conjecture about The Hereafter became commonplace. We discussed both The Unknown for him and the upcoming unknown for me. One of his poems helped me be at peace with his eventual decision to stop fighting.

Oh beautiful Light
Oh mysterious Light
   The light of the Spirit
   That shines within us all
   That shines unnoticed when faith fails
   That beams when there is belief
You are the power that sustains us
Though we are in the dark
You care for us when we are lost
And extend to others in our peace.
Oh beautiful Light
Oh cognizant Light
   The light of the Truth
   That gives the strength to know
   That gives us time to query
   That enables us to love
You are the power that pursues us
Though we try to hide
You share with us your unnatural being
Making us one in you
Oh beautiful Light
Oh celestial Light
   The light of the Light
   That burns complete
   That burns away the pain
   That soothes us in our grief
You are the power that heals us
Though we are mortally wounded
You rest inside us with human purpose
A halo around our world.

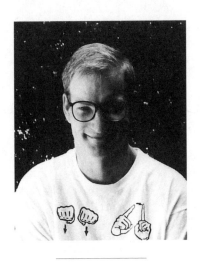

*"To Paulie, your star shines bright
within me."*

*Paul George Hornyak
Aug. 2, 1955–Oct. 27, 1993*

LIFE IS NOT FAIR

JUDITH BLACK

Rachel's Names Project quilt panel is white. It has thirty-two four-inch red satin hearts bordering her calico-appliquéd name, the years of her birth and of her death, and a statement about Rachel and the intense difficulties of living with—not only AIDS—but people's ignorance and fear of AIDS.

Rachel's quilt panel reads:

> Rachel's soul is deep and wide, and if she touched your heart, you *knew* it. She could be *so* difficult, and she is so loved.
>
> One of the hardest things for me about her having AIDS was the dozens of times I shared my grief or fear about her illness or dying with someone and they said, "HOW DID SHE GET IT?"
>
> Rachel *always* deserved more consideration than that. And so did I.

The panel is beautiful. It does not necessarily reflect the five difficult years I was privileged to know Rachel. Her life was hard and her death almost a blessing by the time she suffered her way to it. When she died, I believe she was ready for an end to her agony. She was young—twenty-seven years old—and the world is a lesser place without her.

But it doesn't know it.

Rachel was a drug addict and a sex worker. She was a spirited woman with the defiance of a brush fire. Her mother and I were lovers. When I met Rachel, I found her to be undeniably her mother's daughter. Like Marcia, she was strong and independent and brave. She was loving, sweet and kind. She was sometimes reckless. She was very smart. She had a gentle soul, well camouflaged out of necessity of the life she lived. She was a beautiful woman, a friend and a sister.

She could sure be a pain in the ass, too.

When Rachel was a kid, she hooked up with a guy I would rather not have known. His name was Matt. They ran away together and lived in many cities, the most famous of which was New York. They lived on the streets. They hustled to stay alive. They were wild, sometimes considered themselves free, sometimes trapped—just like we all do.

When Matt was dying, they returned home to California, which is where I met them. Matt was scary, even in his skeletal, PWA, death-warmed-over self. He was steeped in and seething with rage, false pride and insolence. He was a hard man, a malefactor. And Rachel loved him.

Matt died in 1989 and, in many ways, things got harder for Rachel. In many ways, too, they got easier. As a part of her family, I can say that we had more access to Rachel after Matt's death. Eventually, we moved her to San Francisco, the land of resource, and the Bay area we called home.

Rachel struggled to survive Matt's loss. She met and eventually married a man named Richard, who moved with her to San Francisco. Rachel loved Richard, and she also ruled him, much like Matt had ruled her. They created a sad life together, a limited-time offer. Life was not fair.

Rachel and I were friends and peers and family. Our relationship was a mutual struggle. We were both addicts, but I had been clean for several years when we met. Rachel never got clean. (She did, however, get too sick to use.) I never tried to change her. I loved her and accepted who she was.

I did not understand all of what she did, but it was very important to me that I meet her with love, as absent of judgment as was possible. Nonetheless, it was sometimes a source of misgiving and discomfort for Rachel and me. I often disagreed with things she did. She often disagreed with things I did.

Rachel's health declined slowly. She suffered a great deal. San Francisco wasn't the pot of gold for PWA's she might have expected. It was a real city with real pitfalls, a lot of jerks, and a lot of drug addicts. Rachel and Richard didn't get away from much.

Marcia and I broke up after Rachel's move to San Francisco. Rachel never really came to terms with that. She thought I was stupid—and she may well have been right—but we stayed apart and, in some ways, Rachel and I stayed apart as well. There was so much unsaid between the two of us. That is only one of the many things I would deal with differently if I had it all to do over again.

Rachel had dogs and cats the years I knew her. She loved them and struggled all the harder to feed and care for them. And she did. She was a loving soul and regretted many of the events of her youth that shaped her adult life. Nobody grows up with fantasies of being an addict, disenfranchised, and without social skills. Nobody's child dreams of being a sex worker.

I had not seen Rachel in many months when her condition deteriorated and she arrived at the hospital for the last time. I had been away on vacation, and returned to receive a call from Marcia. She said Rachel was in the hospital, was dying, and she thought I should know. I felt shame and guilt and horribly sad that I had drifted away from my family with Rachel and her brother and sisters and her mom. I was also, and still am, eternally grateful for that call. I went to the hospital immediately.

Rachel was in bed, thin and gaunt and pale and sick. She was lucid, and we talked for hours—more candidly than we ever had. We talked about my absence, about our relationship. We talked about my separation from her mother and my new lover and Marcia's new lover. We talked about the many heartaches and betrayals involved. We connected and it was sweet and sad and painful. Rachel told me she was mad at me, and for her, that was just incredible. I felt honored by her honesty. She was right to be angry. I was proud to be present with her.

Rachel's life lasted only six more days. Marcia and her lover tried to get her out of the hospital to a hospice setting, but it was not to be. Rachel's life ended, and with it, her suffering, her sorrow, her years of struggle. And ours continue.

Marcia and I are close now. We're closer than we've been since we separated. We are friends and family, and we share a common grief and many common loves. I cannot pretend to know the depth and entirety of her grief. She lost her child. I lost a friend and a member of my chosen family. We toil onward, and that seems to be all anyone can do.

Six months after Rachel died, her husband's life ended as well. Both of the men in Rachel's life died at Thanksgiving time. I am grateful she didn't have to have that experience twice.

One of the greatest gifts Rachel gave to me in her life, I received after her death. I designed and sewed a Names Project Quilt panel for her, and in the process, I discovered that I could sew. I even like to sew. In fact, I love to sew. I have begun to make clothing for myself, and with every piece I complete, I thank my friend Rachel.

I made another quilt panel after Richard died. It has Matt's, Rachel's, and Richard's names on it. Unlike Rachel's quilt panel, it is only sad and bleak. Their losses are too great, and I cannot help but be aware that as I witnessed these three in their suffering, many others witness many, many others, and the numbers seem unreal. The grief seems unreal. The pain seems unreal. The loss seems unreal.

Life is not fair.

To Rachel, my spirited friend and family.

Rachel Ellyn Hertzberg-Thurman
came into this world Feb. 2, 1966 and
left again June 15, 1993.
Life is too short.

LOVERS

MAUREEN BRADY

James often spoke of his desire to travel to the Badlands, where he'd never been before, but this was only background talk to his real choice which was to buy the next-door studio when it went co-op and affix it to his other one. He set himself to decorating it through most of his last year, going out only for groceries and doctor's appointments.

I saw it once after it was finished. I was staying the weekend with a friend in the city and wasn't planning to see him. Much as he was home, he rarely answered the phone and didn't call back either. Maybe Macy's Furnishings Department, but not me. Yet he wouldn't stop coming into my mind that Saturday so I decided to call anyway. He'd been terribly sick through the night. "I was in N.Y.U. Hospital night before last for my first injection of interferon, in the unit where you have to bring a care partner. Last night I took the second dose by myself.... I had to hire a care partner for the hospital," he added.

"No," I said, "You don't have to. You could have called me. All you have to do is answer your messages and open your mail and see who wants to help you."

He didn't say, *No, I can't,* but I knew it. "I'll be right over," I said, and heard him start to breathe again.

He let me into the new apartment, though I'd rung the doorbell of the other one. It was shockingly pristine, everything in white. A thick white carpet. A gorgeous white sofa. Gleamy white coffee table, its surface free and clear. An abstract, white painting in white frame on one wall, a mirror on the other, reflecting all the white opposite, except for that moment when I stood in front of it, my Chinese red jacket like a stamp on a blank envelope, even my complexion striking too much color.

James insisted on going down to the deli to get us something to eat. "But you're ill," I protested. "Let me go."

"No, you stay here, just *be here*, please."

So I sat on the white sofa and was softly received. In our twenties we were lovers, I in my early ones, he in his later ones, for he had gone from high school to a seminary, then to a monastery, before we met, both in college. He'd been a boy with an appealing swatch of blond hair, elegant eyelashes, skin that looked soft as a female's and was. A strong urge to please his mother. His father seemed not to please her, perhaps not to want to. She was devotedly Catholic, starched and ironed the vestments, the altar garments, even the priest's under-clothes. James, serving as an altar boy, must have felt his closeness to the careful press of his mother's hand on the iron.

He felt sure what would please his mother the most would be for him to become a priest. So Sunday after Sunday he prayed through mass to be called. He told me how hard it had been to keep the con-centration to listen for the calling voice when, over and over, his mind would go elsewhere—to the softball field where he hated himself for repeated ball bungling, to the memory of the priest's hand on his backside reviewing placements for how he was to help him serve mass. He feared the calling might have come and gone and he'd not heard it. Eventually one Sunday, patience exhausted, he'd decided maybe his *desire* for the call was as important as the thing itself and he'd announced after church he was going to the seminary, he'd been called. Even then, knowing it was a strange thing to lie about, but why couldn't his excessive desire for the answer be traded in for it?

I met him a year after he'd come out of the Trappist monastery, the next step up in devotion. He joked he'd left because no one was speak-ing to him. He confessed that silence didn't preclude relationships of a sort. More than one priest had touched him. He didn't say what hap-pened after that, but I imagined him without words, being good, being taken, and this not what his mother thought at all when she stood over the priest's vestments, pressing hard, giving them her tired back.

He did with heterosexuality what he'd done with the calling. Wanted it into being. He didn't really want me, though he proved a good lover, which was confusing enough to both of us to keep us going for several years. He hadn't heard the call to it but he was a twenty-eight year old virgin and wanted to get over that. And I at twenty-three was equally appalled by my status. So with much ado, we did it, and afterwards basked with pride at our angle on normal—*we can be it!* We lay in bed sharing visions, saying none of this for right now but maybe some day. He was in medical school and determined that he wouldn't even consider marrying me until he graduated. A man should support his wife, he thought. This was before the rise of the women's movement. Still I thought it extreme and unnecessary and never felt protected by the surge of testosterone this seemed to imply was going to shield me from the work I'd just finished studying for and had every intention of doing.

We visualized a home. "On a hill," he would say, "looking out over a nice yard and gardens. Everything inside must be simple and exact. Nothing accidental. Nothing slung about. No little figurines or souvenir type things."

"Amen," I would say, having grown up in the knickknack land of my mother, with the impossible job of dusting.

"Everything will be white." Had he said that or do I only hear it now, these twenty years later, sitting here? No hill. I am on the eleventh floor on East Twenty-second Street in Manhattan.

He is back, carrying a bag of groceries in each arm. I follow him to the kitchen where he stands on the small white rug removing fancy deli sandwiches from paper wrappings, putting them out on plates for us. On my last visit here, when I came in for the weekend, we went shopping on the Lower East Side for linens. We found the white rug there, in a linen store. I bought one for my bathroom. He said, "Should I? It's the kind of rug that's no good at all unless it's absolutely clean. But of course it's easily laundered. And what else have I to do these days to distract me from my full-time AIDS watch but laundry?" His career had been aborted the day of diagnosis. He's a facial plastic head and neck surgeon, seven years of residencies, stairs to that title. I think of how he nearly dropped out of medical school when he first had to draw blood—a crisis. "I've faked nearly everything in my life until now," he said. "I may eventually become something, but I always start out as an imposter. But how can you *fake* being a doctor? How can you pretend you know how to stick a needle in someone when you don't?"

Dropping ice in our glasses, filling them with ginger ale and seltzer, I remember the amber potions we drank in our twenties—his alcoholic father, mine, how we determined not to resemble them anymore than our knickknack mothers. But after fifteen years out of touch, when we came together again, our first and best discovery was that we were both recovering alcoholics.

We go to his first living room, not the white one, but the one where food is permissible on the thick glass of the coffee table. He slides down off the couch to the grey-carpeted floor, his legs jutting out straight, pants riding up so I can see the support hose he is wearing. He sleeps with his legs on a wedge, uphill. Otherwise they swell unbearably. I've never heard him complain about this. I have an urge to complain for him, but who would I be relieving?

He wolfs down the sandwich. I suspect he hasn't eaten for at least a day or two. My appetite is upset by how hopelessly young we were together, wandering through those ideas of a house on a hill, a husband supporting a wife, me helping him harden his penis, guiding it into me, our desire for the straight and normal blotting out any inklings that we might be gay.

When the sandwich is done, he downs his glass of seltzer in like manner, full focus on the consumption. He's always been this way— all nor none. We once took a cruise to the Bahamas and finished off a bottle of Scotch between turns puking in the miniature bathroom, the ship tossing in high turbulent water. But we thought we had to down it, for our duty-free liquor had already been purchased to the max.

"Oh, God, Lil," he sighs. "You can't imagine how awful it was last night. I can't believe you called this morning."

"What was it?" I ask.

"Chills, shakes, a feeling I was breaking apart. Some deep heat inside me like a pyre. I didn't...couldn't get to the phone...or if I had I was too messed up to know who to call."

I swallow and nod at him. I wonder how it is that I have come to be, at this moment, here with him, when I'd thought we were finished years ago. I moved to New York to get far away from him, though I pined on a while for the house on the hill, the dreamy after-sex rambling. He moved too, but I never knew where until a year ago, when his face seemed to call me. His sorrow. His questions: "How is it others know so much about how to live? Will I know when I'm finally doing it?" I wrote to him in care of his saintly mother. *I keep having a vision of you ill,* I said. *I hope it is not so.*

It is so, he wrote back, and told me how, while in a weakened state from radiation, he fell off his mother's roof and broke one wrist and three ribs, and then went on to express exuberance over our reconnection. Then he came to visit me and we reminisced about the myths of my family—how my sister and mother made me out to be pathetic and ugly. "And that mole under your chin," he said. "Whatever became of that?"

I nearly wept because of his looking so closely, though perhaps it was only that he'd had the eyes of a facial plastic surgeon long before he became one.

"I need to tell you something I haven't been able to tell anyone," he says.

"Sure," I say, as easy as I can get it out through my thick throat. I am thinking it could be anything. He was raised on weekly confession. It could be that he once operated on the wrong side of someone's nose. It could be that he's planning to leave his mother a fortune in life insurance, but he's realized he hates her.

"It's what I am most scared of."

"What?" I ask, captive, alert. Present time is suddenly startling. The past has fallen away. The air in the room has taken on our pulses.

"What am I going to do when I can't breathe?"

I can't breathe. My eyes pierce through the arch to the white room, the just beyond. I gulp around the lump in my throat, in search of the answer which isn't there. What did I tell him when he called to ask how to proceed in medical school when he didn't think he could draw blood?

He is pale and silent a minute. "I feel better saying it," he says, and I realize it doesn't matter that I have no answer.

It's time to get some help now, I tell him. I lecture him about it. How he doesn't need to doctor himself. He needs visiting nurses. He needs to let himself receive the care of others.

"I've built this whole other apartment for that," he says, "so someone else can be here and not have to stay in the same space with me."

"I know," I say, but I'm not at all sure there is truth to this. I don't think anyone could stay in the white apartment without tainting it. I've worked in the home care system. I explain the various sorts of care available. I visualize for him what he might start with, a nurse to follow up the effects of each interferon injection.

He squeezes his eyes closed and drops his head back over the seat of the couch. "Even though I've done all this, I've been sure I'd somehow be exempt from needing it. Isn't that a bitch. Last night it hit me. I wasn't going to get away with anything."

"Yes," I say, tears sprouting, uninvited.

He, too, is crying. His tears brim and overflow and run down those cheeks that still look woman soft.

My head rocks slowly back and forth. I want to say: I'm really so sorry this is happening to you, but I hold back, fearing that reality speeds up when acknowledged. Then I say it anyhow, my blue eyes locking into his green ones. I see an ocean of color, of life in him in our silence. Then I break it. "How long do you have to take that stuff?"

"That was part of my freakout last night. In my feverish state I decided I needed to read the small print and got out a magnifying glass. 'Terminate dosage when another life-threatening problem supersedes the one this is being given for,' it says."

"Oh," I say. *How impossible and brutal.* Thinking this while my tongue is too heavy to speak it.

I have to leave; I have a date. I fear he will resent this gesture toward my future so I tell him only that I am meeting someone on the hour. He stands up to hug me and his barrel chest heaves. He is sobbing. And so am I. How smart we thought we were, how much we thought we could choose with wishes and fervent visions. And now this. He will be fifty in a couple of months if he makes it.

We cling and cry and the shame of this exhibition of our sadness gradually ebbs with our ignoring it. We have loved, we say. We have loved each other. And especially now, in this parting, there is something solid I know of him. He will breathe. He will stop breathing. Will he hear his name be called?

To Lew, in loving memory,
called at age 50.

Normal Life

James Breeden

O ften, when he comes, he spurts thick webs of himself on my fore-arm. I don't flinch, even though I want to wipe the stuff off as quickly as possible. I let him finish his orgasm, wondering if I have any cuts on my skin. Then I reach for the towel. Me first. But more often than not, there's absolutely nothing on my arm—only imagined cum, phantom semen. He rarely leaks more than a few drops these days anyway. But I always seem to forget.

I'm here. I don't plan to leave him. I just go through the easy motions of the day. You can keep the panic up only for so long any-how. Nine months after his diagnosis, the fear just wore me down. I'm still here. He's still here. We're still here. Forced to return to a sem-blance of normal life.

One night, while sitting in front of our quartz heater, having our little nightcap, I say to him: "You know, I take care of myself, you take care of yourself, but we really don't take care of each other."

He pauses for a minute, taking another toke. The lights on the hillside outside our window are very peaceful. "How else could it be?" he says.

And, of course, he's right. I guess it was a dumb observation. It's just that he's been overwhelmed lately with life insurance problems, new VCR problems, some kind of inflammation on his optic nerve. ("Nothing to worry about," his busy doctor tells him.) Problems. I wonder if I do enough for him. He's always been a take-charge, I'm-in-control, kind of guy. But lately the mountain of details just seems to exhaust him.

Our quartz heater fades to a dim, orange glow. We put out the joint. He smiles and plops his foot on my lap. I wiggle his toes, pulling on them; then I sink into massaging his tender heel, down to his sole.

"What do you mean you don't have tickets?" He's very pissed. "Shanti never called us," the box office tells us coldly.

Jeff leans towards the grating. "I've been very sick lately and made a special effort to get down here."

This isn't true. Actually Jeff has been feeling quite well lately.

"I'm sorry," the box office tells him, though not really.

"Yeah? Well, see what kind of support you get from the gay community!" And he storms off. I follow him, down the stairs to the hotel lobby, where a Black man in overalls spins off elegant Gershwin tunes at a grand piano.

"I'm sorry," I say to him, once outside.

"What are you apologizing for?!" He grabs me and shakes me in mock anger, that's not really mock.

Too restless to go home, he drives up to Twin Peaks. We sit in the car, away from the wind, listening to Roy Orbison on the tape player, and watch the lurid wash of pink and purple twilight fade into city night.

"What I'm trying to say is that I've had a shitty life," he tells me, after giving a long inventory of disappointments.

I don't say much. Really, I'm tired of it. All this constant whining. I just want to go home and watch television. Yet, we rarely talk about how we're actually feeling these days. It's just always in the air.

"What about us?" I say, finally, not really angry, but wanting to make a point. "Are we a part of this 'shitty life'? We have a good, solid relationship. You know how rare that is? Isn't this the primary thing you wanted out of life?"

"I didn't mean—" And he apologizes. He softens, the pain easing. Then we drive home to watch *Star Trek*.

When Jeff was diagnosed, I was sitting on his hospital bed eating from a tray of rare roast beef that had been brought in for lunch.

"Go ahead. I'm not hungry," Jeff assured me, while we were waiting the results of a test for the telling pneumonia.

I hadn't eaten in twenty-four hours, so I was famished. The beef was delicious. But I remember the attending nurse looking at me as if I were some ghoul. Not even her scorching glance could ruin the taste of the meat.

In the beginning, we went to meetings which discussed current treatments, received newsletters detailing drug studies, hooked up to a computer bulletin board which released the latest groundbreaking news. But over the years, nothing has changed much. There was Ribaviran, then dextran sulfate, now Compound Q. "Wonder drug of the month," Jeff would joke cynically. He still pretty much keeps up with the slow progress. I've dropped out. AZT, DDI, CD4, MAI, PCP, CMV, DTC. And on and on. At one time, I could list all the possible major infections and symptoms, recite available social services, break down the blood into its components and functions. Now, I don't think I could remember what drugs Jeff is currently on. "Don't worry," he tells me. "If there's an important discovery, you'll hear about it." I suppose he's right. Why accumulate all this useless medical knowledge?

I have a comfortable routine worked out. "At any minute of the day, I know exactly where you are," Jeff tells me, somewhat amused. I suppose I am fairly rigid about my schedule; Jeff is certainly more secure knowing where to contact me—just in case. Besides, it's easier not having to make any decisions about how to spend my day.

I got a job at the local gay bookstore, which I believed would be low stress while surrounded by sympathetic company, and I go to the gym three times a week.

Actually, I feel more at ease in the gym than any place else, more so than even my own living room.

It's not one of those spotless chrome and mirror vanity palaces. The carpets are frayed, the paint peeling at spots, the equipment creaky and rusted. But the staff is friendly and the atmosphere very casual. I like the mix of people—they really don't know the intimate details of my life. The *alter kockers* speak Yiddish in the locker room and argue over ball games, sleek college kids hash over exams, there's a therapist who talks about his exotic trips, a taxicab driver who tells me of his solitary martial arts discipline. I walk through my exercise routine of weights and the stationary bicycle like a meditation. I find it very soothing. I rarely go up in weights. I just maintain.

Friends and family are kind, but I really don't have much to say to them anymore. When I get home from the bookstore, I think about calling someone but usually end up lying on the bed reading. When they ask about Jeff, I rattle off the symptoms and prescriptions (those I remember) and give a synopsis of his current emotional state. Somehow my testimony usually rings false to my ears, like I'm mouthing someone else's words. Really, I tell the same update over and over again, using the same words, sentences, sighs. Programmed response. Maybe that's why they usually say little after my speech, sensing my own distance. Usually, there's an uncomfortable silence and then we move on to easier subjects.

Once, my sister asked me how I was doing and I told her: "Well, I'm depressed most of the time." And she responded: "So what did you expect?" Then she went on to tell me about the current science fiction book she was reading. I used to get angry that people weren't more supportive, more responsive. But what did I expect? In some ways, they were more frightened and helpless than I was. The trivial, friendly banter at the gym is the best balm. Keep it light. And reading is good company.

The local gay paper runs obits for those who had died that week. It reads like incantations for saints. Those who have passed on were so good and pure and holy. Jeff is no saint, thank God. I have yet to see any golden nimbus circling him. He moans loudly when in pain. Rarely does he have anything nice to say about anybody, though actually he's quite loyal towards his few friends and especially towards me. "So I'm a misanthrope," he tells me, bearing no small amount of pride. I often criticize him for the cynical politeness he displays towards our dinner guests. "Don't worry," he tells me, grinning maliciously. "I'll smile, be nice." I'd almost rather have him be rude. At least it's more honest. But sometimes I see the little boy that genuinely wants to please. "I'll write my own obit," he tells me one day. "None of this phony crap. Tell them how nasty I really am."

We went to Europe the summer before Jeff's illness. It was to be our one last, great trip.

I saw death everywhere. In the astrological clock in Strasbourg where the grim reaper made his rounds every noon. In a deserted piazza at Venice, where a skeleton hung in a masquerade shop. In my dreams, my lack of sleep, I worried constantly about Jeff becoming suddenly, violently ill. Would I be able to handle the emergency, so far from home? Even in Switzerland, surrounded by massive otherworldly mountains, where waterfalls of snow crackled like thunder down sheer rockfaces. Its powerful, elemental beauty brought tears to my eyes. We seemed so fragile.

Jeff's brother arrives in town for a brief, three-hour layover. We rush him out to an expensive sushi restaurant (his favorite). "What do you think?" he asks us. "Should I get a beat-up old Chevy or a forty-thousand-dollar new Jaguar? With all the homeless in this country, you know what I mean?" he laughs. We assure him, in keeping with the joke, that he should get the Jag. After all, he worked hard for it, with an unappreciative wife at home. Meanwhile, Jeff is sinking into debt. He hasn't worked in years (though reasonably healthy) and has been living off Social Security. It doesn't nearly cover his medical expenses. In all fairness, his brother doesn't know this (not directly). And, after all, he did send Jeff two-hundred dollars for his birthday.

Later, over yellowtail and tuna, I tell Jeff's brother how much money the bookstore is making, since I suppose that money is one of the few things that interest him. But as I recite the daily figures, I feel the words drying up in my mouth. Jeff's brother leans closer to hear what I'm saying. But all the words are gone, blown away like dust. There's an awkward silence then Jeff comes to the rescue with family gossip.

"But he really thinks you're great," Jeff tells me after we drop him off at the airport. "A regular saint."

Seven months into the disease, I had joined a support group for caregivers. There was lots of weeping, gnashing of teeth and self-blame. Even I become emotional when describing a close friend whose family had erected a wall around him, so that I was shut out the last month of his life. "I envy your tears," another group member tells me. He runs through his lover's symptoms as if reading a grocery list. "I just can't feel anything," he complains. Several weeks into the sessions, the group leader suggests that we exchange phone numbers.

"No way." I became adamant. No way did I want these people's problems spilling into my private life. I had enough to deal with. Later, after the group had dissolved and I began working at the bookstore, I notice the man who complained of having no feelings browsing through the porno magazines. He sees me, so I have no choice but to talk to him. Actually, he's quite friendly. I can't remember his name so I ask him how Paul, his lover, is doing (somehow it's always easier to remember the lover's name). "Oh, Paul's very sick. He's in a hospice now." He seems almost cheerful with the news.

Now, at present, it has been almost three years since the diagnosis. Jeff finished up his college degree last December. The summer before, we had another last great trip, this time to Hawaii. And just the other day, our friends had sent us plane tickets to visit them in Barcelona. Then one night over dinner, we talk about how long it has been since anyone we knew had died.

Later, while I'm sorting through the household bills, I ask Jeff about these increased expenses.

"Minimum credit payments," he answers irritably, as if I should've known all along. Apparently he's been sinking into debt by about three-hundred dollars each month.

"What? What?" I am angry and amazed, though I shouldn't be. I've simply ignored the financial gloom for a long while.

His plan is to run his credit cards to the limit, then declare bankruptcy.

"What? What if you live for another two, three, four years? What if the social services that you expect to be there collapse?"

But I'm accused of being unrealistic, a prophet of doom, timid in the face of corporate creditors. But I ache with fear and I'm rigid with Midwestern values about unpaid debts, about the burden I'd have to assume after he's gone. So I push for spreading the expenses around to his well-off cousin, and even wealthier brother.

"It's humiliating." He stares at me. "I've always supported myself. This is crushing my spirit."

I tell him that his pride is very expensive.

"What can I do?" he pleads. "I feel helpless, trapped."

Then get a job, I think.

We're off to visit his brother and family in Bakersfield—a suburban city on the edge of the desert. Hot winds blow through the car. The warm air is luxurious on the hairs of my legs. Jeff sighs. "I don't want to fight."

We play an anthology of our favorite tunes on tape, reminiscing, music for apologies and anniversaries. We're struggling to be kind to one another. Bruised and tender from weeklong arguments over finances, we're both on our best behavior.

The trip is long; frequent stops are necessary so Jeff can stretch his back, which has been bothering him increasingly lately. We lie in the shade of wispy trees and talk of Spain. Of windmills and paella and Picasso.

We arrive mid-afternoon, interrupting his brother's wife's siesta. "You've lost weight," she comments, while flipping through television channels in search of her soap opera. Other than that, there is no further mention of his illness the rest of the trip.

Dinner is a bucket of the Colonel's chicken. Afterwards, in the desert twilight, Jeff and I float on rubber rafts about their swimming pool, while his brother's wife conducts a Girl Scout meeting inside. We drift in languid arcs, glancing at the rising moon, glancing through the double-glass doors, nervously snipping at all the bleached hair and pink tops and shorts, suburban manners and styles. We wait for Jeff's brother to return from his big business trip to South Carolina.

"Oh, right, like it's going to be fun," the wife laughs at the brother's suggestion of a short, family vacation to the beach. Her voice is ripe with playful bitterness.

Jeff and I are relentlessly polite, ignoring the tension in the household with meaningless small talk. The brother also good-naturedly ignores his wife's sneers and dashes about the house in a caffeined frenzy, negotiating deals through his tiny home office. Wearing only floral shorts on his tanned fat body, he is like a little boy at play in his sandbox, donning his headphones, relaying faxes, printing up reports, the hushed phone calls.

"I've asked for a few minutes of his time," Jeff says, and asks me to remain for moral support.

We lunch by the pool while Jeff explains our financial dilemma. "I didn't expect to live so long—" he mumbles, almost apologetically. But without hesitation, his brother writes a check for a thousand dollars.

Then he tells us, in the manner of a joke he might leaven at a business meeting, of an affair he's having with another woman.

Sometimes, often, I crave for his death and the terrible wonder of it all. I want to be in the room with him, waiting for the moment of final transition. That moment is mine. I paid for it with my years of devotion. To hear his last breath slip away, feel his spark pass through my arms. Mine. No one else's.

"Let's go get some Japanese food," his brother offers. The last family dinner, thank god. Jeff and I will be leaving the next day. So we pile into his new Jaguar and actually have a decent meal; clean-tasting sushi, free of unspoken anxieties.

Later, after the household is tucked into bed, we sit out by the pool and smoke a joint. The sky is bright with the moon and stars. We listen to the crickets, watch the desert wind gently rock the trees, pushing them on like clouds.

I close my eyes. Jeff is a warm presence beside me; sometimes we seem so close, but other times, like tonight, he's away on some distant planet, far from me. I don't know what's going to happen, or when it's going to happen. But, for a moment, it doesn't matter. The world slips away. I drift.

Waiting.

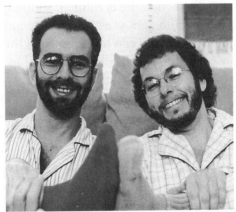

Jeff, left

To Jeff: Honey, it was worth it.
April 14, 1950–May 25, 1991

A Moment in Time

MARISA BROWN

I ditched my traveling companions, thinking I'd be alone with Tom this trip, but the door opened to multiple members of Tom's family, the visiting nurse, his lover—all crammed into a small New York apartment. Tom cannot really move, anyway. With them swirling around us, as if we're in the eye of a storm, I imagine it's just Tom and me.

I sit, holding his hand. It trembles, ghostly pale and bony as it rests in mine, so rosy and warm by comparison. I look from his hand to his face. Each time I come he is thinner, spotted with more purple cancer, his hair more thin and wan. I can never imagine that his face could recede any further between his bones, and then I see him again, and it has. Now his right leg is swollen from a blood clot. His breathing is raspy, his words come in whispers. I think, my God, how much longer can he live like this? Yet the months keep passing.

I have known Tom for nearly seven years, since we met in a sign language class. His gentleness drew me to him, and our shared interest in communicating with the deaf brought us together. Later, we learned we were both musicians and singers. We even share the same last name. In time, we would refer to each other as brother and sister. I moved out of New York City a few years ago and came up to Massachusetts. Lately my visits back have become more frequent.

We talk of small things, a show I went to see, my application to graduate school, the street festival nearby on Broadway. It is a mild spring day in May. Maybe we'll put him in his chair and take him out for some air, we say. Yet the minutes pass and no one moves to do it. Sometimes he seems to hear me, other times he is far away. If the conversation strays too far from his illness, he'll suddenly interrupt with, "It's time for my next pill, you know. I take thirteen of them, now."

"Tom, does it hurt you if we speak about our lives outside of here?" I ask. "Your illness is really consuming you, isn't it?"

"You mean, I'm so self-centered," he replies angrily.

Later, he tells me that he is increasingly losing control of his bodily functions, that now he is a child again. His lover, Frank, overhears. "Tom, you are not a child," he says firmly. "You're an adult who is very sick." Tom rolls his sunken eyes up to look at Frank, smiling with a bitter edge.

Off in the kitchen, I ask Frank, "How are you doing?" He tells me he's got a new job. "Where is it?" I ask.

"Just outside of L.A.," he answers.

"What!"

"Yeah, I'll be starting in a few weeks. I want to be able to support us as soon as possible. I think Tom is really looking forward to moving back home with his parents."

Home!

"Then, you and Tom are moving to California?" I am having trouble speaking.

"Yes, didn't you know?" Frank looks quickly at me, sees my eyes. "Oh, Marisa, I'm so sorry. I thought you already knew."

"How soon?" I ask.

"Two weeks," he replies, then leaves to take Tom his juice.

Alone in the kitchen, I move to the window and lean against the sill as breathing gets hard. I notice the salty traces reflecting in the glass like rain. It had never occurred to me that I might not be with him until the end. It doesn't seem likely that Tom can make it through the summer. Now suddenly, what was just my monthly visit has become my final one. Without the trips down to look forward to, without the giving of myself to him, there is nothing to distract me from his dying. Only the loss of him remains, searing and dark, rushing over me with nothing to stop it.

After a few minutes, I raise my head and go back to the living room. More people have arrived and there is no place to go for privacy. I sink to my knees beside Tom, my back towards them. He notices my red eyes. "You are sad," he says.

"Yes, I just found out from Frank that you're moving," I say. "This is very hard for me. Now I will probably never see you again." He begins to cry. "Tom, is this too hard for you? I want to somehow try to say good-bye."

"It's all right," he says. "But you know, Marisa, there is nothing that needs to be said between us. We know where we are with each other."

"Yes," I answer. "But I want you to know how much I'll miss you."

I tell him about a conversation I had with my father, the week before he died. I had said, "Dad, I believed when I was growing up that somehow, I would always feel connected to you, no matter where you were in the universe. But when you die, it won't really be like that, will it?" And Dad had said, "No, darling, it really won't."

"And it hasn't, Tom," I say quietly. "I've never felt him since he died. Just a lonely void where he once was. So I know how very terribly I'll miss you, because there will only be silence where you are now. I want you to know how much it will hurt me, and go on hurting me."

"But Marisa," he says. "I'll be happy. I'll be at peace. And honey, I want so much to be at peace."

Pain clouds my head. I feel like I can barely see him, smiling at me with such intensity. "And I want that for you too, love, with all my heart," I say.

Gazing at him silently, I realize how much I am connected to him, just as I am losing him forever.

"Tom, I believe that you will be happy," I finally say, touching his face. "I'm only sad for myself, because I won't have you with me. But who knows? Maybe when it's my turn, I'll be able to come and find you again."

He puts his head in his hand, sobbing openly now. "Oh shit," he says.

Postscript: Less than two months later, the doctors discovered a tumor in Tom's brain stem. Frank called me and said, "I think you should come." With the miracle of a frequent flyer trip from a family member, I was able to fly out that weekend, and spend a few days by Tom's bedside. Although he could no longer remember my name, he kissed my hands and pulled me close for hugs often, telling me he knew I was someone he loved. I sang him old show tunes as he lay dying and shared the letting go process with his parents, sisters, friends and Frank.

Three days after I left, Tom died. The missing does not dull with time. Yet always, I treasure our last visit in New York, when we got to say what we wanted to, while we still could.

Tom Brown died that summer in California on July 24, 1992. He was thirty-four years old.

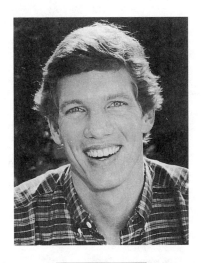

For my friend, Tom Brown:
I will miss you always.
June 11, 1958–July 24, 1992

VISITING TED

JILL CAGAN

I felt a great sense of relief as I sped along Nineteenth Avenue in my red Mazda toward Sausalito. I had just taken a difficult essay test at San Francisco State, on a hot, humid August afternoon. My thoughts centered on my six-year-old son and what to feed him for lunch. Exhausted, I threw an Enya cassette into the tape deck and blasted my air conditioner.

As I approached the Golden Gate Bridge, my body stiffened. A shudder crawled up my back like the legs of a spider. I watched in amazement as my hands turned the steering wheel sharply to the right and away from the bridge. I twisted my car through the wide avenues of San Francisco. Images of Ted flashed through my mind. An incredible urge to visit him overtook me. It had to be now, since there wasn't much time left. I had to complete this mission today.

I didn't have an exact address for the hospice where Ted had been living for the past two months, but I knew what street it was on. So I headed for the Castro, the heaviest populated gay section of town. The orange sun pierced my exposed flesh as I navigated through the light traffic. My throat felt dry. I clutched the wheel to try and stop the shaking in my fingers. My heart pounded in my chest. This would be my first visit with someone dying of AIDS.

After driving around in circles, my Mazda zeroed in on a short, narrow road, filled with rows of houses which looked like they were stuck together with glue. Gay men, selling lamps and books, covered the sidewalks. They strolled together hand in hand, loving each other with their eyes and claiming their space. There was little place in this world for my female energy.

I pulled alongside two men sitting together on the steps of their white-shingled house. One of the men, dressed in a black tank top and cut-off jeans, looked at me with amusement and shook his head when I asked him for directions to the hospice. I stopped a pair of lovers with the same question but they told me that they had never heard of it and hurried down the street. Shocked and confused, I wondered how in the midst of the AIDS epidemic no one knew the location of the hospice.

I drove up and down the street in despair, searching for a large structure, like a hospital, as I had no idea what a hospice looked like. Finally, a bearded man pointed to a small blue house across the street.

"That's it, right over there."

"But there's no sign on the door," I said.

He nodded in acknowledgment.

Unable to find a parking space, I settled for a twenty minute green zone and walked up to the entrance of the hospice. I stood and faced the pale blue door for what seemed like hours, but I just couldn't bring myself to ring the bell. Finally, I stepped back and hid my face in the frills of my pink blouse. Then I turned and ran away. Oh well, I thought, at least I know where the hospice is. I'll come back another day.

As I rushed to my car, I bumped into a telephone booth. The same force that had taken hold of me at the bridge overpowered me once again and compelled me to pick up the phone. After fiddling with my long auburn hair, I dialed the number of the hospice. A deep female voice answered.

"Is this the nurse?" I asked.

"Yes, it is."

"I'm a friend of Ted's and I want to visit him."

"Sure, that's okay."

"But you see, I may have a cold." This was true, as I had been up half the night with a sinus attack, probably due to my anxiety about the exam.

"Honey, in his condition, that's not going to matter."

"Well," I continued, "maybe he doesn't want to have visitors anymore."

"Come on over. I'm sure he'd like to see you."

I hung up the phone and took a deep breath. As I walked back up the street toward the house, I thought about the first time I met Ted. Two years ago he co-facilitated a bereavement group at the Center for Attitudinal Healing in Tiburon. My father had just died in early July. I had watched his body and mind deteriorate slowly and painfully over the previous six months from progressive heart failure. This was my first major loss. Waves of grief rolled through me like the tides of an angry sea. Some days I cried. Other days I lay in bed and stared at the ceiling in disbelief. My husband tried to help me but I needed additional support, so I called the Center and decided to join their bereavement group.

I remember, that first night in the group, the way Ted leaned forward in his armchair and listened attentively with his heart as I poured out my sorrow and my tears. I noticed how thin and frail his body was. He wore a striped shirt, baggy jeans and a plaid cap which partially covered his wispy blond hair. His face, drawn and pale, had an ageless quality but I figured he was probably around my age, forty-something.

A few weeks later he told us that he had AIDS. I shifted my body in the green leather chair and stared anxiously at the other participants. Was I in danger of catching it from him? I had been sitting in this room with him, week after week, breathing the same air. I had even hugged him after the group. These thoughts ran through my mind, in spite of all the education I had received and literature I had read assuring me that I could not get AIDS from casual contact. I felt deeply embarrassed because I was convinced that no one but me had these uncomfortable feelings.

A sharp pain of grief ripped through my body. Relaxing my stomach, I drew in a deep breath. I stared into Ted's sad brown eyes. Oh no, I thought, am I going to lose you too? I needed him to be here for me. He understood my grief. He always knew what to say. Now all this might be taken away from me. I felt so angry at this plague for stealing away the good people.

I continued to attend the group, even after I found out about Ted's illness. One evening Ted smiled broadly at us and pointed to a shiny gold medal, with an American flag hanging from it, pinned to his blue shirt. His eyes brightened as he explained that he had just returned from a ceremony in Las Vegas, the culmination of President Bush's "Daily Points of Light" program established to recognize Americans who have enriched their communities. Five-hundred people, including Ted, had been singled out from the entire country to receive a medal of honor for their contributions to humanity.

After the group, I grabbed the other facilitator and dragged her into the corner of the room. I wanted to find out more about Ted, who he was and what he did when he wasn't at the Center. She leaned against the balcony door and answered my questions in a hushed voice. Ted volunteered, not only at the Center, but at the United Way and many other charitable organizations. He had done this even before he developed AIDS. He gave and gave of himself. She knew little about his family except that he came from the East Coast and his mother and father were still alive. She didn't know if he had a lover but he had many friends. Everyone at the Center loved and respected him.

I darted over to Ted and hugged him like a proud mother. When I opened my mouth to speak, he raised his arm to silence me, resting his hand on my shoulder. To my surprise, he thanked me for all the support I had given to the other members of the group. He urged me to become a facilitator, assuring me that I would be very good at it. My face turned apple red. He winked at me and walked away.

Four months later, right after Christmas, Ted dropped out of the group due to his failing health. Our paths had crossed only twice since then. The first time I saw him was at an afternoon orientation meeting that he conducted at the Center. I sat on a stiff plastic chair in the back of an oblong room crowded with men and women. Ted was about to start the group when his eyes connected with mine. He pointed to an empty space next to him on the couch and asked me to come and join him. After hesitating, I got up and slipped into the soft beige cushions by his side. He sneezed, blew his nose into a crumpled white handkerchief and held my hand for the opening meditation. When the group ended, I raced to the bathroom and scrubbed my hands three times with Ivory liquid soap. Collapsing on the tile floor, I shoved my head between my knees. Here I go again, I thought. Is this fear ever going to end? I exited the Center in shame.

Last year, in the late summer, I ran into Ted again at the Center, on his way to an AIDS support group, this time as a participant. I held up a membership roster and clipboard and waved it in his face. Largely due to his faith and encouragement, I had finished a two-month training course and was now an official co-facilitator of the bereavement group. He raised his thumb in a sign of approval.

When the Center warned us, a few months ago, that Ted's health had deteriorated fast, I made plans to visit him. But it never happened. I became obsessed with my own life. I found a small lump in my breast during a self-exam. Although it eventually went away, I ran frantically from doctor to doctor. When thoughts of Ted did pop into my mind, shivers of anxiety coursed through my veins, as once again my dread of being around the AIDS virus emerged.

So I forgot about Ted. I pushed him out of my mind until I found out that he had moved into the hospice. A facilitator at the Center informed me, kindly but directly, that it was too late to visit him, that he had no strength left. Could I send him a card, I asked. Of course, she said. So I sent him a note. But it wasn't enough. I had missed my chance to be with him, I thought. Disappointment became my solace, as it has always been. I drowned in my self-pity.

One afternoon I broke down and called the hospice to ask if I could see Ted. His home visiting counselor answered the phone. I heard Ted's soft, tired voice in the background mumble, "No, not today." I had been rejected. But I called again a few days later. This time a nurse picked up the phone and told me to "come on over." Still I hesitated. My mind said no. My heart said yes. And here I was.

I rang the doorbell and waited. Then I saw a white piece of paper tacked to the door. Typed in bold black print were the words, "Please press this bell gently. Residents are sleeping." I rang another small bell beneath the note. An elderly gray-haired man opened the door and greeted me with a smile. I stepped into a warm, quiet house with rooms downstairs and upstairs, filled with people with AIDS, all waiting to die.

The man led me into an alcove that, at one time, must have been a den.

"There's a visitor here," he said.

A plump woman, with brown skin and bushy black hair, wearing a pink t-shirt and tight red slacks, sat at a desk strewn with papers and books. She stood up, grasped my hand and grinned at me. This nurse, to whom I had spoken on the phone, was far too cheerful to be working at a hospice. She belonged in a florist shop. She chirped continuously as she led me up a steep staircase.

We turned right at the top of the stairs and entered a spacious bedroom. My heart fluttered and my eyes grew larger as I made my way through the still, dark interior of the room. Ted lay motionless in a hospital bed. He rested flat on his back with his arms folded across his chest, his tiny body buried under a mound of soft gray blankets. The nurse called to Ted and told him he had a visitor.

Although half asleep, he responded to her booming voice and turned his head in our direction. Blinking his heavy eyes, he glanced at me with a vacant stare. He did not at all resemble the Ted I once knew. He had lost an enormous amount of weight and looked like a skeleton. His skin had a pasty pallor. Sunken cheeks made his nose appear bigger. A very large purple lesion covered the tip.

For a brief moment, I felt sorry that I had come to see him. I had no idea if he really wanted me here or if he even recognized me. Then he gazed at me and remembered. His eyes lit up like a shining star. Sensing his warmth, my body relaxed a little.

The nurse joked with Ted but he could not speak. While his frail body no longer possessed the strength to create sounds, he did make a brave effort to communicate by moving his lips.

"Don't you want to stay awake for your visitor?" she asked. I noticed that she took care of Ted as a florist tends to a very special plant, giving it water, nurturing it in the hope that its leaves would thrive. I admired her spirit because all three of us in that room knew that Ted was not thriving and was coming perilously close to the end of his journey.

"I can't believe he's all alone here," I whispered. "Where are his family, his parents? Why aren't they here with him?"

"His folks are in their eighties, honey, so he asked them not to come. He thought the trip from New York would be too hard on them."

"I see."

"Well, I'll be downstairs if you need me," the nurse said and left me alone in the room with Ted. I had no idea what to do next, so I started talking to him. I told him that I loved him. His soul resided in his eyes now and he shared as much of himself as he was able. Then, turning his head, he shut his eyelids. I peered closely to see if he was actually going to die right now with me standing next to him. But he fell into a quiet sleep.

I mumbled to Ted, who couldn't hear me anyway, that I was going to sit down for a while. I dropped into the arms of a hard brown chair. Plopping my leather purse on the fuzzy rust carpet, I looked around his room in awe.

This was his dying place, the last room he would live in. I rested my elbow on a pile of rumpled woolen blankets spread over an oak table next to me. A big black TV sat mute in front of the bed which took up a large area of the room. Paintings of country scenes covered the walls. My foot brushed against the metal leg of a shiny, beige portable potty whose useful days were over.

I pressed my trembling fingers together. My flowered rayon skirt stuck to my legs. Then I jumped out of the chair. I couldn't stay in his room any longer. I swallowed a couple of times and cleared my parched throat.

"Ted," I murmured, "I know you're tired and I don't want to bother you. I'm going to let you sleep." I walked to the side of his bed and debated what to do next. My fear of touching someone who is infected with AIDS bounded to the surface. Then my mind reminded me that I couldn't catch this virus like a common cold. The time had come to put an end to this conflict and face my fear head on.

I reached out and picked up Ted's puffy white hand. Another purple blotch of Kaposi's Sarcoma, partially hidden under his blue silk pajamas, enclosed his wrist. I gently squeezed his fingers.

"Ted, I love you. You mean a lot to me and I think about you all the time." He opened his eyes and I blew him a kiss. He smiled at me like a ray of sunshine. Then he pursed his lips and threw a kiss into the air in my direction.

"I'll come back soon," I promised.

I let go of his hand. Grabbing my purse, I walked out of Ted's room. I knew this might be the last time I ever saw him. Descending the narrow staircase, I rushed into the alcove and skidded to a stop. Two young men sat on a chair together in the far corner. The one with fluffy reddish hair massaged the shoulders of the other. They laughed loudly. Once again I felt they belonged in a health club, not in a hospice.

I blurted out my sins. I had only stayed a few minutes. It had been so hard to be there with Ted. I hadn't known what to do.

"Why don't you go back up there and sit with him and watch TV for a while?" the man receiving the massage asked.

"No, I don't think I can."

The more I said, the more disgusted with myself I became. The guilt, having planted its seed inside of me, was growing and flowering.

I began to feel as if I had committed a crime. I slinked down the hallway, out of the front door and into the bright blinding sunlight.

I jumped into my Mazda and drove up Eighteenth Street, past the gay couples, the yard sales, the tree-lined sidewalks. Racing toward home, I began to indulge in my favorite pastime, beating up on myself. I didn't know if I could bear to visit Ted again. Was it a lie to have told him that I would? Twenty lashes. Why didn't I stay longer? Twenty more lashes. Why had I only managed to visit him once while he was in the hospice? Twenty more.

My heart sank deep into my chest as I contemplated what Ted had left to experience: sadness, abandonment, pain, loss, emptiness, fear, and finally, peace. Plowing my way through heavy traffic, my heart slowly started to lift. And my mind began to empty itself. A white light hovered around my car. I had fallen into the hands of God.

As I turned the corner onto Van Ness Avenue, I turned a corner in my life as well. I felt a shift in my perceptions. I forgave myself for my fear and confusion and thanked myself for having the courage to visit Ted. I thanked Ted for welcoming me into his last moments on earth and tried to imagine a better place for him.

I prayed to God as I drove through the thick fog across the Golden Gate Bridge. Then I blessed Ted's soul. If he had the courage to die, maybe I would find it too, some day when it was my turn. I promised myself to go back and see him again. And I wished him good-bye.

To my friend and mentor, Ted, with love.
Sept. 15, 1946-Aug. 18, 1993

WOOL

C.A. CARMEL

The last thing he did was walk out of his apartment in his pajamas and bare feet. He walked along Thirty-fourth Street, walked purposefully, I was told, while his lover followed him, begged him to turn around and go back home. It must have been a weird sight, a tall emaciated white man, distinguished even, walking across Third Avenue in his pajamas and bare feet with a fat, young black man following him, pleading with him to turn around and come back home. *Please, Pat, please, please.*

Later, when Al told me this story, he said he'd been afraid white people would think he was trying to mug Pat, so he had not dared grab hold of Pat's arm and drag him back home, which is what Al thought any white man would be able to do. Al said Pat seemed too light and floaty, like something you could pull along behind you, like a pull toy or a helium balloon. Except for Pat's strong will, Al said, except for the strong will that pushed a man running a fever of 104, maybe 105 degrees out of his bed and onto the street.

Well, I know all about Pat's strong will. Pat was my husband's brother. I knew Pat for nearly thirty-two years. We fought a lot. He didn't like me until nearly the end. But during the last few years we became good friends. I can picture him now, on that last day, stepping into heavy traffic against the light on Park Avenue. He is wearing the blue pajamas we gave him for Christmas, and his huge flat feet are bare. His long straight toes are filthy. His mind is so befuddled with fever he has forgotten about traffic lights, he doesn't know green from red, but he knows there is somewhere he has to go. He has to go *there*, but where is *there*?

"Pat!" Al shrieks, yanking him back onto the sidewalk. "Where do you think you're going?"

"I don't know," Pat says. He tries to keep on walking. The light has turned green. He walks into the street, makes it to the center island.

Al keeps plodding doggedly beside him, his determined body-guard. Al says, "Is it your office you want to go to?" He says, "Have you forgotten the way to your office?" He says, "Listen, I'll take you to your office. Let me lead you there."

Pat relaxes. He takes hold of Al's arm. Al turns Pat around and steers him east toward Third Avenue. Slowly they make their tottering way downtown. It's a balmy morning in early June, but Pat is shivering. A tremor—a kind of lightning flash—flickers down one side of his face.

At Twenty-ninth Street, Pat urinates into his pajama bottoms. A rivulet of urine streaks the length of a pajama leg, splashes onto Pat's bare feet. Pat does not seem to notice. He does not seem to notice anything. He just keeps on walking.

It occurs to Al that maybe people will think he is just leading home an old drunk. That he is just a sweet black man helping out a sick old drunk and nobody will care much. It is true; nobody seems to notice them. It is ten o'clock on a Monday morning and the sidewalks are packed with passersby and the streets with traffic, but nobody even glances at them. Or maybe people are just being polite. Good old New York.

At Twenty-sixth Street, they arrive at Pat's office. Pat heads straight for the beat-up leather Eames chair. This is Pat's "psychoan-alyst" chair, the chair he sits in when he listens to his patients—or "clients" as he calls them. Now Pat is *there*. He is exactly where he wants to be. Now he can fall into a feverish sleep. He closes his eyes. He is fast asleep.

Al sits on the edge of the low-slung leather couch—the couch Pat's clients lie down on—and waits uneasily for Pat to wake up. He waits and waits while Pat dreams his feverish dreams, maybe dreams he is doing what he loves best to do: listening to his clients' secrets, analyzing their dreams, coaxing them into discovering the most useful versions of their lives.

Once Pat analyzed one of my dreams. It was Christmas, and Pat and Al had come out to our house for Christmas dinner as usual. As we were picking up festive paper and ribbons from the living room floor, I told Pat about a dream I'd had that morning. I'd dreamed I was visiting the home of a woman whom I admired, even envied. I saw a basket containing three balls of orange wool sitting on a table. I picked up two of the balls and somehow got the skeins unwound and hideously tangled up. I was so embarrassed. I said to myself in the dream, *I can never do anything right.* After Pat listened to the dream, he said, "You're afraid of your own messes." I was so upset I had to leave the room. I did not want Pat to see me cry. At the time I did not understand what he meant, but I understood that he was right. Precisely right. I could feel it.

Sometimes the dream of the orange wool floats to the surface of my waking mind. It appears when Al calls me to complain that his apartment is such a mess, it's so cluttered up with Pat's things. He still hasn't got the guts, he says, to throw them out. His voice sounds funny; I suspect he's been crying, is probably drunk. Just the other day, for instance, Al called me up, his voice crumbly and faint, saying that whenever he opens the door to the hall closet, the first thing he sees are Pat's huge old running shoes bent to the shape of Pat's feet.

He said—he always says this twice—"What are your thoughts about this? Carol, what are your thoughts?"

I was thinking about the tangled-up strands of orange wool. I was picturing my fingers picking at the knots, working at the snarls, trying to wind the strands of orange wool back to their original shape. As in the dream, my task seemed hopeless—my trying to stop the mess, to stop the inexorable and inescapable unwinding.

For Pat, brother and friend. R.I.P.

To Ray Ray, Little Raymond, Mi'jo

Kim Christensen

I

Most of the time, I can't believe that this is happening to you, to us. When I let myself think about it, my lungs fill with water. No scream is loud enough to touch this pain, this fury.

It was such a short time ago, Ray, I remember you running around City Hall with your video equipment, sticking the camera in our faces while we yelled at Koch. I remember you admonishing the rich white men in ACT UP for their racism. I remember you sitting at the Village Star eating one of those enormous, gross, hamburgers you love, and kvetching about Anthony, your lover, about love, about life. "Do relationships ever really work?" "If you want monogamy, baby, marry a swan."

Six weeks ago, you outlined for me an article you wanted to write on semiotics and modern visual art for some German magazine. (I have to admit, I didn't understand half of what you were talking about.) Six weeks ago, you and I were having discussions about what you'd say to my AIDS class, as if this were happening to somebody else, Ray, as if this wasn't your life, your taut little body we were talking about.

Why the hell did we think we'd be exempt; we'd be the ones who wouldn't really be hit? Did we think your politics would protect you? Did we think that the love from your many friends—your ACT UP family— would somehow make you immune? How many preciously-loved PWAs have already died, Ray? Why weren't we more ready?

But how the hell could we be ready for what's happened these past few weeks? Screaming in pain at the top of your lungs for hours on end? Your gorgeous, muscular body alternately blown up like a balloon and emaciated as a Dachau survivor? Losing forever your artist's eyes, your artist's ears? Tied to a bed so you won't hurt yourself; being forced ever more inward into a world full of pain, and terror, and hallucinations? "Who's the lady in blue, Kim?" "Ray, honey, there is no lady in blue. There's just you and me here." "Oh, shit." "Kim, turn down the music—it's too loud—I want to sleep!" "Mi'jo, there is no music." "Oh, Christ, not again."

There are funny moments. When you started singing "Party! Everybody gotta party!" and danced—lying down—all over your bed. Or when, terrified, you asked for the priest. When he got there to give you a blessing, you looked him right in the face and said, "Father, you know it's really hard to fuck when you're sick." You later claimed hallucinations. But I don't believe a word of it.

You're still in there somewhere: sassy, campy, irreverent. But you're going farther and farther away every day. And I don't know if I can reach you and bring you back. More and more, I don't even know if I have a right to try.

What bothers me most is not the fact that you might die. (You told me before the crypto meningitis hit that when you thought about the flux of the universe, about how little we arrogant humans really know or understand, you're much less scared of dying.) I'm not even bothered by the fact that you're being so hideously mistreated by the too small, too scared hospital staff.

What bothers me most is the fact that you who six weeks ago were writing semiotics articles for a German magazine, are now crying tears of joy when I teach you to sign your name into my hand: R-A-Y. R-A-Y. KIM LOVE RAY. RAY LOVE KIMBA. LOVE YOU. Love you, love you.

The last time I left, you roused for a minute, put your skinny, IV'd fist in the air as far as the restraints would allow, and yelled "To Freedom, Sister!" Yes, Ray baby, to freedom.

II

Well, here we are again, Mi'jo, seventh floor, St. Vincent's, the AIDS ward. When I get on the elevator and push seven, the hospital staffers look down. Other visitors with bright yellow seventh floor passes smile sadly. They travel in strange pairs to the seventh floor: women in their sixties and men in their thirties; the mothers and the lovers.

The monster came back so suddenly, Ray Ray. You'd had so many good days lately: listening to tapes from your friends, painstakingly learning Braille, taking walks in Tompkins Square, even going on a carriage ride around Central Park. You wrote prolifically: pieces on racism and the politics of language, each word dictated into your little green Sony boombox. You even hosted a People with Immune System Disorders (PISD) Caucus meeting at your house. I was so proud of you that night, Baby. You came walking out of your bedroom, slowly, on a cane, but with much dignity. Your gorgeous black and purple Guatemalan pants were drawstringed to your tiny waist. You'd dressed up for them, Ray Ray. You'd dressed up for them.

When the KS spread to your mouth and throat, the doctor gave you thirty to fifty days to live. With chemo, you might have ninety, but you'd vomit the whole time. You decided against chemo, saying you needed time to gain weight first. We both knew what you were doing. Sixty days later, your mama called from the seventh floor.

I sat with you for six hours last night. Thirty seconds did not go by in which you didn't cough. Anthony and I ran back and forth to the bathroom, emptying the basins of vomit. During one too short respite, you said that if you ever got out of here alive, you wanted to open a nightclub for PWAs, The Cough and Puke Club. You'd have a unique door policy: Sputum specimen required for admission.

Ray Ray, I don't know whose idea of a bad joke this whole thing is, but it ain't funny anymore. Two years ago, Michael McGrath discovered that Compound Q killed infected T-cells and macrophages. But he waited to release the information until he had a patent. Before the San Francisco AIDS conference, Robert Gallo announced that he had developed a nontoxic cure for KS, but he couldn't get a patent, so he refused to disclose the formula. Anthony Fauci of the National Institute of Allergies and Infectious Diseases delayed the testing of aerosolized pentamidine for PCP for eighteen months, because he said he couldn't find the staff to conduct the trials.

Ray Ray, I want Robert Gallo to empty your next vomit basin. I want Anthony Fauci to put on gloves and help you piss. I want Michael McGrath to hold your hand while they poke your pincushioned little arms for a vein. I want George Bush (who couldn't be bothered to address the San Francisco AIDS conference) to fetch Miss Sally, your stuffed chipmunk, and sing to you while you cry yourself to sleep.

Back in June, you said you wanted to be wheeled in Gay Pride if I would come and hold your hand. Over potholes and rough roads I held your hand. You were resplendent that day, baby, posing for the cameras in your Audrey Hepburn hat, waving to your fans like a sixteen-year-old Homecoming Queen. You had thousands of friends that day, a virtual Ray Ray Fan Club. Forgive me, Ray, but I had to wonder where they'd all been during the days of the bedpans and the vomit basins, pity for the sick being so easy to come by, the patient labor of love being so hard.

In the space of a year, I've watched you transformed from a feisty filmmaker and disco dancer into a blind, mostly deaf old man who writes on cassette. You have borne it all—the pain, the terror, the losses—with an almost unbelievable grace. I am so fucking proud of you, Mi'jo. Whatever happens now, baby, you have won.

III November 9, 1990

West Side Highway again, on my way home from you for the last time. They came and put your still-warm body in a grey plastic bag today. They wouldn't let us put you in your Audre Lorde t-shirt or your tie-dyed pants; hospital gowns only were allowed for those with AIDS.

This is all so unreal to me, Ray Ray. I held your hand until your pulse got weaker and weaker and finally stopped. I held your hand until it turned cold and purple, and then colder and white. (Your sister Christine said, "Mi'jo, you're turning into a gringo!") And I still don't believe it.

I kept staring at you, waiting for you to wake up and make a smart remark. You never got to the ocean, Ray Ray. You never got that pumpkin pie I promised you for Thanksgiving. We couldn't even take you home to die. ("Kimba, I know that I'm not going to make it home. But, please, could we call the ambulance and have them drive me around the block a couple of times? I really don't want to die in here.")

Kimba; Kimba the Lion Cub with the Soft Padded Paw; Kimba from the Babar stories of your childhood; my name now: Kimba.

It wasn't supposed to end like this, Ray Ray. Seventy-nine pounds, bed sores the size of my palm, gasping for breath for sixteen hours, drowning on your own blood, struggling in death as you had in life. You were supposed to take a pill, hug Miss Sally, roll over, and go to sleep. That's how we had envisioned it when we talked about your death.

Three weeks ago you told me there was a man who had come down from a mountain who had been following you around for a few days. He wore a black hood and a purple cape. ("A purple cape, Ray Ray?" "Hey, I'm a fag; what do you want!?") "Talk to him, Ray Ray; find out what he wants." A long pause. "He wants my life, Kimba." "Are you ready to give it to him?" "No, not quite yet, but soon, I think. He told me to remember that I am a brilliant, shining white light, in the universe. Do you think that sounds crazy, Kimba?" "No, sweetheart, it sounds perfect."

Just a month ago, you threw a great birthday party, complete with *Wizard of Oz* invitations and Aldo's tunes. Many of your gifts were in loving recognition of your disabilities: a backgammon set for the blind, wonderful stories on tape, and a pair of very cool dark glasses. Wow. Dark glasses. There was a slight pause. You put them on, leaned back, banged on an invisible piano, and started crooning, "Georgia, Georgia on my mind." You cracked us all up.

In the middle of a circle of friends, you danced that night. ("*The Reader's Digest* version of dancing," Catherine called it.) Danced until exhaustion forced you to sit. You refused to go to bed, until you fell asleep in a chair. "I never want this night to end," you said. Neither did we.

I have learned so much about courage from you, Ray Ray. Battling crypto, toxo, KS, and more pain than I can fathom, you always asked about my joints, my lungs, my father's heart. After fighting so hard for so long, you decided it was time to go. Gasping for breath, you told the nurse to get the damned suction tube out of your throat; you wanted to die.

I hope that you found that man in black with the purple cape today, Ray Ray. I hope he was cute. And I hope he took you to that light, that last station home. I miss you already, baby. Good-bye.

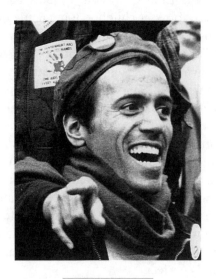

To Raymond Navarro,
Oct. 6, 1964–Nov. 9, 1990
Political activist, video artist, author and
beloved friend. Te amo, Ray Ray.
I shall never forget you.

Valentine's Day

Cynthia Lee Clark

One year ago today
I brought you
Flowers and chocolates
I wore red
For the holiday, you know
Also so that you would find me
In your dark and crowded hospital room
I sat in my red dress
Held your hand
Remembered that when I was six years old
I believed I would
Marry you and we would be
Together always
On Valentine's Day, one year ago
I held your hand and pledged
Myself to you
Sister to brother
Love and cherish
In sickness and in health
'Til death do us part
Valentine's Day, this year
I hold my own hand

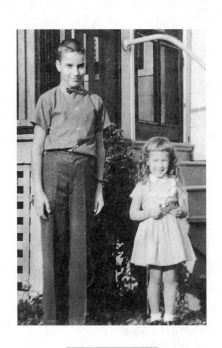

To my brother, Oren Clark, Jr.
I miss you.
Oct. 16, 1949-April 3, 1993

BARRY AND ME AND THE ANGELS

LOUIE CREW

B arry died last night and nobody much cares.

When I was last with him at St. Michael's, he said, "My family doesn't come anymore. They think they'll get it by breathing the same air."

Barry was twenty-eight, brilliant, black. Barry and his Puerto Rican lover were together for eight years before his lover died, three years ago. Both families were always hostile. With his grief, Barry went berserk for a while, ran up enormous debts, lost his catering job, and had to sleep on the streets for several months before he got a bed in a shelter for PWAs, the only one in all of Newark, though we have the highest HIV infection rate of any city in the USA. The shelter was for HIV-positive drug addicts, most of them macho straights who "know how to handle a sissy." To escape their abuse, Barry found one of the addicts, a straight man who still liked to cuddle, especially if it could get him a hit or two. They moved out to splurge in a motel on some back social security payments that came through for Barry. When that money ran out, they got a welfare apartment.

Barry loved music and the smells and bells of my religion, so I took him to church occasionally, but he stayed away most of the time, saying it made him feel guilty. "A third of the parish is gay; several on the vestry are gay. Why on earth do they make you feel guilty?!" I asked.

"It's not them!" he told me, shocked that I had misunderstood. "It's me; it's God; it's the way I was brought up…"

"Barry, do you seriously believe that the God who made the universe, who placed the sun, moon and stars in place, who made a sweet and compassionate man like you, has nothing better to do with Her time than to run an Almighty Data Base to record every time you upset some fundamentalist?"

"Well, I wouldn't put it that way, but yes, in my heart of hearts I believe God hates me. He has to. I don't live the way I was taught to live. My parents hate me. Society hates me. When I was young I tried every way possible to live right, but I'm me; I'm gay. And, Louie, I'm scared of God."

No matter how good the meal, whenever I drove him home, he would always bring the conversation back to God. We both realize we were talking about a different God. He seemed to like my God more than his, but wasn't convinced. "Convincing" wasn't the issue for either of us. Speaking candidly was. He testified to his experience and I to mine. I am an atheist to the God he feared; I believe that kind of God is a fraud and not worth my belief. If that God turns out to be real, let the sucker burn me. I will not yield. I have no use for patriarchs. None whatsoever. But the God I believe in scares me, too. She/He knows all secrets. She/He is completely righteous and just and patient and compassionate and vulnerable... And I know I cannot ever be worthy—not because I love Ernest, but because I could never possibly love Ernest enough, not even as much as I love myself ... So I understand awe.

I understand awe all too well. I've got more awe than any God worthy of the identity would ever be comfortable receiving.

At St. Michael's the last time we were together, Barry asked me, "Do you believe in angels?"

"I've heard them."

"Really?!" His fever was 104 and had been at least 102 for eight days but he got very excited.

"I don't talk about it, though," I said awkwardly. "At least I haven't talked about it to more than two or three people, and as much as I write, I doubt that I will ever write about it. When other people talk about things like that, they spook me. I don't want to be a spook. Some people talk about seeing angels as if to say they're better than anyone else. The fact that the angels have come (and only a few times many years ago, so far as I knew or remembered) says little about me, but much about God..."

"Angels have come to see me several times here at St. Michael's," Barry interrupted, as if to confirm, as if safe for the first time to tell someone. "One sat right there on the edge of the bed this morning, but he did not say a word."

"How did you know it was a He?" I teased. "Are you sure it was not that pretty Portuguese orderly..." He wasn't in the mood to camp. "Right there on the edge of the bed and he did not say a word."

I said, "That's like the way mine behaved, though I never got to see them. I just knew that they were there. It always seemed like a pair. It also seemed to happen when I was in danger, like when Ernest and I lived in Georgia in the seventies and integrated the neighborhood both racially and sexually. Whenever a white kid sprouted new pubes it seemed he had to announce the fact to the world by throwing rocks at our window shouting, 'Nigger! Faggot! Nigger-loving faggot'. We would squeeze tighter, and sometimes I would hear their wings. I'm not absolutely positive. Not a lot hangs on it, but I was very conscious of it at the time, heard the flutter quite distinctly. And then I could go to sleep."

"Another one sat right over there a few days ago," Barry said, pointing to the other side of his bed.

We sat silent for several minutes.

"Barry, they wouldn't come if God hated you," I said.

If Barry heard, he did not say so. I think he had drifted off. His eyes lit up when we kissed goodbye, though.

Now his family has whisked his body away for a private funeral.

Tonight I don't give a tinker's malediction about what straights think about us and our visitors. They'll let the whole world die before they notice or care or understand.

Goodbye again, Barry. My close friend's nephew went into the hospital today. Looks like PCP, but it may be tuberculosis instead. That will take longer and be more painful. I'll give your kiss to him and to his lover who has tested positive, too. Goodnight, sweet angel. Goodnight. Goodnight.

For my friend Barry Godfrey.

Ave Rizza in the Hospital Room

DONNA DECKER

Each moment died to the next
while we hung on your last apnea breath.

Then your dead body's love swelled,
and rose to fill the room, pushing us down to our knees.
There was nowhere else.
    In that grace-soaked room, I lived to kiss your arms.

Done now, the years of searching for the perfect word to
    release you,
The many hours of lotus sitting and praying through oceans
    of breath,
    trying to empty your mind.
Believing food and mirrors stuck your path to heaven,
never knowing your ecstatic heart
        was already there.

While we collected the details that had been you,
you lay, your skin still weeping and warm, and continued
    to wake us.
One of us placed your silenced fingers in a white clasp,
for your mother loved your fine hands, but she never came.

He worked to close your lazy eyes,
while your stained lips relaxed, growing pink again,
the long horse teeth now yours too.
Two hours later, your arms still bled
when the nurse finally withdrew the I.V.s,
    the three machines clicking their green neon.

In the last-week slow motion beginning of this end,
an insane mage's charms had blossomed your penis
    into a giant pale pink hothouse tomato,
stiffened your legs to river logs,
fanned a barrel of bark inside your chest,
fun-house mirror doubled everything but your face and arms.

Showering you with whatever we thought was holy,
we chanted *Om Namah Shivaya*, prayed the Hail Mary,
read from *The Tibetan Book of the Dead* to cover all our bases.
Whispering "head for the white light"
    as your clumsy spirit-guides,
    we tried to calm the rushing waters.

How can I tell them how death
delivered me to rest my lips on your fingers,
trace the sides of your concave face,
whisper love and secrets to your dead ears,
stare till I had my fill,
    witnessing your deliberate transformation into stone.

The oven would be your next lover
Your ashes would fit in a 6 by 12 inch box
you were beyond numbers

_____

To my brother in poetry and spirit
Gerard Anthony Rizza

Taking You to Forever

Helen Decker

I
From the plane window—
that which is soft & brown,
then windswept dunes
the size of a hill.
Straight through the brown,
a highway,
the lifeline of the earth
I follow
until I can no longer see
its distance.

II
The ashes of Gerard Anthony Rizza,
poet brother journeyer
are at the feet of my red cowboy boots.

III
Did I hear you?
Did you speak
something soft and old into
my once ear?

IV
Security stops us.
They cannot identify the large, green mass inside Gary's pack.

Is it explosives
of a spirit
that once
was the size of the willow,
the colors of autumn's high time?
"It's our friend's ashes," Gary recites.
I, once again, tear—
my eyes droop green—
the ruins they are building
glisten as storm.

V

I continue that way for over an hour.
The takeoff scares me.
The large lift to the sky
finds me weeping with more reason than ever.
Gerard Anthony Rizza is dead,
& I climb the sides of the sky in an airplane.
We are taking him to the coast of Oregon,
to scatter
the grey fine remains
of what was once
the sign of ebony
in the hair & eyes.

VI

I read Gerard's first book *Regard for Junction*
on the plane.
A tear between the physical and heaven.
Only for a moment I am allowed to hear him,
the way he said his words,
his feet, dogs,
the rearrangement of morning pieces
& classrooms.

VII

To walk the clouds would be to slip into your arms.

For Gerard Rizza, poet, journeyer
Oct. 20, 1959-April 4, 1992
32 years of age

DAVID LEMIEUX

DENISE DUHAMEL

My first boyfriend is dead of AIDS. The one
who bought me a terrarium with a cactus
I watered until it became soft. The one

who took me to his junior high school prom where I was shy
about dancing in public. The one who was mistaken
for a girl by a clerk when he wanted to try on a suit.

In seventh grade my first boyfriend and I looked a lot alike:
chubby arms, curly hair, our noses touching
when we tried our first kiss. My first boyfriend

was the only one who met my grandmother
before she died. Though, as a rule, she didn't like boys,
I think she liked my first boyfriend.

My first boyfriend and I sat in the back seat
of my mother's car, and on the ledge behind us
was a ceramic ballerina with a missing arm.

We were driving somewhere to have her repaired
or maybe to buy the right kind of glue.
My first boyfriend was rich and had horses

and airplanes he could fly by remote control.
My first boyfriend died on a mattress
thrown in the back of a pickup

because the ambulance wouldn't come.
There was a garden in my first boyfriend's yard.
One day his mother said to us,

"Pick out some nice things for lunch."
My first boyfriend and I pulled at the carrot tops,
but all that came up were little orange balls

that looked like kumquats without the bumps.
My first boyfriend and I heard ripping through the soil
that sounded close to our scalps, like a hairbrush

through tangles. We were the ones who pushed
the tiny carrots back down, hoping that they were able
to reconnect to the ground. We were the ones.

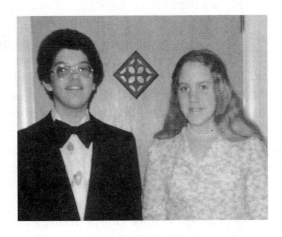

in loving memory (1960-1992)

CHARLIE

SANDY DUTKOWSKY

At seven, I stumbled around in my mother's six-inch pumps, singing the theme song to Mister Roger's Neighborhood. At nine, while my mother vacuumed the family room, I gently applied to my quivering lips September Harvest Lipstick. At twelve, I burned my thumb and my bangs with my sister's curling iron. At fourteen, I developed a hard-on after peeing while sitting down on the toilet. At sixteen, I had sex with a girl my age and it was a complete drag. At seventeen, I danced to "Midnight at the Oasis" in front of a full length mirror in the first pair of pumps I paid for with my own money. At eighteen, I went to the prom in a tuxedo and pictured myself in pink taffeta. At nineteen, I moved to New York City. and had all unnecessary facial hair removed by electrolysis. At twenty-one, I entered nursing school. At twenty-two I started wearing a slip and pantyhose whenever possible. At twenty-five, I completely understood that Cherry Red lipstick was not only a great color for a sizzling Saturday night, but a state of mind. At twenty-eight I decided I needed to be a woman.

Now don't get me wrong. At this point in my life I was more of a woman than most of the women I know. I had a fabulous figure, I understood the art of makeup, I had great hair and a flawless complexion. I got to wear a little pure white nurse's outfit with optional hat, which I opted for, for forty hours a week which I was paid very nicely for. I personified the ultimate woman, from a man's point of view, and I played it to the hilt. I would do things like wear stilettos and run onto the subway and just as the door shut I would feign twisting my ankle and wince. I would slowly remove my shoe as the subway pulled away and stroke the full circumference of my ankle. Then I would glance upward to look for reactions. Imagine, even in a New York subway, this stunt would have men clambering to assist me. Unfortunately, I never knew what to do with the attention that I demanded from men. Two penises in bed was one too many for me.

In public, you couldn't stop me. At home, in the deep recesses of my mind, I viewed myself as a freak. I would come home from work in my little outfit and look at myself in the mirror and a shriek would fill the folds of my brain. What the hell is a guy with a dick doing in white pantyhose and a bra filled with rubber falsies?

One night I finished my shift and returned him to my apartment. I looked at myself in the mirror and I expected my mind to yell something like, *men have greasy fingernails, you have red fingernails!* But this night, I looked at myself and I really liked the way the humidity was making my hair wavy. I removed my work clothes, my stockings and even my false breasts. I picked out a very nice greenish jumper and put it on. I looked at myself in the mirror and I had the urge to go into a public place and wince as I dribbled ice cream down my front and watch for reactions. I felt good. But I didn't get ice cream. Instead, I improved my figure by stuffing my bra with tissues, which are much more comfortable in the humidity, to about a C cup. I applied a soft spritzer of juniper perfume to my pressure points and set off to make myself a nice dinner.

As I rummaged through my cabinets searching for what would soon be a fantastic dinner, my dog Simpson began frantically running around the apartment. Mind you, Simpson is not a mellow creature, but this was unusual. She was chasing her tail, rubbing up against the wall and doing my all-time favorite: the butt to carpet rub. Now, I've had pets all my life. A novice pet owner can tell you that those behaviors coupled with a warm summer evening add up to one thing only. Fleas. A novice could also tell you what happens to an apartment when a flea is left alone.

So, I coaxed Simpson into the bathtub and gave her the flea bath of a lifetime. I dried her and sprayed her with a powerful pesticide. A few dead fleas floated to the surface of her fur. I victoriously picked them off her and flung them into the toilet. I flushed with glee and returned to the kitchen to make my dinner.

I must say in retrospect I made a fine dinner that night. I didn't get to eat it, however. I believe I was eating a tomato in basil vinaigrette when I had the strange sensation that a caterpillar was walking on my upper lip. I checked, of course, and there was no caterpillar. A few minutes later the caterpillar turned into a low electrical frequency. My lip was burning, tingling, and tickling all at once. I returned to the mirror and was shocked to see that my lips had swollen to twice their size. I realized that I was having an allergic reaction to the flea stuff. So I jumped in the car and drove myself to the hospital.

I walked into the emergency room and it was absolutely packed. I mean, if I didn't know better I would have thought that a 747 had crashed or something. Every chair was filled with some sort of casualty. People were on stretchers, kids were screaming and my face was the size of a balloon. I checked in, the nurse gave me a Benedryl to tide me over, and I looked for someplace to set my body. Under normal circumstances, I would have used my body to its full advantage. I would have played this thing up to the point where men would be begging me to take their seat. But I really didn't feel good. I spotted a radiator that looked like it might work as a chair. I meandered over to it and claimed it as my own. It actually was surprisingly comfortable.

I began to feel the effects of the Benedryl. My lip felt pretty good and I was so relaxed. The emergency room was calmly swaying in my head and I was thinking about how much I liked Benedryl when my tranquility was shattered by the sound of someone vomiting. I suddenly sobered up and became the nurse that I am. I removed a pair of latex gloves from my purse, applied them to my hands, and with the snap of rubber, I was ready to go. I located the victim. He was lying on a stretcher. I knelt down to him and realized he wasn't vomiting. He was gagging and dry heaving. He was shaking, sweating and curled up into fetal position. I asked him if he wanted some water and he nodded that he would. I went to the bathroom and I got him some water and a cool paper towel for his head. I returned and he sipped the water. For a moment his trembling subsided. He looked at me and said, "Thanks. My name is Charlie." A few more moments of calm passed. Charlie began to tremble again and with one big whoop he threw up the water he drank all over my lap. A few seconds later he threw up again, this time expelling his false teeth in the explosion. I acknowledge, this is a gross story, but this is how I met Charlie. So I'm there, my lap is soaked, there's a pair of false teeth sitting in a puddle and I am very aware that I'm in the presence of a very sick man. So, I reached into my bra, removed the wad of tissues from my left breast and padded my lap. I picked up the false teeth and wrapped them in the wad of tissue which I removed from my right breast. Seconds later, Charlie was whisked away by a couple of orderlies.

A couple of Benedryls later, the vast majority of my face returned to its normal size. My lips remained puffy, but that was okay with me. There was more space for lipstick that way. A few days later, upon the completion of my own personal trauma, I realized that I still had Charlie's teeth in my purse. So, I returned to the hospital hoping I could find him. No one should be without their teeth for Godsake. I discovered there were three patients named Charles in the hospital that day, so I went from room to room until I found him.

He looked so pathetic, lying in that bed. However, when he put the teeth into his head, I caught a glimpse of the man he must have once been. I imagined his grayish green skin was once olive. I dreamed his listless, greying black hair was once wavy, jet black and tousled on a salty beach. I saw his mangled, scaly hands lifting a newborn child strongly and securely over his head. I saw his dull green eyes blazing with passion as his feeble voice bellowed out his love for someone. I realized I romanticize everything. On this day Charlie was not a poetic vision. He was a pathetic, sick man lying in a dingy hospital room.

In return for the help I gave Charlie that night, he reached under his bed and gave me of all things a First Aid kit. Now this was no ordinary First Aid kit. This was a bright red steel box which encapsulated surgical grade instruments, gauze, antiseptics, tapes, you name it, it was there. Now I knew this stuff had to have been stolen from the hospital and how Charlie managed to acquire it all, I'll never know. Regardless, that First Aid kit absolutely endeared him to me. I just thought it was the sweetest thing. After he presented the kit to me, he gave me a little lecture. He told me that the world is a dangerous place, especially for a beautiful woman like me. Oh, my ego was soaring. He told me that what I did the other night was very nice, but also very stupid, as I could catch some terrible disease. He then told me he is an intravenous drug user in recovery and that he has AIDS. A powerful feeling overwhelmed me. My ego was flattered by a very sweet man who was also very sick. All of my caretaking instincts poured out of me. I felt so feminine. Charlie needed to be taken care of and I was the one to do it.

For the next six months I spent most of my time with Charlie. He had a fairly sizeable disability check as well as a lot of money coming from another source that I was never able to identify. We spent every cent of it. I was given anything I wanted. Charlie bought a lot of clothes and jewelry for himself. He had a passion for fish so he bought himself a number of salt water and fresh water tanks and watched them for hours. We saw a lot of movies.

In retrospect, I realize I'll never have that opportunity again. I stumbled upon a rich guy who was dying and had the desire to grab life by the balls with whatever he had left and all I had to do was go along for the ride. Not bad at all. Charlie had never forged any lasting relationships with anyone over the course of his life, and he wanted to rectify this. So while we enjoyed material pleasures, he told me everything about himself, things he hadn't told anyone.

Charlie was once a high-class drug runner. He had Cadillacs, houses, he hung out with stars at Studio 54 and he had a different woman every night. Unfortunately, he couldn't resist dipping into the product he was delivering. He did this once too often and fell out of favor with the people he worked for. He lost everything and became a typical street junkie. He moved from place to place, sticking people up, sharing needles with a lot of people and using women left and right. I never wanted to meet that side of Charlie. Nevertheless, he trusted me to tell me these things and I in turn trusted him enough to be vulnerable with him.

One night I told him I had something I had to let him know about myself. I blurted, "Charlie, I'm not a woman, I'm a man. I just really want to be a woman. I don't want to mislead you."

His reply was quintessential Charlie. I'll never forget it. "I figured something was up when you cleaned up my puke with your tit. Let me tell you something, when I die they're going to put something like, 'Here lies Charlie. He's had more ass than toilet paper.' I don't want to screw you. I probably couldn't even if I wanted to. I just need you to be with me right now, that's all." And that was that. Afterwards he took me out and bought me a fantastic maroon dress.

Towards the end of our time together, I noticed Charlie was sick an awful lot. He was either having diarrhea or vomiting. Now mind you, at this time, Charlie had five T-cells so I wasn't surprised when he started getting sick. I was willing to face what I knew was inevitable. I could support him through it.

Charlie went into the hospital and the doctors told him they thought he had MAC. When they explained to him what MAC was, a frightening change came over him. He ordered me to leave him alone, which I did. When I arrived at his room the next day, he was gone. One of the nurses told me that he said he was going to Las Vegas to invest in property and get himself a showgirl.

I reeled in anger until two months later when I got an anonymous phone call from someone saying that Charlie was dying in a hospital room in Nevada. The anger subsided and I called every hospital in Nevada looking for him. No one had heard of him. I decided that he must have died and no one would tell me.

Then a few days later the phone rang at three o'clock in the morning. It was Charlie! He was calling from a bus station in L.A. He was sick as a dog and needed to come home. He said he needed me. My sadness melted away. He asked me to wire him money, which I did.

He arrived a week later and admitted himself to the hospital. When I hugged him I could not believe how thin he had become. Shortly thereafter, I lost all respect for him. As soon as I sat on the edge of the bed he handed me an address. He said a taxi would be coming any minute for me. All I had to do was go to this house, knock on the door and pick up a package and bring it back to him. I couldn't believe what I was hearing. My heart went into my throat when I realized the old Charlie was back. The Charlie who hurts the people who care about him. The Charlie who used and abused everything in his path. I told him I wouldn't buy him drugs. He replied by saying cocaine took his pain away. I told him again that I wouldn't do it. He swore at me and told me to get out of his room and started rolling a joint.

I never saw Charlie alive again. He called me months later to say he was in a nursing home in the Bronx. He couldn't walk anymore or feed himself. He wore diapers. He spent the majority of the conversation crying and saying how scared he was. On the flip side, he was happy because his estranged sister had found him and visited him daily. This was the fulfillment of a relationship he craved his entire life. He told me he loved me and that I was the only woman he ever trusted.

He called me a few times after that but I didn't understand what he was talking about. He babbled. I called him one more time and was told he could no longer talk on the phone. I wasn't surprised to learn that a few weeks later Charlie died. I went to a bar that night and had a few Rolling Rocks. I wasn't too upset because I mourned the loss of the Charlie I loved when he left for Las Vegas.

Charlie has been dead now for a little over two years and I still grapple with what our relationship was all about. It was so bizarre, a transsexual and a former tough guy forging a friendship. One thing I'm clear about is my anger. My anger isn't directed at AIDS. I could have cared for Charlie as he died of AIDS. I could accept his decay, his weight loss, his chronic diarrhea, the smell of his vomit. I could not accept his addiction, his lying and his blatant disregard for my feelings when he used drugs. AIDS didn't take Charlie from me, his addiction did. Charlie was thirty-seven at the time of his death.

For Patty and Sally

My Son Mike

ALICE E.

Nobody in my family is very big, and my Mike wasn't much over five feet tall. His favorite things in life were eating, his cars, and shopping for clothes, especially shoes. Mike and shoes were a trial sometimes. He hated to polish his shoes. If they needed to be polished he "lost" them and had to buy a new pair. If I got to them first I polished them just so he wouldn't throw them away. He wanted his clothes to be just so. He was kind of a little tiny peacock and, because he was so little, finding just the right clothes—and they had to be *just right*—wasn't easy.

Mike didn't have an easy time growing up in our little Illinois town. When Mike was growing up, the other kids in our town and in our church were mean to him, and teased him, and made fun of him and bullied him. I remember they'd play hide and seek and when he was "it" they'd just quit playing and leave him looking for them.

Mike got sick in June of 1987. My mother was ninety-five years old that year, and I was staying with her in her house in another town as I had done since my father died in 1979. When Mike got sick I had a terrible time finding somebody to stay with Mother so I could come home and look after Mike.

At first we thought Mike just had a summer cold. When he didn't get any better, I took him to the local hospital and when he still didn't get better, we went to a larger clinic about an hour's drive from home.

They evaluated him and kept him. He had pneumocystis. After all the tests were back the doctor called and told me, "You son has AIDS." I'd never heard about AIDS until Rock Hudson died. Then, in 1986, one of Mike's classmates died from it. But it still didn't seem like it would be something that would ever be in my life. Now here it was: "Your son has AIDS."

I can't tell you what an effect it had on me. When my other son and I went in, Mike was just lying there. I didn't know what to say.

I talked to the chaplain and he was nice. Then I went to talk to the doctor. He was very sympathetic and told me just what to expect. Only, to experience it was so much harder than I imagined. Mike was so sick. All I could do was say, "I love you, honey."

When he finally came home, he stayed only two weeks before he had to go back. The doctor told me not to be surprised if we had a lot of quick trips back to the hospital. After that Mike was in and out of the hospital. The doctor didn't exaggerate.

Most of his nurses were wonderful, but every once in a while I had to get kind of ugly with a nurse to get him the right kind of care. There was one who didn't want to cover him up even though he was cold. You can bet I settled her! I think that's one thing other people need to learn. You can't always just take whatever they do in hospitals. Sometimes you have to fight. And when I had to, I did. This was my boy lying there!

In spite of being sick, Mike was able to work about a year and a half after his diagnosis. The people he worked with were very kind and supportive of him.

But that was at work. Our hometown was a different story. I can truthfully say out of that same town there was one true friend, named Clara. When Mike was in the hospital, both of our cars were down. Clara took me to the hospital. She was a rock. She was always there, until God called her away three years later.

From the very first, Mike worried about me. He wouldn't let me kiss him because he was afraid that I could get it, too. I told him you couldn't get it that way, but he was afraid that a few years in the future they'd find out you could. He wouldn't let me give him any vein injections because he was afraid I might get his blood on me. He made sure I wore my gloves when I was doing things for him.

After one hospital stay that was about a month, I closed up my mother's home and she came to live with Mike and me in the trailer.

She hadn't lived with us very long before she started to fail and soon was bedridden and blind and senile and had to wear diapers. It was nothing for me to wash her sheets and clothes a dozen times a day. Mike was thoughtful of her, too. If she hollered for me while I was doing something for him, he would tell me to leave him and see to Grandma.

Having Mother so bad off and Mike so sick was a terrifying experience. Just the trauma and worry about both of them was enough, but we had to put up with the attitudes toward Mike, too. So many, many remarks, and discrimination, and persecution.

The churches in this town were rude and inconsiderate and unchristian. One preacher told me that other people would not come to church if Mike and I went there. We went to three different churches before we could find one that would accept us. One church woman brought some brownies to our trailer. She had two dishes—one glass and one paper. She said the ones on the paper plate were for Mike. I told her we didn't want them. Sometimes I would have given anything if just one Christian in that town had said, "Why don't I sit with your mother so you and Mike can have some time alone together?" But no one ever did.

Prejudice showed up in odd places. When our cars broke down I wanted to rent a car from the place where we had bought cars several times. They refused to rent me one because of Mike. You can bet I won't buy one of their cars ever again! And we were not welcome in the only restaurant in our town, either.

The only real encouragement and support we got was from the GCAP (Gay Community AIDS Project) Buddies in Champaign (Illinois), and the doctor and nurses at Carle Hospital there.

In the last year, as Mother got worse and worse and she was out of her head most of the time, and I had to be at the hospital so much with Mike, I had to do something I didn't want to do—put my mother in a nursing home. It made me feel terrible, but I didn't have much choice. I had to fight with the nursing home, too, because they didn't take very good care of her.

Mike was in and out of the hospital, which was a long drive from our home. By February he was only 102 pounds.

It got to be like a roller coaster. Mike got sick and got better, got sick and got better, over and over. I called him my little Timex because he "kept on ticking." He went from 102 pounds to 60 pounds.

In August, Mike felt well enough to go to Florida and came back about nine days later. Mike and I took a trip through some rural counties to see the sights, but he was not feeling good at all.

November 22, 1990, Mike's lungs collapsed and they put a tube in his lungs. February 21, 1991, his lungs collapsed again.

Mike came home May 13th. He had a feeding tube in his nose and once a week it had to be taken out and cleaned because it got clogged. Several times we had to go back to the hospital to have it replaced because it got clogged up.

He had a shunt put in his arm. A nurse trained me to put the infusions in the shunt every six hours. Once I had to do it in the back seat of our car.

We went to Indianapolis to see the Names Project quilt panels that summer and Mike said he wanted a panel of his own after he was gone and he wanted to design it himself. And he did. He wanted balloons on it, of all different colors.

Through the years he was sick, he never stopped trying to educate people about AIDS. He was interviewed on TV. Mike and a public health nurse who became a good friend talked to college students. A high school student interviewed him and wrote a paper for one of her classes. She got an A on it, too.

My mother died in September 1992 at the age of 101. I sometimes think God took her then to make it easier for me to look after Mike, because soon after that he went downhill so terribly fast.

The Names Project was in Washington, D.C. in October 1992. Mike was very, very weak. He knew his time was about over. But he said there were two things he wanted to do. He wanted to be baptized by immersion and he wanted to go to Washington to see the Names Project. He got his first wish and was baptized. I was happy at that, and it was a beautiful ceremony.

I was afraid to take the trip to Washington. I thought the long trip would be the end of him and I wasn't ready to give him up. But I didn't say so and we went. We went to Washington on a chartered bus, on October 11th, a thirteen-hour trip. Mike lay on the back seat the whole trip. He was carried on and off the bus by friends and had to be pushed in a wheelchair. He had to be helped to the bathroom.

And then the long, long trip home. I was so afraid. I knew I was losing him bit by bit. We were not home a day before Mike had to go back to the hospital. This was on Monday. We got there about 2:30 in the afternoon, went to the emergency room, and he did not get in a regular room until 11:00 at night. He was on I.V.s.

Wednesday, they put a feeding tube in his stomach. Mike had said time and time again that he never wanted a feeding tube, that he couldn't live with one. Thursday, the doctor said Mike had pneumonia. He told the doctor, "Just make me comfortable and no life support except oxygen."

Mike's sister and brother came over and his sister stayed. Mike just kept getting weaker but he was still able to enjoy company. A friend called from California but Mike didn't have the strength to talk to him. Among the friends and relatives who came was Mike's friend and buddy, Forrest. Forrest was there many times when nobody else was and he helped us so many times when there wasn't anybody else to help. Two other special friends were mothers who had lost their sons to AIDS. He called them his "other mothers." They were wonderful to us.

Near the end, Mike said, "Mom, before you say goodbye at the last, will you kiss me and cover me up?" I said I would. And I knew he didn't mean the everyday goodbye. He meant the very last one. He died on October 20, 1992.

After the funeral service, when everybody was gone, I told the funeral director who had been so nice through the whole thing what Mike wanted me to do. He said of course and left us alone. So there we were, just my boy and me, and I covered him up and kissed him goodbye.

His suffering was over and he looked so beautiful.

I made the quilt panel with felt balloons just like he wanted, and a couple of months after his funeral we had a memorial service where his friends came and said a few words. They talked about his sense of humor and about his shopping sprees. It was a happy time, really, remembering Mike when he was alive. There was laughter and funny stories about Mike. Mike would like that. Then everybody signed the balloons on the quilt panel. Then we all went outside and when we felt we could let Mike go, we released our balloons. It was a gray, cold day, and the balloons sailed up against the clouds.

There isn't a day goes by that I don't miss him.

A newspaper did a story with a picture about me and Mike's quilt panel. Not long after that I got a call from another mother whose son died of AIDS. "I don't know how you do it," she said. "I tell everybody my son died of cancer. I'm too ashamed to tell them the truth." It made me feel very sorry for her. And it made me sad for her son. I told her, "I have never been ashamed of my son."

If some of those people who treated Mike bad were just half as respectful to him as he was to them, it would have made his last days more pleasant. If people would get more educated they wouldn't be so cruel. They don't know what kind of trauma it puts a mother and family through. Maybe they don't care. They should care, since they call themselves Christians. And yet there were other people who were supportive and made up for the uneducated ones.

Mike was a very courageous person. He took abuse, cruel remarks, and rejection from a lot of people. My prayers and hopes are that people will get more education. Until they get educated it will be hard for all our sick ones. Don't these people ever think they could be a victim of this dreadful disease?

One of the unfinished things Mike wanted to do was to help start an AIDS Task Force for education in our county, because there isn't any at all. So I have been one of the people trying to do this but it is very, very hard. It is an uphill battle.

People must get educated to avoid getting AIDS. And they must learn to practice the Christianity they talk about. They must learn to be kind

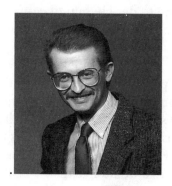

To the caregivers and all the friends who
helped make Mike's life more enjoyable in
the last few months.
Michael Robert Kindred
Feb. 23, 1952–Oct. 20, 1992

GOODBYE

JENNA A. FELICE

They all knew in 1986. I found out in 1988. They told me in 1989. Mommy died on November 21, 1991.

Mommy died on November 21, 1991. Sometime in the mid-eighties, they took out her adrenal gland, her gall bladder, and something else; she had a FEO, some sort of tumor thing, obviously a result of her weakened immune system. I remember when she went into the hospital for the operation. She had to drink this awful, chalky orange stuff before she went in, and the next time I saw her, she was totally zonked out on painkillers, with an ugly red line running from her cleavage to her navel. It took months to heal; every time she went to get the tape changed, she would come home in so much discomfort, all she could do was lie in bed and sigh now and then. When the stitches came out, there were these horrible holes on either side of the gash, with some nasty beginnings of scar tissue down the middle. You could tell that if you tugged at both arms, it would split apart.

That was when I started to take over for her. I was twelve. Of course, I always assumed it would only last until she got her strength back. I never relinquished my position; she never got strong enough to recover it. Looking back, I suppose she lost her strength early, because she had no adrenal gland; but it would have happened eventually.

I was twelve. I fell into a routine: up, school, home, housework, bed. I was the head of the family, with three children to look out for.

My sister, five years younger, couldn't match her own clothes. My stepfather wouldn't even move away from the television unless he thought we were doing something wrong. Mommy was simply too weak. She would always feel bad about not helping around the house, and would try to do something; my stepfather would yell at me for not doing it first.

At least she appreciated it all. And no matter how sick she was, she was determined not to be treated like an invalid. She loved to go shopping. But whenever we went, she would have trouble with the stairs in the subway stations, and we would end up having to take a cab home. That was expensive. She was taking about five different pills at that time, for asthma, blood pressure, the operation stuff, and the virus. But they still hadn't told me. One day I went snooping around, found the medicine bottle that said "AZT" on it and thunked onto the floor, stunned. I knew she was sick, but it had never occurred to me that it could be so serious. I didn't cry.

I didn't cry. I just gritted my teeth and determined to be a better housekeeper. I read recipe books, got a subscription to *Redbook*, and hid the one-subject reports that came in the mail from school saying, "She is not living up to her full potential." I became a pretty good cook, learned to despise ironing, and let my grades slip further; the choice between homework and dishes became simple once I figured out which one would keep my stepfather's belt in the closet.

Mommy developed Kaposi's Sarcoma, and all the little "lilacs" bloomed about her face, neck, arms, and legs. In and out of the hospital she went. One day she slipped under, and they put her on a respirator for two weeks. The decision to unplug her or not was left up to me, so I decided. The next day, when I went to say goodbye, she sat up and smiled at me.

It was then that they finally told me. I said I knew; they got upset at me; she cried; I told her that it would be okay, that I would take care of her. I guess I lied.

I guess I lied. She got pneumocystis pneumonia, and there was a three month stay in the hospital. My stepfather and I both snapped at my sister, who grew more sullen and wild each day. Everyone at school thought I was a "weirdo" because I didn't hang out with them after classes, or go to movies or parties. I wasn't allowed to stay over anyone's house, because I would be "too far away." I hid my report cards from my classmates. I wasn't stupid; I was just busy.

She came home. One night the ambulance visited at three o'clock in the morning when she was pissing blood, puking blood, breathing once every thirty seconds, each breath reeking of blood. I wrapped her in a blanket after rubbing her with alcohol, trying to bring her temperature down from 104°. This time she was only at Maimonides Medical Center for a month.

She got a lot stronger, and we would go to the park with friends. She started to gain weight when I made her shakes from mixes I bought at the health food store. But soon she started to lose it again. Her belly got bigger and her arms and legs were sticks, like those of the children you see on television commercials that ask you to spare the price of a cup of coffee. Now the KS was a permanent thing; she got weaker, bruised easily, and would sleep until noon. She never used to be able to sleep past 8:30 in the morning.

She got PCP again, and was back in the hospital. Things got worse, but she wanted to come home anyway. She started alpha interferon treatments, and I learned how to give her shots when her coordination wasn't too good. She got a little better, but she was miserable. My stepfather left, taking his bad vibes with him. Now things were okay. She was getting a little better, doing more things around the house—things I probably shouldn't have let her do.

She got PCP for the third time, and it was back into the hospital. By now the I.V.s wouldn't even stay in, her veins were so weak. After some discussion, she and I decided to go ahead with a bone marrow transplant, and I got ready for my own first hospital stay. She got a little stronger. We postponed the transplant. It looked like she would come home. But the day before she was scheduled to leave, her fever shot up. She was too weak to move. Her bedclothes were constantly drenched. She couldn't breathe.

She died.

I didn't even say goodbye.

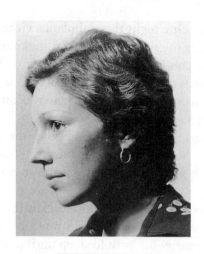

*For my mother, who was forty when she
died, but who will always remain
ageless in my memory; and for RKJK:
This is why I have such sad eyes.*

ANNIVERSARY 2

MIRIAM FINKELSTEIN

I
A year ago this December
They took my blood and told me
They would let me know
Whether or not I would
Live and die as my husband had
Shriveling, burning, shivering
Unable to walk, eat or
Breathe.

II
The counselor from the Board of Health
Was very nice.
"These are the support groups," she said
"If you should need them.
Call us on Thursday.
We might know by then."
They did, but couldn't tell me
Over the phone.
I took my daughter with me
In the cab and into the office
Of the counselor (a different one
But also nice).

When she said Negative
I didn't believe her
Until she showed me
My secret number and the word
Beginning with an N.
Then I burst into tears.
My son was waiting for us
We celebrated in a nearby coffee shop
The children were joyous
They must have been so worried.

III
Preoccupied with grief
and fear of positive knowledge,
Often tempted to shout,
"See what you did to me!"
Or to whisper, "Reunion may be imminent,"
I had put off the test
For months.
The cab ride back was different, but
Not as different as I had thought.
I had been resurrected
My life no longer tantalizingly
On hold. Why was I not
Ecstatic?
On that cold grey afternoon in December
Unable
to give him the news
I was for the first time alone.
In my head a neon sign
Blinked on and off
NOW WHAT?

To Jim: Feb. 14, 1930-July 22, 1989

MY LIFE WITH SCOTT

CARIE FORD-BROECKER

At twenty-one, I found out my fiance had HIV. At twenty-two, we married, at twenty-four I tested positive for HIV, at twenty-five, I was widowed, at twenty-seven I was diagnosed with AIDS, at twenty-eight, I am alive, happy, in love, and full of hope!

My name is Carie Ford and I am the widow of a man who died of AIDS, and I am a person living with AIDS. I married Robert Scott Ford in 1988. I was twenty-two years old. We already knew Scott was positive, but I had tested negative.

Scott had been through the Care Unit drug rehabilitation clinic a few years before we met. He had never been addicted to any one drug. He had sampled a wide variety of drugs since his youth, and at one point (around the age of twenty-three) he tried cocaine intravenously. He only shot up a few times, usually at parties, but it was enough to get him infected with a virus that he wouldn't know he had until five years after contracting it.

After our third date, I was in love with Scott. We had never even kissed, but I loved him and wanted to spend my life with him. I admired his directness and honesty. He had done a lot of work to become the person that I met. I never knew the "addict" Scott, the party animal, the manipulator. When I met Scott, he was at a point in his life when he was being the most responsible he'd ever been, and he was determined to live his life with love and integrity and to do it without drugs or alcohol. Scott had developed a profound spirituality and a simple philosophy of life. And all this before finding out he had a life-threatening illness. His recovery from addiction and his new outlook were the foundation he needed to cope with his positive test result. Finding out he was HIV-positive did not faze him. He was grateful to have lived as long as he had and to be experiencing the rewards of a sober life. Our commitment to each other only deepened and for two years we kept his diagnosis a secret from everyone.

By the time I tested positive, Scott had already begun to show some symptoms of the disease. We decided it was time to let our friends and family know what was going on to get some support. Scott's health continued to decline. Two and a half years after testing positive, Scott's health became very unpredictable. Some days he felt great and other days he couldn't get out of bed.

Scott's first major setback was a fungal infection of the esophagus. He would vomit all night and have fevers and chills almost every night. At first, I would get up with him whenever he was ill, to be with him and comfort him, but it got to be too much for me. I needed to take care of my own health, and I needed to get enough rest. The symptoms would subside for a few days or even a week, but they would always return.

After numerous blood tests and a spinal tap, we found out Scott had something more serious than the fungal infection. He had a bacterial infection called MAI (Mycobacteria Avium Intracellular). At the time (1990), there was no effective treatment for MAI. The medications were very toxic and even with treatment his prognosis was only a matter of months. After Scott began the anti-MAI medications, he felt a little better. He was still having chills at night and not sleeping well but during the day he felt okay. That lasted about a month and then he had a total relapse. He began the fevers, vomiting, and the coughing. And he was losing weight again. His illness became more and more like a roller coaster ride for both of us. He would start to feel better, have a relapse, take new medications, start to feel better, have another relapse, and on and on.

It was very difficult for me to get a full night's sleep. I would wake up in the middle of the night and listen to Scott coughing, shivering, and moaning, and I would feel so helpless, angry and tired. All I could do was put a pillow over my ears to drown out Scott's misery.

One of the most heart-wrenching days of his illness was the day his legs went numb. For months he'd had mild neuropathy which caused a tingling numb feeling in his toes and feet, but one morning he woke up and the numbness had spread to his knees. He called me at work to tell me, and he started sobbing. I went home right away, and we just hugged each other and cried. It was the first and only time I'd seen him scared. It was also the only time I ever saw him shed tears for himself. He learned to accept the neuropathy, and began walking with a cane and occasionally using a wheelchair.

Scott's MAI seemed to be stabilizing, but he began experiencing dementia which caused memory loss, confusion, and personality changes. He was becoming irritable, easily agitated, and often confused. He began getting lost on routine outings. He once ended up driving 100 miles away from home while trying to find the post office that was half a mile from our apartment. There were some rough times and thankfully, I eventually learned to stay calm, patient, loving, supportive, and caring. At times, it was difficult because some of Scott's actions were so frustrating and infuriating.

The most frightening experience of Scott's illness was the morning he had his first seizure. I was talking to him and all of a sudden he started shaking, having convulsions, and his eyes rolled up into his head. I called 911 immediately, and by the time the ambulance arrived, he had already begun to regain consciousness. It took him ten minutes to regain his memory as to how old he was, who I was, where he was, and what year it was. Once we got to the hospital, they ran numerous tests on him, but never did figure out what caused the seizure. He got a prescription for anti-seizure medication and we were sent home. That day, we decided I would stop working and stay home with Scott. The fear of what could have happened if I hadn't been home was overwhelming.

From then on I tried to never leave Scott unattended, but sometimes I had to leave him alone for a few hours to go run errands or just to get out and exercise or meditate. After the seizure I never could sleep well. If I wasn't watching Scott, I would imagine that he was having another seizure or that he wasn't breathing. I'd have to wake up and look at him and make sure he was okay.

Two weeks after the first seizure, he had another seizure. I didn't even call the ambulance this time, and I wasn't scared. I'd been through it before, and I knew he'd be okay. I just put his head in my lap, stroked him, and waited for him to regain consciousness. I didn't want him to get up too quickly or he'd be confused like the last time. When he came to, he didn't even remember that anything had happened. I actually had to convince him that he'd had a seizure. Then we called his doctor. He was told to increase his anti-seizure medication and to go in the next day and get a brain scan. The brain scan came back clear. Still we didn't know the cause of the seizures.

Over the next few weeks, Scott's body became racked with pain. He would wake me up screaming in pain two or three times a night. He had pain in his back, his legs, and his knees. I would rub whatever was hurting, which usually would help to minimize the pain. Massaging his body was like massaging a bone. There was no muscle or fat tissue, just bone covered with skin.

One morning Scott said, "I'm getting almost so miserable that I don't want to live any longer, but I'm not ready to leave you yet." I wanted to take away his pain. I didn't want him to die because I would miss him, but I didn't want to be responsible for holding him here in this life of pain and misery. I told him that I would be okay when it was time for him to leave and that he was not to stay for me.

Scott began getting bed sores and many different skin irritations all over his body and on the bottoms of his feet. Then he began to lose his hearing. For three weeks he ate very little. A bite here, a bite there. I did everything I could to keep Scott comfortable. I massaged him, stroked him, and put lotions and ointments on his bedsores. I helped him to get from one room to another so he wouldn't be in the same bed, in the same position constantly. I did a lot of research and made a lot of calls to get advice about every one of his ailments. I found out that, through a Buyer's Club in New York, I could purchase an antibiotic that was not approved by the FDA but seemed to be effective for treatment of MAI. I immediately sent away for the medication even though it was five-hundred dollars for a four week supply.

A week after sending away for the new MAI medication, Scott was rushed to the hospital in the middle of the night. At 3:30 in the morning he started having a series of small seizures. I called his Home Health Nurse who came over right away. I also called his doctor who said I should call an ambulance. By the time the ambulance arrived, he had lost consciousness. At the hospital, the doctor discovered that Scott's blood sugar level was extremely low. He was given an injection of glucose which immediately had him feeling better.

Once he was stabilized, he was admitted to the hospital for more tests. He had numerous blood tests, a spinal tap, a chest X-ray, and continued to have his finger pricked every four hours to check his blood sugar level. He was put on a constant glucose drip to maintain his blood sugar. I stayed in the hospital with Scott for over seventy-two hours doing everything I could to care for him and to keep him comfortable. Oftentimes, I slept in his bed with him and sometimes I slept in the spare hospital bed.

Scott's primary physician was out of town but would be returning on the fourth day of his hospitalization. The attending physician suggested intravenous feeding, but Scott wanted nothing to do with it. At least not until he could talk with the doctor he knew and trusted. That night Scott was given an injection of an anti-nausea medication. Immediately after the injection, he began hallucinating. He was very confused and very uncomfortable. He couldn't function. He was knocking stuff off his bedside table, and kept trying to get up and move around even though he was hooked up to I.V.'s. He tried to take a sip of water but didn't know how to swallow. I stayed up watching him all night to be sure he didn't hurt himself.

At about 2:00 a.m. he started having trouble breathing. The nurse hooked him up to some oxygen, which made him feel better, and he finally fell asleep. At 6:00 a.m. he woke up and said "Carie, are you alive?" I said "Yes, honey, I'm here." Then he asked "Am I alive?" I said "Yes, you're fine, you're going to be okay."

He was still hallucinating, and he knew it. He thought he was going crazy, but I explained that it was a side effect of the medication he'd been given the night before. I got in bed with him, and he put his arms around me. I lay on his chest. I cried silently, but he could feel the tears on his chest. He said, "Don't worry, I'll make it." I fell asleep in his arms praying he'd live. When we woke up at 8:00 a.m. his regular doctor was back. When he arrived, he was very concerned. He said that Scott should start intravenous feeding to build his strength, but that most likely Scott was coming to the end of his disease. Scott agreed to accept the feeding, but asked for some pain medication to make him more comfortable.

A few minutes later, the doctor came back and said that Scott was bleeding from his intestines, and the intravenous feeding wouldn't do any good. He said there was nothing more he could do, and he gave us the option of taking Scott home to die. I began making arrangements to get him home. Scott said he wanted something to make him as comfortable as possible right away. Then he asked the doctor to give me a Valium, and he asked me to call my mom to have her with me. Even moments from his own death, he was concerned that I would be okay and have the support I needed to survive him. I turned down the Valium. The strength we shared and the support of my friends and our families were all I needed to get me through.

Scott received three shots of morphine and then stopped breathing. I was by his side, and I stayed calm. I told him I loved him, that I'd be all right, and that I knew he'd be all right. I stroked his hair, his face, and his arm. His doctor turned off the oxygen and said, "Bye, Scott." Dr. Troll listened to his heartbeat which became fainter and fainter. I kept talking to Scott to make it easier for him to let go and to let him know I'd be okay.

After Scott's death, I rationalized and intellectualized to the point of not letting myself grieve. I told myself this was a natural process. People die every day, Scott was in a better place, and grieving would only harm me. At times, I would let my feelings of anger and sadness out, but mostly I just told myself I was okay. When I finally began to feel the pain of the loss and the yearning for him to come back, I never wanted the pain to end. I was afraid that if the pain ended, I would have to let go of Scott.

Three weeks after Scott's death, I began to have dreams about him telling me to take better care of myself. I hadn't been sleeping well, eating, or exercising. I kept going over and over his death in my mind, trying to make sense of it or trying to figure out what I could have done to make things different. At times, I wanted to stay in bed and fade away. I couldn't imagine moving through everyday life: the laundry, the dishes, preparing food, going to work. When Scott came to me in my dreams and meditations, he told me there was a lot I needed to do in this lifetime. He told me it was okay to let go of thinking about him so I could concentrate on myself.

I began to come out of a fog. I tried to remember the last few months before Scott's death, and it was extremely difficult. I had refused to believe he was that sick. He weighed only 115 pounds and much of his skin was not normal texture, but all I saw was my beautiful husband. There came a point where I no longer saw his disease. I only saw Scott. I was essentially living with his soul. And that was so alive to me, I didn't think I could lose it.

Scott and I had a wonderful love here on this physical plane, but what we have now and what he has left me with is more meaningful and more beautiful than anything we had before. I thank Scott for this precious gift that I am left with. My life is better for having loved and lost him.

When I met Scott I was looking for the meaning of life, and I found it. There is no better way to learn about life than experiencing death. Most of the time, my life doesn't seem out of the ordinary to me. I don't wonder why this is happening to me. It all feels all right.

I remember talking to Scott when he was sick, and saying, "What am I going to do without you?" He said "You're going to run and play and have joy." I didn't believe him, but now I know I can feel joy, and I know he wants me to.

It has now been two years and nine months since Scott's death and I'm engaged to be married. I am happier than ever and very much in love. My fiancé is an old family friend whom I've known for over ten years. He is HIV negative and is truly supportive of me, my AIDS activism, and my struggle to maintain my good health. Three years ago, I never could have imagined this to be possible. I'm in love, I'm happy, I'm healthy, and my memory of Scott no longer brings me pain, only the joy he wanted me to have.

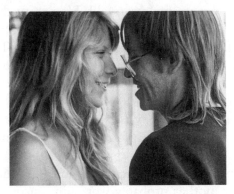

To my husband and friend, Scott Ford
Feb. 9, 1960–May 23, 1991

NEVER CAN SAY GOODBYE

WILLIAM H. FOSTER III

Not long ago, my younger brother, Timothy, died from AIDS. I received my share of sympathetic gestures from friends and wellwishers; flowers, plants, fruit baskets, kind notes. But these expressions of empathy gave me very little comfort. How could I possibly be consoled, when with every breath I drew I was trying to absorb the reality that my brother was dead?

He was only twenty-five years old. He deserved better. Better? Hell, he had just started living, only just begun to pull his life together. He was intelligent, fun-loving, a good brother. Tim was a kind, thoughtful and loving person. He attended church regularly, and even made sure that younger members of our extended family attended as well.

In a family of nine, he, my two youngest sisters and I were the closest. Because we were the last four kids "left at home," that seemed only natural.

I was the first to go away to college, and I am sure, although he never said it, my mother probably wore him out with reminders to follow his older brother's fine example. But Tim had ideas of his own. Even though he did manage to go to college for two years, he dropped out to find his own path. He started his own small hair salon and was doing well.

It was his apartment I stayed in whenever I came home. It was one of the few places I felt completely relaxed and comfortable. I often wonder if that was because we were both clean-freak Aries babies.

When I received word that Tim was in a hospital dying of AIDS, I was immediately struck by a wave of helplessness. I rushed to him to spend whatever time I could with him, fully expecting to see him as I last remembered—tall, laughing, glowing with health. I was led into the isolation ward to see him and was instructed on how to put on the protective gloves, gown and footwear. Seeing him hooked up to all those tubes and wires was shocking, heartbreaking, and made me mad as hell. I wanted to rip it all away from him and carry him back home. As he was down to not much more than 100 pounds, it wouldn't have been too hard.

We talked, that is I talked with him, and he nodded or shook his head, for as long as his strength held out. All he could manage at his best by this point was to write in a shaky scrawl, that yes, he loved me, too. He died about a week later.

At his memorial service, I tried to speak about the goodness of Tim's life, about the admirable type of young man he had turned into, and how our parents would have surely been proud of him. The words failed me. It hurt too much that he was gone.

The same thoughts kept whirling around and around in my brain: *It's so damn unfair! It isn't right! This is in no way just!* Where the hell was all that "Divine Justice" that I'd heard so much about since I was a child? How come God wasn't there to watch over my baby brother and keep him from dying? How the hell does the death of my youngest brother fit into God's Cosmic Plan? I had too many questions, too much pain, and no ready answers.

I cried a lot for Tim—loud, long, and frequently. Yet somehow, I still had the feeling that something, some part of my mourning was left undone. This seemed only to increase my anguish. However, the last memory I have of my brother occurred the week after his memorial service.

I dreamed I met my brother. In the dream, he appeared to me the way he looked when he was only about nine or ten years old. As his family-appointed guardian and babysitter, it is a time I remember well. Tim asked me if it hurt to see him again, now that he was dead. I said yes, and I missed him very much, and I started to cry. He went on to say that from where he was now, he could look down on me, as well as visit all the places our family had lived while we were growing up. He told me that our mother (who had died some six years earlier) was impressed with the writing I was doing. The exact phrase Tim said was, "You were always the one who was heavy at the typewriter," an expression he would typically use. It was also like Tim to ease my curiosity about what my mother would think of the work I was producing after she passed away. Suddenly, the pleasure and pain of receiving a message from my mother, delivered by my deceased brother, became too much for me. I fought my way out of the dream and clawed into wakefulness, tears streaming from my eyes.

The experience left me physically and spiritually drained. But as the days passed, I began to experience a long-awaited sense of relief, a feeling of completeness in my mourning. I finally realized that until his dream visitation, I had never said aloud, "I miss you." And speaking those words was very important, something I needed to say to him.

I will never truly recover from Timothy's untimely death. I will always feel that he was unfairly taken away before his life had really begun. But I am told by people who have experienced a similar loss that while the jagged hole in my heart will never heal, it won't throb so much after a time.

That's all I have to share now, except for one last personal lesson, and one final irony. The lesson? That love, particularly family love, does not end with the grave. It can reach out and touch you with warmth and caring from surprisingly far away, thank God.

Of all the realities that I ever imagined for myself, none included surviving the death of my younger brother. And yet, with his help, somehow I have. Not easily, to be sure. But somehow. The irony? It's that while I used to watch out for him, Tim is now watching over me. And somehow, sometimes, that knowledge eases my sleep. Thanks, baby brother. I love you, too.

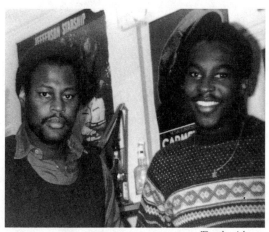

Timothy, right

To Timothy Harold Foster
brother, movie partner and shining spirit;
you'll always be a part of me.
March 29, 1960–Jan. 30, 1986

Frozen in Time

Suzanne Fried

1956

The little boy falls to the sidewalk as an older girl pushes him. Like a bolt of lightning, another child hurls herself at the girl. "You Rona, you! Get off him, leave him alone." She pushes the other girl to the pavement, sits astride her and begins pounding her back. "You jerk, you leave my brother…"

Her words are interrupted by an adult's shout. "What are you doing to her? Suzanne, stop that this minute."

The mother pulls her daughter off the girl. "Why is Richard crying? Why were you hitting Rona?"

Tears are streaming down the seven-year-old's face as she looks up at her mom. "But Mom, she was hurting him. No one hurts my baby brother, no one." This last pronouncement is accompanied by a vehement shake of her head and fists.

Later that night she hears the grownups laughing as her mother recounts the story to her father and her aunt and uncle. "Why are they laughing?" she asks herself sleepily. "What's so funny? He's my baby brother and I always keep him safe." Clutching her dolly to her chest she falls asleep, secure in the knowledge that whatever happens she will always be there to protect him.

Fast Forward to 1986

The little brother is now a busy executive with Walt Disney Studios. He has won national video awards for his directorship of the Home Video Department. He flies to London on the Concorde for business and he is about to be made Director of International Video Marketing. Life is good and sweet. His sister lives in San Francisco, an hour away by plane. She is in graduate school getting her Master's Degree in Counseling Psychology and she is waitressing to make ends meet. She has flown to Los Angeles for their birthday weekend. He will be thirty-four on February 19th and she is turning thirty-seven on the 26th.

She is waiting for him in his condominium and he is late coming home from the studio. Finally she hears the front door open.

"Hi, Suzie."

"Hi, Richie, where've you been?"

He is standing in the room, his tie in one hand and a crumpled piece of paper in the other.

"What's going on?"

He extends his hand. "Here, read this."

"What..."

"Read it!" His sharp tone startles her. "Sorry," his voice softens. "Suzie, please, read it."

Puzzled, she opens the paper. The words swim before her eyes. She reads it once more. "No, Richie, this can't be?"

He looks at her, blue eyes filled with tears and shock. "Suzie, I have AIDS, what am I going to do?"

August 17, 1986 (six months later)

The hospital room is hushed. It feels like a chapel. Richie is lying unconscious in the bed. His sister is holding him. He is dying and she cannot save him. Something bigger than both of them has knocked him to the ground and her hands cannot grasp and pull it off her baby brother's back.

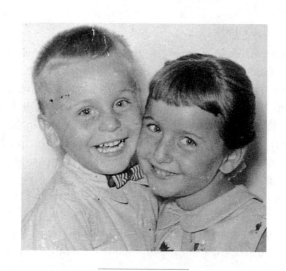

To Richard Bruce Fried, my baby brother
who lives on in my heart.
Feb. 19, 1952–Aug. 17, 1986

WHEN THE NIGHT HAS BEEN TOO LONELY

JANE FUTCHER

Octber 20, 1991, Mill Valley, CA. Steve called this morning. "Ruffin's in the hospital," he said. "He's very weak. He's got lesions in his brain. Don't tell him I told you. He doesn't want anyone to know."

"Thanks," I said, and hung up the phone.

Ruffin is my third cousin, my Texas cousin. We're bonded by the fact that we're both gay, both artists, and both children of mothers who grew up in the same dusty little Delta town in Arkansas. I've known for some time that Ruffin is HIV-positive, but this is new. This is AIDS and a disease called toxoplasmosis. It can mean only one thing—pain and sickness and probably death.

I drive to the hospital in San Francisco thinking of the night we first met, in 1977, when I was thirty and had just moved from New York to San Francisco with Catherine, my lover. Ruffin invited us to an opening of his photographs at a gallery off Union Street. My cousin was short, with a big personality, a huge smile, and a bald head. "Do you think he's gay?" Catherine whispered.

"Maybe. Let's have him to dinner." A few weeks later, at our apartment in Pacific Heights, he told us his story—about growing up gay in Texas, about going to college in Boston, about starting in 1967 an avant-garde nightclub called Cerebrum in New York, where guests were asked to leave their inhibitions and their clothes at the door.

Since that time, he'd been a theatrical agent and a hippy on the Hog Farm. His career as a fine arts photographer was just taking off.

"Do your parents know you're gay?" I asked.

"No," he said. "They wouldn't understand."

I arrive at the hospital. Ruffin is asleep. He opens his eyes. I put a flowering cactus on the table next to his bed. "Who told you I'm here?" he asks.

"A little bird," I answer nervously, hoping he won't be angry. "How do you feel?"

"Headache." He rubs his forehead and closes his eyes.

"I love you," I say.

"Love you, too," he whispers, and falls back asleep.

I sit for a few minutes, watching the I.V. drip into his wrist, listening to the rattle of dishes and dinner trays being carted through the halls. I feel sad and disoriented. This docile man next to me is not the Ruffin I know. *My* cousin is always "up," always a cyclone of activity, always planning something extravagant, like photographing the Statue of Liberty from a helicopter or installing giant pennants in the Port Authority building in New York. The Ruffin I know is in control, driving me crazy with his ambition on my behalf. He wants all his friends to achieve, to go for their dreams. Tonight, he is quiet, and it's disturbing.

I call Steven when I get home. "Will the lesions go away?" I ask hopefully.

"I don't know." Steven's voice cracks. Ruffin is his best friend. They have known each other since their hippy days together on the Hog Farm. Ruffin was Steve's first gay trick. "He's very sick, Jane. I think he might be dying."

"Now?" I say, catching my breath.

"Even if the lesions get better, it's just a matter of time."

"Does his mother know?" His mother, Edwynne, is a small, strong Southern lady in her late seventies. Ruffin is her only son, and they travel together several times a year. Her husband is dead, and her other son, Ned, was killed in Vietnam.

"She knows," Steve says.

"Is she coming?"

"Ruffin doesn't want her to."

I shake my head. This is all so sudden. A month ago, when I last saw my cousin, he was planning for a show at the Comedie Francaise in Paris. Now, Steve says he's dying.

I call Edwynne in Texas. "I saw Ruffin today."

"Did you?" Her voice is cautious; she is disconcerted that I know he is sick. His AIDS is her secret, too.

"He's very weak," I say. "But he recognized me."

"Thank you for calling, honey."

We say goodbye awkwardly.

At forty-nine, Ruffin is still not out to his parents. As far as I know, he has never taken a gay friend home to Texas. Once, in the eighties, he had a boyfriend, Bruce, for an entire year. But he never told his parents the nature of their relationship. His family has played a grim little game for years—don't ask, don't tell.

January 4, 1992. Today is Ruffin's birthday. Incredibly, he is in Costa Rica, vacationing with his mother. It is hard to believe that the man I saw in the hospital in October is well enough to travel in Central America. But the drugs have reduced the size of the lesions. "He insisted on going," Steven tells me on the phone. "I was sure he was too spaced out to make his connecting flight. He can't remember anything. But he's down there. Called me today. Says everything's great."

February 27, 1992. I am forty-four today. Erin, my lover, gave a birthday party for me at a bowling alley in San Rafael. Steven and Douglas, his lover, brought Ruffin. The three of them gave me a slinky silk nightgown from Saks. Ruffin looked pale, his eyes huge, his skull dangerously close to his skin; a small red lesion tipped the end of his nose. When he spoke, finding words was very hard.

"This is my cousin Ruffin," I said, introducing him to Robin, a psychotherapist friend whose specialty is hospice counseling. She took his hand, and as she stared into his eyes, I felt a circle of calm surround them.

"Why, you're not rough at all," Robin said gently. "You're very sweet."

Ruffin smiled a beautiful Ruffin smile. "Thank you," he said, his eyes reaching into hers.

Steven pulled me aside. "We absolutely cannot allow him to drive anymore. I've hidden the keys to his car. He can't remember anything."

April 2, 1992. Ruffin is in the hospital again and Douglas, who has taken over the administration of Ruffin's life, has asked me to sign a power of attorney which gives me the authority to write checks in his name. We must do it quickly, Doug says, before Ruffin is too disoriented to write his name.

"Why don't you be power of attorney?" I ask, nervous about playing such a key role. I feel like I might be trespassing.

"You're family," Douglas explains. What he means, I think, is that Edwynne wouldn't approve of Ruffin's gay friends signing her son's checks.

"Why doesn't Edwynne come?" I ask. "Surely it's time."

Douglas sighs. "She's got some wedding in Texas. She can't come till it's over."

At the hospital, Douglas explains to Ruffin that he's signing a paper that gives me permission to sign his checks. I'm afraid he will be furious. "Fine," he says pleasantly, as Douglas places the papers in front of him. I start to cry. This is a man who has never been happy with anything less than total control. He is signing away his life, and he is not in the least bit concerned.

That night, I call his mother. "Ruffin's terribly sick," I say. "Can you come soon? He won't be coherent much longer."

"Thank you, honey," she says. "If it weren't for the rice bag party I'd be there."

"Rice bag party?"

"For the bride."

"The bride?" I'm still confused. Edwynne adores Ruffin. How can a bride in Texas be keeping her away? "What's a rice bag party?" I say finally.

The ladies, she explains, will come to her house for coffee and dessert, at which time they'll wrap little gauze squares around bundles of rice, which they'll tie with ribbons and then throw at the bride and groom as they leave the church. "Her parents are old, old friends," Edwynne says, as if that explains everything.

"Do they know how sick Ruffin is?" If they're old friends, I think, surely they won't mind if she cancels the rice bag party.

"They know absolutely nothing," she says coolly. "And they never will. I'm going to tell them Ruffin has a brain tumor."

Easter Day, April 19, 1992. Ruffin is home from the hospital and we had a wonderful, joyous party at his apartment in North Beach overlooking the San Francisco Bay. His friend Randy flew up from L.A. for the weekend and ordered a turkey dinner from Safeway. Doug and Steve were there, and Erin, and Erin's mother Maggi, and Ruffin's friend Ruth, and Randy and me. We had such a nice time. Ruffin had no idea what was going on, but he seemed very happy as he lay on the couch, his head propped on a pillow, the top button of his jeans undone. He has gained weight from the appetite pills he's been taking, and we all laughed at his little belly poking out. For one thing, it means he's still eating, and for another thing, it's poetic jus-tice—he's always been critical of us when we have weighed an ounce more than we should.

Steve and Doug and Erin and I are becoming very close friends. It turns out Erin and Steve travelled in the same hippy circles in the six-ties and know some of the same people. Steve is very funny and smart and pessimistic and hysterical, the way I often am. And Doug, a set designer who's known Ruffin since college, is quiet and gentle and strong. Although he's on a tight deadline—finishing a set for a George Lucas multimedia road show in Japan—Doug still handles all the details of Ruffin's life—doctors, hospitals, insurance companies, friends.

Edwynne called to say that she is coming on April 28th. Having her here will make life easier for all of us. She can oversee Ruffin's health care and run his household, which Doug and Stephen have been doing for almost two months. In preparation for Edwynne's visit, Steve and Doug removed all of Ruffin's sex toys, which he kept in a closet under the stairway. There was so much paraphernalia that they had to hire a taxi to drive them to a dumpster, where they ditched five bags of dildoes, harnesses, nipple clips, and pornography.

May 10, 1992. Edwynne is here! And Ruffin is in Pacific Medical Center. We're relieved that he's back in the hospital, because Edwynne fired the night shift nurses when she arrived and then got frightened about what she'd do if Ruffin wandered around in the mid-dle of the night or had a convulsion. Edwynne is great with Ruffin, goes to the hospital every morning at nine and doesn't leave until the evening, when Steve and Doug, or sometimes Erin and I pick her up and take her to dinner. She bathes and feeds Ruffin and badgers the nurses to change his sheets and cut up his food if she's not there to do it. His mind is completely confused. But, to our amazement, he had one very clear moment the other day. Steve visited after work, smiled and said, "How are you, honey?"

Ruffin sat up, opened his eyes wide, and said, "Scared!"

Steve looked startled, then squeezed his hand and said, "I know, honey. This is really, really scary. I'm scared, too." I started to cry and so did Steve.

Having Edwynne here has created some new problems for us, the worst of which is her homophobia. A few days ago, two friends of Ruffin's from his HIV support group came to visit him. They are both very thin and weak, and Edwynne shooed them away, making it very clear that she did not want them to come back. "What horrible people," she said to me, after they'd gone. "How dare such sick, unattractive people visit Ruffin?"

"Edwynne," I said. "Those are Ruffin's friends. They're from his support group. They love him. They came because they care about him. How can you be so unkind?"

"Unkind? I'm not unkind. If it weren't for their terrible ... lifestyle, none of this"—she glanced at Ruffin—"would be happening."

May 18, 1992. Stephen finally exploded at Edwynne. He'd had a long, exhausting day at work, and when he got to the hospital, Edwynne complained that those awful men from Ruffin's support group had come again. Stephen went ballistic. "Goddammit, Edwynne," he yelled. "If you don't like gay people, at least have the courtesy to keep it to yourself. I'm gay," he said, "and Douglas is gay, and your son is gay, and all the people who are taking care of Ruffin are gay, including Jane and Erin. So you'd better shut your mouth. We love Ruffin, but we can't cope with his illness and your homophobia at the same time."

Douglas listened in silence, half appalled and half relieved, and Edwynne became very subdued and was absolutely quiet all the way home. Today, when I spoke to her on the phone, she said that she and Stephen had had a little "run-in" last night, but it wasn't until Stephen called that I found out what really happened. Stephen feels better and says he can handle Edwynne now because he's not holding back so much anger. Edwynne is such a mass of contradictions. She loves hanging out with Steve and Doug and Erin and me, but our sexual orientation terrifies her. I wonder why.

Memorial Day, May 31, 1992. Edwynne and Steve and Doug were supposed to come here today for a holiday barbecue. This morning, after playing racquet ball with Erin at the Y, I burst into tears. "What's wrong?" Erin led me out into the sunshine.

"I think Ruffin's ... I think he's dead."

At home, when I phoned the hospital, no one answered. I called his house, but no one answered there. Then I rang the nursing station. "Your cousin passed away early this morning," a nurse told me. "His mother was with him, and his friends came and picked her up a few minutes ago."

The sound of my sobs startled me. Erin put her arms around me. All the pain, all the confusion, all the strain is over. But so is the good stuff. The cousin who encouraged my writing, who fought for the best in me, who entertained me with stories of his travels abroad, is dead. So is the docile, helpless child-man he had become.

When Stephen called, I cried again. "Come on over. Right now. We all need to be together. Bring the food," he said. "We'll cook on Ruffin's deck and have a party. There's nothing else to do."

The day was clear and warm and the luncheon was wonderful. We ate grilled lamb and sat out in the sunlight, on the back porch, away from the wind, and talked. Edwynne insisted she does not want a funeral. She will cremate Ruffin and take his ashes back to Texas.

Two Years Later

March 10, 1994. "I can't take much more of this," Stephen said to me today.

"More of what?" I asked. "What's happening?"

"I lost two more friends this week. Neither as close as Ruffin. But it's fucking painful."

"You miss Ruffin?" I said, knowing that these new deaths had brought back the pain of that other one.

"I miss him all the time. He was my closest, gayest friend. I miss his energy. I miss that frenzy of activity that happened wherever he was. He forced me to try new things. And he always knew what was happening in the gay world—what was in and what was out. My life is really flat without him."

Doug, who's often absorbed in his work, nodded in agreement.

"I spoke to Edwynne last week," I said. "She says she has her group of lady friends, that they do everything together, and they see each other every day. But she feels terribly alone without Ruffin. She says she misses us a lot."

"She doesn't miss us," Stephen roared. "She hates our queer guts."

"That's not what she said. She says she misses us a lot."

"She better miss us," Stephen fumed. "We saved her ass. Her son's ass, too." Then, after a long pause, he said, "Shall we call her?"

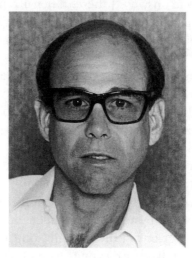

To my cousin and friend, Ruffin Cooper, Jr.
Jan. 4, 1942–May 31, 1992

To my Son, Tim

Joyce Gallegos

My journey with you was a learning experience. I learned patience, unconditional love and courage...a lifetime of all emotions that will stay with me forever. In all its pain, it will strengthen and guide me in your pathway when the time calls. I feel changed in a way that words cannot describe. What an honor to be at your bedside when you very gently took your last breath. At that moment I truly witnessed something that very few will experience...a complete circle of a lif ...birth, growth and death. It all seemed so orderly and right at that moment.

My fondest memories of your love and courage occurred a few weeks before your transition. I'll never forget the soothing hug and reassuring words you spoke to me when I was in a panic over your rapidly dropping temperature. We were alone in the city with a paralyzing snowstorm outside and could not get help. Another time, during the night, I asked if you were cold and wanted a blanket. You indicated you were okay and I said I was freezing. You reached out with your very thin arm and hand and softly rubbed my arms to warm them. And the most memorable moment...just twenty-four hours before you left this earth, you were able to gather enough strength to turn your body and roll down next to me from the top of the trundle futon to the lower part where I slept. At the time I didn't get it, but later I realized that was your only way to say goodbye to me. How you could do that feat in your frail and weakened condition was true testimony of your grace, strength and courage. These special moments are the richest gifts I shall ever receive and will never ever forget.

Thank you, my son, I will always love you and carry you close in my heart forever.

With Loving Gratitude,
Mom

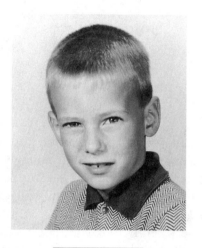

To my son, Tim, whom I carry in my
heart, with all my love, Mom
March 29, 1956–April 4, 1994

RECUERDO...I REMEMBER

DAVID GARNES

June 28, 1992—Manchester. Luis died at 6:30 this morning, peacefully, in our bed. His hand was still warm when I went back into the bedroom just before the funeral people came. We had to move some furniture so they could get the stretcher in and out. These are the two things I keep thinking about.

December 3, 1990—Hartford. Today Luis was given the State Commissioner's AIDS Leadership Award. He's a cynic regarding public recognition, particularly in a political context, but he's also a performer and somewhat of a ham. I know this pleased him. There were a lot of cheers and whistles from the audience when he walked to the front of the room.

November 26, 1992—San Juan. I am spending Thanksgiving here, my first trip to Puerto Rico since Luis died. I'm staying in Isla Verde, near Santurce where Doña Mery lives and Carolina where Luisa and her family have a house. Luisa who is eight years older than Luis lived in the apartment upstairs when they were growing up. Luis always called her his sister, and her two boys once stayed with us in Connecticut for a few weeks when they were little. It is all wrong that I am here without Luis. I remember the first time he showed me around the island. This is his country, not mine.

July 1, 1992—Manchester. I asked Catlina if she would help plan the memorial service. I think she is glad to do this, but I also need to remember that this is a hard time for a lot of people. I've never known anyone who engendered more intense affection in his friends than Luis. It used to bother me that I had to share him with so many people, but that was a long time ago.

October 24, 1981—Storrs. I've been at my job in the library for a couple of months. I think I'm going to like it here in Connecticut. The other day I just happened to be working at a colleague's desk during her lunch break. A quiet voice above me said, "Excuse me, I'm the grad assistant working with the bilingual program, and I have some books for you to order." I looked up and saw the smile. What is it about this man's smile? It's gentle, confident, open. It's the first thing I noticed about him. His name is Luis Felipe. His family calls him Willie.

May 16, 1986—Hartford. Yesterday the doctor asked me to wait outside while she spoke to Luis. About five minutes later he called me in and I knew right away what she had told him. We didn't say much, just held each other. Today we had a long and good talk. He is off the oxygen and recovering quickly, and I just want to get him out of the hospital.

September 25, 1982—Mansfield Center. "Hi, I'm home," I shouted as I closed the door one night last week. From downstairs I heard footsteps running, and then I saw Luis' head as he turned the corner on the landing. He still couldn't see me from that angle, but I will always remember the joyous, expectant look on his face. Can I really be making someone this happy? Me?

November 26, 1992—Santurce. When I opened the black iron gate to Doña Mery's patio, I thought of all the times Luis must have walked these steps and greeted the cats who were forever waiting to be fed. How many of the cats I saw today did he know? In the back bedroom of the apartment—Luis' old room—I noticed some textbooks, neatly arranged on a high shelf from his days at the University in Rio Piedras. It's noisy all the time around here, and Doña Mery told me that Luis used to study every night at the library, a long ride away, to escape the boomboxes and the neighbors shouting and the kids playing in the street.

April 12, 1992—Boston. Luis sang "Gracias a la Vida" at José and Larry's service of union. I was a little concerned that he hadn't recovered from the pneumonia completely, and he is still really thin. But his voice was strong and true, and everyone came up to him at the reception and told him how beautiful his song was. It's been almost eleven years since we met.

March 24, 1989—Hartford. Luis was on television again. He's been interviewed so many times as an AIDS educator that it's not such a big deal anymore, but I recorded this so he can see it later on. I'm always amazed at how at ease he is and how perfectly he speaks English. Maybe that's why my Spanish is still so lousy. I am so proud when I see him in public, and I always think, yes, and after the show he's mine!

June 22, 1992—Manchester. The hospice staff who come to the house are good people. I really like Liz, the nurse, and I know that she and Luis have taken to each other. A lot of friends want to visit and I am trying to balance what is good for Luis, for me, and for them. I admit that I lean more to those who were there for him always. Yesterday he played cards with Mary and won. We've gone for a few rides in the car. Today I asked him if he was glad to be getting out in the fresh air. He looked at me with that sweet smile and just said, "Oh yes!" His hand holding mine felt so strong and warm.

February 8, 1993—Santurce. Today I met Luisa at her office and we walked for ten or fifteen minutes through the crowded streets to visit Doña Mery. Luisa pointed out two empty movie theaters where she and Luis used to see Saturday matinees, and a pizza house where they ate after the show. "Willie was always talking, talking, talking when we were little," she said. "He was always looking up when we were walking and asking me questions about this, about that."

July 12, 1992—Willimantic. The Hispanic Church was the right setting for the service. Luis' heart was really in this community. I turned around at one point and it was a shock to see so many people. I am glad I wrote in the program instead of speaking. We ended with a tape of Luis singing "Gracias a la Vida." I tried not to feel the irony.

January 17, 1994—*Manchester.* Today Dan and I were talking about Luis, and I said I felt that he had been my partner, my friend, and maybe even a bit of my child, inevitable, I think, when there is a

14 year age difference. I wonder where I feel the greatest loss. He was first of all my partner; my life companion and lover. But I think I also understand the helplessness a grieving parent must feel. I would have done anything to make him live. This pain never goes away.

February 1, 1993—Manchester. I have hundreds of photos from the trips we took: Luis entering the main gate at Disney World. Luis a tiny figure in front of the Queen Mary in Long Beach. Luis laughing next to a guard at Buckingham Palace. Luis in New Orleans, leaning on the Bourbon Street sign. Luis barely visible in a sea of grass on Block Island. Luis standing in front of a steamboat in Nashville. On that trip I had met him after an AIDS conference, and he's wearing the white and yellow t-shirt that says "Remember Their Names."

July 11, 1992—Willimantic. From program notes to *A Celebration of the Life of Luis Felipe Pereira:* "I am honored as Luis' partner to be able to share with you in this celebration of his life. To have known Luis in any capacity is to have experienced a warmth and love we all look for but do not often find. When you were with Luis, you knew that he was there for you at that moment with all his humor and honesty and caring. Whatever I was able to do for Luis was returned to me many, many times over. Rest in peace, Love, and know that you have given me a lifetime of joy."

November 30, 1993—Manchester. I'm back from my fourth trip to Puerto Rico since Luis died. Why have I gone running down there so many times this year? This morning in San Juan as the plane taxied for the takeoff, I had a sudden and overwhelming image of the cemetery in Bayamon. I felt the sun beating down on the bronze plaque, and I heard the constant buzz and drone of the cicadas in the burnt grass. I will go about the business of my life, such as it is, and the sun in Bayamon will keep scorching the ground, the rains will come and go, drenching the artificial flowers, and still Luis will remain in that marked plot, locked in time. I am beginning to know that what I am looking for is really in my heart. There he sings and laughs and holds my hand. There he is always smiling, running up the stairs to greet me when I come home.

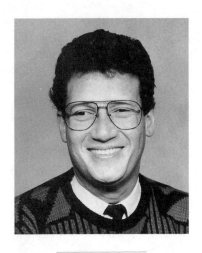

For Luis Felipe Pereira
Jan. 4, 1955-June 28, 1992

LUIS

KIMBERLY GEROULD

"Butterflies count not in months but in moments, and have time enough."
–Tagore

The phone rings on a warm spring morning, and a man with a soft accented voice introduces himself as Serge. "I'm a friend of Luis' and he asked me to call you. He's in the hospital, and found out yesterday that he has AIDS." Silence. I feel his quiet presence on the other end of the line.

I think of myself for a quick moment: could I get it too? What do I really know about it? But I tell Serge I'll be there.

Luis. I haven't seen him for a while. Now I understand. He wants to protect me.

That afternoon I prepare for my visit. I am afraid, afraid of what I'll see, afraid of this disease, for him, for myself, no matter what they say about not getting it from casual contact. Afraid of witnessing death. My mother's is so recent and I know that Luis has thought of that. I take him a tape of Silvio Rodriguez, the Cuban singer/poet we both cherish, cut some zinnias from my backyard plot, and go out into the now hot afternoon and catch the bus for the hospital.

The hospital is a monstrous building with tall, dark windows. I enter to the shock of cold air, muffled voices and bells over loudspeakers, families coming and going with packages. I try to read their faces; do they have tragedy, too?

I come off the elevator onto the floor Luis is on, feeling nervous, breathing deeply, trying to look calm. I read the room numbers—203, 204, 205—his room. A sign on the door says "Contaminated blood products: use gloves." So cruel, so primitive, I want to take him out of here, I want to run away. But I push through the closed set of double doors. "Luis?" He lies on the bed looking very thin and tired, skin sallow, a tube in his nostrils, and there is an older woman by his side. He sees me and slowly turns up his lips slightly and crinkles his eyes. Ay, Luis, you still have your magic. "Kimita…" is all he says. I sit next to him in the chair the woman has offered and take his hand.

I first met Luis Armando Valdes soon after my first long-awaited trip to Cuba. I was bursting with the experience, a revolutionary society full of wonderful and terrible things, but had no one here who could quite comprehend the contradictory picture I brought back with me.

I've been asked to translate for a Salvadorean man speaking at a Harvard forum on Latin American refugees. Next to me at the speaker's table is a thin, dark-skinned man with a slightly pockmarked face. He's neatly dressed in tight, creased jeans and a tan leather jacket. He speaks to the woman next to him, and my ears pounce on his Cuban accent.

The forum begins so there's no time to grill him. How did he end up here in the U.S. and this forum? I like the way he talks, gesturing with his long-fingered hands as if he were conducting music. Even though he's speaking seriously, in keeping with the scholarly room we're in, I can easily imagine him joking. In fact, I think he'd like to. "The local block Committees to Defend the Revolution are really neighborhood spying and gossip organizations. They keep track of who you're mixing with, how you dress, if you sign up for so-called volunteer work." It is refreshing to hear this said so matter-of-factly, but I can see faces looking at one another in the small audience, as if to say "Ah yes, we know what kind of Cuban this is."

Luis played the game in Cuba, tried to be "correct," participated in his local political organization, but felt stifled. To be openly gay meant at best certain ostracism and losing his job and at worst imprisonment. Luis wanted more in life. He wanted to be himself and so he made the irreversible decision to leave.

He packs up his papers when he finishes his talk, and I am unable to speak to him since I am still on the panel. I urgently scribble him a note. "We must talk. I understand what you're saying. Please call."

Four years later this tattered piece of paper is returned to me with other cards and letters I have written Luis.

It's moving day, a bitter, blustery January day, and Luis has to leave this subsidized apartment to go to another: his roommate who also had AIDS died last month.

I run in out of the cold, up the dirty stairwell, pass someone I don't know carrying a box, and go into the apartment, now dismantled and filled with people. The inner core, Luis' adopted family—Sharon, José, Ray, myself—are there, plus others from the AIDS Action Committee. Some are packing, others loading the cars and van out on the street. There's a festive air, as if all our combined energy could infuse Luis with strength. He is in the back room now empty except for the bare mattress he lies on, huddled under a blanket. Barbara, his old ESL student who's adopted him (her sons are in Colombia), wipes his forehead with a damp cloth. "Ay, yo no sé, I don't know if I can make the trip," and he looks as if he's going to cry. But Ray and Jose come in with his overlarge winter coat, bundle him into it, wrap a soft wool scarf around his face and put on his fedora. They gently embrace him into a chair they've made with their arms and carry him down the stairs.

Luis' new place, his own place, is exquisite. It's on a grey treeless street in a neighborhood surrounded by factories, but inside his apartment is an oasis. Every artwork has been carefully hung, plants and candles and ceramics deliberately placed, his tapes neatly organized by the bed, which is underneath a mantel that holds an intricately carved candle and a painting of pastel stucco houses in old Havana. The kitchen is bright with a lush fern in the window, a blue table and yellow trim around with white walls. Luis has a special affection for butterflies, "mariposas," and there's a delicate print of a butterfly on the wall.

Barbara, ever present, except when she's cleaning a city office building at nights, is stirring a pot of black beans and rice that fills the air with the fragrance of garlic, cilantro and cumin. Luis is in a frenzy because Stephen and Luis met at Christmas, and now, a month later, Stephen is coming from California to live with Luis. It's insane, Luis is dying, how can Stephen pick up his life and move here? Why do any of us do this? I dread coming each time, but as soon as I enter his house I'm in the charmed place, Luis' web.

"Kimita, ¿Cómo tu estás, mi hija? Te ves tan bella, tan radiante." Only Luis can make me believe I look radiant. "Estás enamorá…I knew this was the man for you. Right from the start," he says, laughing, lying back in his propped-up pillows. "And he had to be Latino, of course."

Luis believes in his own odd mix of astrology, Buddhism and Santeria and makes pronouncements about me that I'm inclined to believe. "Chica, you had a past life, there's some African blood in you —must've been old Havana. I can see you dancing a guanguanco in high heels and a red satin dress."

"Seguro, Luis, and you sang at the Tropicana, crooning boleros and rumbas to Havana socialites, in one of those tight shirts, you know, with the ruffled sleeves." Luis has a rich, romantic singing voice and would like to sing professionally.

"And now we're ESL teachers…where did we go wrong?" he asks and closes his eyes for a moment. I know it's the nausea, but he doesn't like to go on about it. "Ay Kim, me hace falta Cuba, I miss Mami, my little brother, I miss Mami's picadillo and rice, the coffee. It's so strange that you've been able to go and see my family, and I can't. You know, you're like a bridge for me."

Luis is a bridge for me, too.

Cuba. Luis and I are going to tell his story of Cuba—of his leaving, coming to the U.S., being a "Marielito"—"Scum" to the revolutionary Cubans there, "worm" to the Cuba lovers here. Yes, we'll write about it, a book, like an autobiography. Luis has the stories and I have the language and the understanding. Though it remains unspoken, Luis is aware of his mortality. He wants the world to hear his story.

Except that it's my story, too. I've been a Latinophile for a long time, somehow melding bits of Latin culture into my Swedish/Anglo heritage. I lived in Puerto Rico, work with Spanish-speaking people, dance salsa, and now have children who are half Puerto Rican. I came of age during the Vietnam War and my sense of the world's injustice became painfully clear during the year I lived in Puerto Rico. Up close, I witnessed people taking huge risks to change their society. I was nineteen, and it was a turning point.

Cuba has a special pull. Cuba had had a revolution. What a thought—could a liberated society really exist, so close to us, and a Latin culture on top of it all? Sounded like utopia. But I knew enough to distrust the starry-eyed reports of U.S. leftists who returned from revolutionary guided tours of the island.

During my first visit I dutifully attended the tours of carefully chosen farmer's cooperatives, a meeting of the national women's organization and centers of official culture. But I also wanted the streets of old Havana and partied at night during carnival. I started to meet the "underside," people who didn't volunteer to cut sugar cane, who weren't members of their block committee, their union, the Young Communist League, people who grew up in the revolution and loved it for all the good it had done, but now wanted the freedom to be different—to be gay, to be a hippie, to call Fidel Castro power-hungry, to read the great Cuban counterrevolutionary writers. These people's faces stayed with me long after I left, and I was indebted to them for trusting me with their forbidden stories, stories that broke the confines of "left" or "right."

I felt alone with the weight of their words until I met Luis. He, too, needed to share his story with someone in this new land he had escaped to. He missed his country terribly, suffered with the knowledge that he could not return and that he had not been able to say a proper goodbye to his mother and little brother.

I decided to make a second visit to Cuba, to reconnect with friends I had made the first time, and to visit the families of Luis and José, his childhood friend who left Cuba with him. My big red backpack was carefully packed on the bottom with gifts from Luis and José - a pen set for Angel, Luis' brother, a pipe for José's father, some reading glasses for his mother, medications, colorful scarves. I also had two books of Reinaldo Arenas, the once-famous, now banned Cuban writer, for a writer friend, packed beneath underwear and tampons, in the hope that they would distract the vigilant customs officials.

Upon arrival in Havana, I call Estrella, Luis' mother, who invites me to come for dinner. I ride the crowded bus several miles through the city, amidst stares of Cubans unaccustomed to seeing foreigners in this section of the city, and get off where she has told me. Walking down the street, people smile at me knowingly—clearly the neighborhood has been alerted. Friends and relatives of Luis' family happily guide me to the house, or actually the two rooms of the house in which Estrella and Angel live.

She hugs me as if I were her own daughter, her head barely reaching my chin. We sit in the only chairs in the house at the small kitchen table, and I tell her about Luis— his job, his apartment, his friends, what he does—he isn't sick yet. Yes, he cooks great Cuban food. Yes, we go dancing, to the movies. Yes, he talks about Cuba and his family all the time. There is no mention of how he left, of the conditions in Cuba.

Does she know he's gay? Somehow I sense that she deeply accepts her son as he is, whatever she says to herself.

She has prepared rice and black beans and picadillo, a rich mixture of ground beef and raisins and olives. Only I eat; she refuses, insisting she has already eaten. I imagine that this is the meat ration for the week. Upon leaving, she gives me an old family photo of herself and her two young sons to bring to Luis.

I am the courier of her pain and loneliness.

"I came here to be free," snorts Luis, "and look at me now." He's recovering from his second bout with pneumocystis pneumonia and is starting to get some color into his face again. "Yes, yes, I'm gay and I'm proud. They're just going to have to wheel this loca through the Gay Pride March."

It's a relief to see him rallying again. We all feared that this time might have been the end, and we're all tired from spending nights on mattresses on the floor in his hospital room. There simply isn't enough care: he needs someone by his side—to wipe the sweat off his face, to clean up after he vomits, to hold his hand.

Luis is also angry, another sign of his reviving energy. Interns and other hospital staff have been coming in with masks and gloves looking scared and treating him like an untouchable, even when they're not about to have any physical contact. He has made formal complaints to his health plan and to the hospital, and he's asked us to write letters, too. His treatment changes: clearly the staff has been alerted to treat this man with respect.

I'm preparing to move to western Massachusetts, after a year of commuting on weekends to be with Roberto, my partner. We decide to take advantage of the early summer warmth and go camping on Mount Greylock. Each evening, we trek up to the tower on the top of the mountain to watch the sunset and to call the hospital to check on Luis. It doesn't look good this time. The beauty around me is heartbreaking. How can such cruelty exist alongside this perfect place?

Luis wanted so much for his life, he took such great risks, and look where he is.

Each evening I enter the stone lodge and dig out change from my pocket, trembling, my stomach churning. Tonight José, his childhood friend, answers the phone. "Come now, Kim." This is it. We pack up our gear and head toward the city.

Miraculously, Estrella has been allowed to leave Cuba in time and is also on her way. After many setbacks with the Cuban government, meeting with a lawyer, pooling our money, and a great deal of help from Mel King, a local political leader, Estrella is on a small private plane from Cuba to Miami. It's a media event: "King's Cuban Connection Unites Mother and Dying Son." Poor Estrella, the only time she left her island nation is to see her son die of AIDS. AIDS has not hit Cuba yet in force, although the Cuban government knows of it and wants to keep it out of Cuba.

We all meet at the hospital. Luis seems to be in his own world now. It's hard to know if he is aware that his mother has arrived, that his loved ones are all around him. But we tell each other he must sense our energy, our love. And we are there for each other. We gather in a plant-filled solarium near his room overlooking the city, and discuss what must be done. Luis wants to die at home, so arrangements are made to take him home, with twenty-four hour nursing care, along with his mother, Barbara, Stephen, and shifts of the extended family— me, Sharon, Alice, Jose, Ray, the rest.

I am at Luis' for the day. I dread coming, but once I'm in his home, I feel better. Even the medical apparatus cannot diminish the warm spirit of his place. The nurse is a tall, soft-spoken man who talks to Luis in a matter-of-fact voice as he holds Luis's retching body. "Yes, there you go, that's fine." He soothes us all. He must have lost someone to AIDS, too, I think. Barbara and Estrella, the mothers, sit vigil by the bed. Stephen and I tidy the apartment, chat, help the nurse clean Luis and dispose of the blood that he continually spits up. Oh, please God, let him go.

Estrella tells me he opened his eyes yesterday and said, "Mami, I'm ready. I'm at peace." This is a gift to us all.

Stephen and I walk up to the store to buy some food, to do some everyday thing in the midst of this dream/nightmare. It's amazing that we have appetites, but we are hungry, and the sun feels good on our faces as we walk down the row house-lined street, carrying grocery bags.

As I open the door to Luis' house, I can feel it. I know. It's over at last. Luis has died.

It is a brilliant, hot June morning, and I awake feeling drained physically, yet peaceful. Today is the day we say our public goodbye to Luis.

But first I must greet a newcomer into the world. My close friend gave birth to her first child last night in the very same hospital where Luis last stayed. I put on a turquoise blue summer dress and a light woven blue-green shawl my mother gave me, and drive to the hospital. I enter the familiar lobby, wrapping the shawl around me against the air-conditioned chill, but go into a different wing this time. My friend and her husband are exhausted, dazed and happy. The baby is a cherub with fat cheeks and sharp blue eyes. I hold her gingerly at first, unsure of myself, but little by little allow myself to feel her weight, her warmth and her perfect newness.

I then drive to the city cemetery where we will bury our friend. We are a motley group—friends, coworkers, students form Haiti, Puerto Rico, Colombia, old and young, teachers. The grave site is sandy, with a gaping hole and the grey coffin next to it. The work crew and bulldozer are nearby, looking impatient. Luis' mother sits in José's apartment in the city; she cannot bear the ordeal of his burial.

José invites people to share their thoughts; I act as translator. A few students speak. José reads a poem Luis wrote called, "Friendship." Stephen places a yellow rose on the coffin from the backyard bush; it bloomed the day after Luis died. Ray reads Luis' favorite selection from *The Little Prince*: "It will seem like I am dead…But I will be living in a star, and laughing…you will look up in the sky and want to laugh with me."

Luis Armando Valdes died two months before his thirty-fifth birthday. Poet, singer, dancer, teacher, lover, friend. Eight years later, I still talk with him in the stars.

A la memoria de Luis Armando Valdes,
mi querido amigo
1952–1986

HE WAS LIGHTNING

HARRY GIPSON

He was lightning
And how often does lightning strike in the same place
Illuminate the same face
With eyes full of him
Seeing him in a crowded room for the first time surrounded by
    seemingly grey, shadowy people
Shining there for me like an incandescent light into my eyes,
He was lightning
And my heart ricochets everywhere looking for him, looking for
    him,
I want to see him
I want to hear him
I want to touch him
Just one more time, just all the time
But no!
His journey continues in mystery
And how often does lightning strike in the same place?

It was frightening
That grievous journey with him through AIDS
It devastates as it raids
The body and the mind
But he handled his illness with great dignity and courage

An inspiration as he helped me face my own inevitable mortality.
It was frightening
And my heart ricochets everywhere looking for him, looking for
    him.
I want to hold him
I want to kiss him
I want to ravish him
Just one more time, just all the time
But no!
His journey continues in mystery
And how often does lightning strike in the same place?

It was tightening
That death grip that AIDS had on him for so long
On all of us like a macabre song
Whispering in our ears of HIV or some other mode of departure
He is us and we are him
He just went sooner into forever.
It was tightening
And my heart ricochets everywhere looking for him, looking for
    him.
I want to cuddle with him
I want to play with him
I want to laugh with him
Just one more time, just all the time
But no!
His journey continues in mystery
And how often does lightning strike in the same place?

He was lightning
And our lives sparkled much of our happy ten years together
It does not matter whether
I know this kind of profound love again or not
What matters is that I loved passionately
And was loved passionately in return.
He was lightning
And my heart ricochets everywhere looking for him, looking for
    him.
I want to talk with him

I want to sing with him
I want to dance with him
Just one more time, just all the time
But no!
His journey continues in mystery
And how often does lightning strike in the same place?

I have read that someone dies of AIDS every seven minutes, so
while you were reading this poem, somewhere on this planet a
human being died of that disease.

Someone's lover
Someone's wife
Someone's husband
Someone's daughter
Someone's son
Someone's sister
Someone's brother
Someone's aunt
Someone's uncle
Someone's niece
Someone's nephew
Someone's friend
Someone's enemy
Someone's someone
Someone's human someone.

Let us wonder who it was this time.

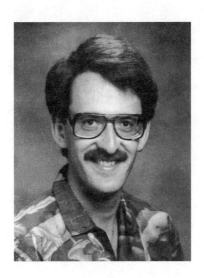

For Gary Roberts, my beloved life partner
June 18, 1949–March 7, 1993

THE QUESTION

JEWELLE GOMEZ

Day after day, side by side for seven years
like being married or the better part of being married—
we still remembered to look in each other's eyes
over coffee.
In that first office we shared, architectural wedge
along a Dickensian corridor. What was it
drawing your gaze to mine?
That I'd just read a book of stories
from Latin America that made us want to sing?
Or the way my flesh plumped inside a too small jacket
vulnerable and wise?
For me it was the steadiness of your pale blue eyes
not openly afraid of me, but curious.
I was afraid of you
and curious. That became our bond.
Fear and curiosity, embattled, overcome, succumbed to,
reignited each day and still we glanced
in comfort and surprise, knowing we were never meant
to see each other at all.

I've just been to one of those readings
where all the poems were written for the ghosts
of long-dead white men

who stand guard over the canon:
Words so tightly wound
around the in-joke of prosperity
and white-skin privilege
even I can hardly bear to let them down.
But I don't care if they've travelled
to the south of France
or vacationed in Third World countries.
or that they know what the insides of words look like.
I smile the smile you've taught me—broad mouth
drawn into a noncommittal curve, marked by dimples
I do not have
and the pale blue of your eyes shining through.
I sit, you inside me, both content.

I've been to a reading where frightened men
have taken on the mantle of forgetfulness.
The only metaphor they have for life is sex and that angers me
Our metaphors were so many, so large. A berry pie, oozing
    purple,
damaging, enduring. A berry pie eaten by the dog you loved.
Just one berry pie that lived forever.

Each weekend you drove north with your beloved.
Twisting pavement of ill-repair, then told me the terror
of sleeping truck drivers and the sweetness of mundane tasks
done together.
I want you to have a poem filled with these things—
precisely sharpened pencils lined neatly on a desk
the planted trees and fallen leaves
scattered gleefully by your dog,
the corn fritters you stopped to buy
on the way up
the mysterious door to the attic
which would never stay locked.
the silent belfry

You introduced me to your neighbors
so warmly. Did they in their moneyed ease

know what it meant for us to be friends,
to embrace fear and curiosity?

One afternoon you returned to our office from lunch
full of yourself in a coy male way.
Cheeks flushed, prepared to tell a story as we both loved.
Lunch with a young woman…acquaintance waiting to ask
a question. Tentative and enthusiastic:

Will you father her child?

You said, no, of course not!
As if it were not a question
balanced on much thought.
As if you are not proud. But I see in your eyes
you might have wanted to be the father of a child.
If you could.

Neither of us expected death. A foolish optimism
Yet optimism was there in the tone of your answer.
Not there in dark with me
after you'd left the office
and they waited to turn out the lights.

I'm listening to the tape of "Sweeney Todd" you gave me.
Pies more pies!
A metaphor for life. Harsh chords and fearful passion
digested into cool murder: madness made bureaucratic.
Music made to force you from your seat.
Ask why a love might be so great.
You would say, "To create an opera, clearly."

There is a futile innocence in the questions asked:
why me? why now?
As if the world was a perfect place before the virus hit.
As if those children starving in India our mothers used as
persuasions to our vegetables
were only a myth, as if they do not have
counterparts in North Virginia or the South Bronx.
As if there had been no Middle Passage, no Trail of Tears,

no Holocaust.
No railroad built on Chinese bones,
no California internment camps.

But you spit that innocence back,
traded it for things more useful
I want to remember them: peace in the morning
to write letters:
ideas to wrestle to the ground,
a man's hand firm at your back, the surprise of flowers,
a good scotch, the music of Spanish spoken aloud
and questions.

Day after day
side by side
for seven years, the spirit number.
Like a marriage
like the better part of marriage.
Todas son preguntas.
Abrazamos la curiosidad
y el miedo.

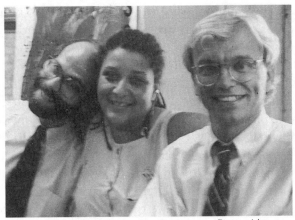

Gregory, right

for Goyo

DENE

NORMAN C. GREENOUGH

D ene Ralph Greenough was born September 16th, 1960. If only it could end there and still be a life story unfolding.

Our family moved to Auburn, Massachusetts in August of 1962. Our daughter Meg was born the next month. Here, Dene grew up with his baby sister and his two older sisters, Dorene and Jody.

The next several years were relatively uneventful. Four children growing up in a middle-class neighborhood with a working Dad and a Mom at home.

In 1982, Meg and Dene decided to pack up and try another part of the country. Because of other particular, unrelated events, their sister Dorene and family had moved to Duluth, Georgia, so this seemed to be a natural place to start. Meg lasted about three months and came back home. For Dene it worked. Atlanta was his place to be.

In 1984 Meg took some vacation time to visit with Dene, make a side trip and spend some time in Florida. While in Atlanta, because of a previous bout with hepatitis, Dene was having his blood tested. He and Meg went to the clinic where the blood workup was being done and was told that he was HIV-positive. Dene told Meg, but assured her that it was nothing and not to concern herself about it. She took him at his word, never telling anyone. Not even family. For Dene, just plain ignorance (which I can't even imagine) or heavy-duty denial.

In the September of 1989 we got a call from Dene telling us that he had to go into the hospital for a catheter implant. He had come down with CMV Retinitis and it was the only way the drug used to combat this virus could be administered. This was our wake-up call to AIDS. He urged us not to come down. This was a relatively simple procedure and in no way life-threatening. No need to panic.

The next couple of years was relatively quiet. We would visit in Georgia a couple of times during the year and have Dene home on occasion, keeping in touch by phone quite often, making sure that everything seemed to be under control. His T-count was continuously falling. In the beginning, it was approximately 85. He went on AZT and it jumped to 120. It was downhill from there on out. In January of 1992 he told me his count had dropped to 36. I never bothered to ask after that.

In retrospect, January of 1992 was the beginning of the end. His catheter implant became infected and had to be replaced. Something that usually takes place after a year of use, not two plus. During the spring, Dene had to quit his job. Primarily so he could qualify for Social Security benefits although his job was tiring him out more than usual. During the summer he developed aplastic anemia which is usually taken care of only by a bone marrow transplant but other therapy was attempted to no avail. There was also a bout with renal failure which was eventually overcome with treatment (keep in mind that this doesn't happen overnight and is expensive, time-consuming and does nothing to cause the virus to go into any kind of state of remission). There were other nuisance things that happened during this summer of 1992, HIV-related, that were as usual brought under control by whatever means were available at the time. It's our understanding that on Monday morning, September 28th, 1992, Dene had an appointment with his doctor. Apparently nothing was functioning anymore. The CMV had migrated to his bloodstream as well as cessation of red blood cells or white blood cells. Nothing more could be done. Dene went home and, I believe, decided that it was time to go. The battle had been fought and he was tired. The virus had won again. He died that night watching *Northern Exposure*, surrounded with the love of his sister Dorene, Floyd (his companion) and friends.

During the time frame from January of 1992 until Dene left us, his mother and I were able to get down and visit on three occasions. Once in March for a week, a visit over the Memorial Day weekend and another visit over the Labor Day weekend. In looking back, we wish it could have been more but because of the way this virus works and because of Dene's constant "up" attitude (at least for our weekly telephone conversations), only on our last visit did we really notice a radical change in his appearance. He was a lot thinner and his skin coloring was unusually darker. We were given to understand that this was related to medication side effects. Even then we didn't realize just how sick he was because as always, he was "up" as usual for Mom and Dad, never complaining and doing things with us to make our visit a pleasant occasion.

We've come to realize that Dene was a very special person in his adopted home town. There were an awful lot of friends at his memorial service, a lot of nice people said some pretty nice things about him. I only wish that his mother and I had been closer geographically so we could have gotten to know him as well as others had. The occasional visits we made were the kind that you tried to jam six months of casual visiting into a few days and it just don't work!

I wish I could be more eloquent in expressing how I feel about my son but for some of us of my generation, this is an almost Herculean feat. Just to have told him, as I do his sisters, that I loved him was a hurdle of sorts but I'm so glad that I was able to do it. Able to look into his eyes and say, "I love you," and with a hug to let him know that I meant it.

From September of 1989, when Dene came down with the CMV Retinitis, until he finally succumbed to the havoc the virus had wreaked, he (like so many others) fought the most valiant fight that anyone could, never giving up, always a ray of hope that something would come along to put this virus in its place, always there to help or counsel others in what to do or not to do.

Dene was my son, I loved him more than words can express and will miss him forever.

I love you Dene,
Dad

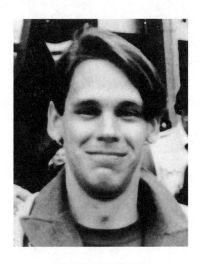

To our son, Dene Ralph Greenough
with love,
1960–1992 He was an evergreen!

"There are trees that seem to die at the end of
autumn. There are also evergreens."
—Gilbert Maxwell

I honor the memories of those who are gone, and
I bless and honor the presence of those among us
who stand like evergreens.

PASSOVER WISH

ROBERT H. GROSS

D uane was a Jew by choice. That fact, revealed to me shortly after
we met, was one of the things that drew me to him in some inex-
plicable way. Perhaps it surprised me that someone would spend years
to become what I, given as a gift at birth, had taken so for granted all
these many years.

Of course I had known others who had converted to the Jewish
faith, but those cases were more conversions of convenience, done for
the sole purpose of being able to marry someone from the tribe in a
traditional ceremony, with little if any desire to truly accept the tenets
of my ancient religion.

But Duane was different. After feeling rejected from the Christian
church of his childhood due to his being gay, he still felt a deep need
to find spiritual support and acceptance of who he was. His search
eventually led him to the Jewish faith, and after spending several years
of study he was inducted into that faith by being immersed in the traditional *mikvah* bath.

However, even that simple yet meaningful ritual wasn't easily
accomplished. For not only was Duane a gay man, but also a Person
Living With AIDS, and the community where he resided was not
comfortable letting him enter the sacred waters of the *mikvah*.
Although his Rabbi worked hard within the local Jewish community to
address their fears, hoping to make them understand that they would

not, in any way, be putting themselves at risk, her pleas could not convince them, and the ceremony was not permitted to take place. But so great was his commitment to complete the conversion, that ultimately Duane settled for a private ritual in a homemade *mikvah* of collected rainwater, finally becoming a Jew on a warm Spring day in 1991.

Within six months of this ceremony, Duane was dead of AIDS-related complications at the young age of twenty-six. He spent those last few months of his life as he had lived: traveling to the places and spending time with the people he loved the most. Exploring this precious gift called life with all the passion, joy and faith he could muster, exuding a wisdom far beyond his years.

At his memorial service, the Rabbi spoke of Duane's special love of and rapport with children. She recounted how when she would stop by Duane's house with her kids in tow, he would always get down on the floor with them, no matter how ill he might be feeling and join them in their games, sharing his own extensive collection of toys and the ever-present bowl of candy with his young admirers. And they loved him in return. Never before had they known an adult who could so completely and effortlessly relate to them on their own level.

She then recounted a special Passover memory that touched all of us in attendance that afternoon: Shortly after completing his conversion, Duane was invited to celebrate the Passover *seder* at the Rabbi's home. As was their family custom, they went around the table during the *seder* dinner and each participant was asked to share a special Passover wish with those assembled. As it came time for Duane to share his special wish, he looked over at the children gathered around the dining table richly set with the traditional objects of the holiday, symbols to remind everyone of God's miracles and ancient covenant with the Jewish people, and quietly said to them: "My Passover wish is that you never forget me."

I can't know for certain whether or not the Rabbi's children will, through the years, continue to remember Duane, but I do know that each Passover, no matter where I am, or whom I share the *seder* meal with, I recall my friend, Duane Kearns Puryear, his courageous battle with AIDS and most of all, I remember and honor his Passover wish.

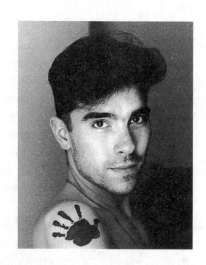

In loving memory of
Duane Kearns Puryear
Dec. 20, 1964–Oct. 8, 1991

AUTHOR, BROTHER, HERO, BAROSAURUS

MARNY HALL

It's the size of five giraffes stacked end to end," I told my brother, Richard, hoping to entice him out to see the Barosaurus at the Museum of Natural History just two blocks away from his Manhattan apartment. After stopping every few steps so he could catch his breath, we finally made it. Contemplating the beast's three-story neck gave us both vertigo. Richard commented that it must have had to stoop in order to dine on treetops. How, we wondered, could such an incredible creature ever have existed?

As a child, my brother's head had also seemed to graze the clouds. Well over six feet tall, seventeen years older than I, his weekend visits were incandescent events. First, there was the thrilling trip to the train station to pick him up. Then there would be a special meal followed by homemade blackberry or pumpkin or rhubarb pie. After these feasts, I would make a beeline for Richard's lap. Ecstatically ensconced, I might press for further favors. Could I comb his hair? (I still have a fourth-grade essay entitled "My Hansom (sic) Brother.") Would he toss me, swing me, hoist me up on his shoulders? Could we go exploring? Could I show him how I could chin myself or ride my bike with no hands? Could we play Parcheesi or Monopoly? Could I wear his shoes?

Usually he indulged me, a hoyden with scrawny braids who must have seemed sadly deficient in everything he valued. How must he have felt when, instead of showing the slightest inclination to read a book, I rushed out to play cowboys or soldiers with the neighborhood kids, or worse yet, sat glued to the TV? A gifted musician himself, he had to suffer through my wretched piano lessons. My long tapering fingers notwithstanding, I had not a glimmer of interest or talent. The only time Richard ever lost patience with me was when I was noisy in the mornings. Chastened by the sudden and uncharacteristic expression of fury issuing from the upstairs guest bedroom, I would quietly occupy myself drawing portraits of Richard as an exploding atom bomb. It was, after all, the fifties.

I parlayed my artistry into a bigger project when my mother, who had some extended business away from home, packed me off to Richard's New York City apartment. Kellogg's cornflakes had announced an outer space drawing contest. Richard got a huge sheet of butcher block paper and taped it on the wall of his apartment. My practice with bombs transferred easily to rockets. I had also mastered the depiction of Saturn's rings, particularly proud that they disappeared, as the rules of perspective dictate, around the far side of the planet. When this project dragged on for some days, Richard never hinted that he might find intergalactic travel with me less compelling than the literary gay life he had had to put aside during my sojourn. Later, I think, Richard came to regret the provision of such a comfortable asylum for me.

When I was fourteen, my mother sent me away to an upscale boarding school for which I was temperamentally, socially, and academically unsuited. A year and a half later I was expelled for lesbianism. Back home in disgrace, desperate to prove I wasn't queer, I was dallying with the local boys. One night, when I'd come in particularly late (I'd gone to "third base" in the cemetery with Frankie Cox), Mother asked me where I'd been. It wasn't a casual query. Standing by the kitchen stove, her hair a silver blizzard, she looked like an avenging angel. "None of your business," I retorted. She slapped me. I slapped her back. A donnybrook ensued. After two days of stony silence, I took my small stash of cash and caught a train to New York.

Years later Richard told me how torn he had been when I appeared on his doorstep almost simultaneously with a telegram from Mother: CAN NO LONGER TAKE RESPONSIBILITY FOR MARNY. He had always been my advocate, but he couldn't imagine parenting a rogue teenager full-time. I was sent away to a school for wayward adolescents.

Years later, after I had finished high school and college, Richard and I found each other again. By now, a full-fledged lesbian, I had been sending him postcards from my travels. One of these cards was a photo taken in an Aegean harbor cafe. A group of rowdy young dyke—we imagined ourselves world-weary rakes, old beyond reckonin—leer at the camera over a pile of thoroughly descanted ouzo bottles. On the back of the card/photo I wrote, "Having a very gay time." The next time I saw Richard, he came out to me. It was 1965. I was twenty-two. He was thirty-nine.

Over the following decades, Richard was my friend, mentor, editor and boon gay companion. We talked frequently on the phone. Even after I moved to San Francisco in 1969, we saw each other at holidays or birthdays, usually with our respective friends or lovers. His support was unequivocal, his advice impeccable, except in fiscal matters. When this shortcoming became obvious, I still sought his counsel. Bad advice from Richard was, apparently, more valuable to me than good advice from anyone else.

After Richard got sick, I visited him a lot. We had wonderful talks. Though I'd become more scholarly and literary over the years, I was still in awe of his talent and erudition. Sitting in Central Park a few months ago, I told him how much I had always admired him, how I'd wished that I could have taken after mother, as he had, instead of the mediocre *other side* of the family. Good brother that he was, he immediately launched into a laundry list of my talents. Yes, I said, I knew I was good at certain things, but I wasn't really gifted like he was. He was quiet for a moment and then he said he knew how I felt…that everyone probably felt that way about someone. He, himself, felt that way about E.M. Forster.

Richard died as he had lived with great discipline and grace, wisdom and wit. He chose to discontinue the regimen which had kept him alive, but which had reduced his life to an unendurable round of transfusions, catheters, and toxic, nauseating medication. During his last bout with AIDS, he managed to fashion the hospital into a hospice, refusing—against medical advice—all intravenous medication and nutrition. He died peacefully on his own terms. He was a model for me in this as in all else.

I have his ashes on my mantle. Somebody brought me flowers. My favorite vase also just happened to be on the mantle. Almost reflexively, I've retrieved some of his old photos and put them by the flowers and ashes. Without premeditation, I see that I've enshrined Richard. But then, what's new? At some moments, looking at the makeshift shrine, I feel—can it be—happy, even euphoric. I cannot, in good faith, expect the psychotherapy clients I work with to explore and accept their own less-than-ideal motives without subjecting myself to the same scrutiny. Could I—perish the thought—be happy that Richard has died, that the Barosaurus is extinct, that we lesser creatures can finally get a shot at the sun? Probably. And there may be something else. I am one of Richard's heirs. Do I believe, magically, that now that he is dead, his extraordinary gifts will be part of his legacy to me? Probably.

I have brought his shoes back, the great pirogues that I used to clop around in as a child. Down at the heels, one missing an instep, they are nonetheless his shoes. But they don't help me edit this piece —don't, with the deftest touch, turn dross into golden, timeless phrases. Oh, Richard, how I loved you. In a time when the whole idea of "family" is unfashionable unless "chosen," you represent the best that contested term could ever offer. You were my brother, my chosen one.

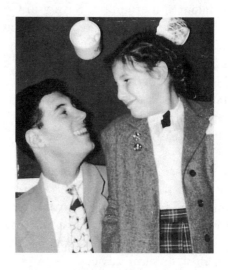

For Richard Hall: 1926–1992

WHAT I DID ON MY SUMMER VACATION

NELS P. HIGHBERG

Summer is over. I am back in school. Summer was very, very busy. I did a lot. I got married in May. I loved a man. His name was Blane. Blane loved me. I am also a man. We decided to have a wedding ceremony even though it wouldn't count. My friends from high school came. My friends from work and college came. His friends came. He said he loved me and wanted to live with me in front of everybody. Then I said it. Then we all ate cake and drank Coke. It was fun. We were very tired. We went to our home. I slept very well. I had my arm around him all night.

I moved all of my stuff to our home. I bought a desk and a bookcase. I bought a washer and a dryer. Blane was still very tired. He sat in bed and watched television. He saw many game shows and soap operas. At night we watched television together. We ate dinner in bed. Then he would sleep. I would go downstairs to work.

My mother wanted us to go on vacation with her and my family. Blane wanted to go but he was still tired and wanted to stay in bed. He told her he couldn't go. He told me to go and I went. We went to Washington, D.C. I saw the Washington Monument. We went to the zoo and I saw monkeys and panda bears. I called Blane many times. I told him about the monkeys and panda bears. He was happy I called. I missed him very much.

He was in bed when I got home. He was more tired. He could not walk to the bathroom. He had to wear diapers. His mother and brother flew all the way from Philadelphia. His mother was very sad. They sat downstairs and talked about him. I sat with him and fed him and watched television when he slept. They took him away to Philadelphia.

My mother came to Houston to take me home. I had to move my desk and my bookcase. I put everything in my bedroom. I put my washer and dryer outside with a sign that said "For Sale." There was a lot of stuff in my room. I could not walk around. I tried to help my mother. I cut the grass. I put wet clothes on the line outside so that the wind would dry them. I fed our dog, Pugsley. He is very cute and very fat. He likes to run and jump. He was glad I was there. Every night he slept in my room with me. He slept on the floor.

It was July. It was very, very hot outside. Blane's brother called. Blane was dead. I walked around outside for a very long time. I could not go to the funeral. It was too much money. The airline said I was not family. I could buy a special ticket only for August. I sat at home. I watched television. I watched *The Price Is Right*. Klondike bars are $2.99. I watched *As the World Turns*. Evan slept with Emily. He told Courtney. She broke up with him. I watched *Where in the World Is Carmen Sandiego?* I know where Albania is. I sat in front of the air conditioner and watched television every day.

In August I flew to Philadelphia. I saw a pile of dirt covered with dead flowers. Some ribbons on the flowers said "Son." Some said "Brother." It was Blane's grave. I sat in front of it for a long time. I sat under a pine tree. The wind was blowing. Then I walked around Philadelphia. I saw Independence Hall and Benjamin Franklin's grave. Then I rode a train to New York City. I liked the train. I walked down Broadway. I sat in Central Park. I watched the Hudson River. I sat at a table on a sidewalk and ate something called Middle Eastern. It was green. It was good.

I flew back to Texas. I packed all of my stuff into boxes again. I moved to an apartment. I said goodbye to my mother. I said goodbye to Pugsley. I went back to my job. I am back in school. Summer is over.

8 February 1993, 12:13 PM

Bill Clinton is president. Pugsley died. Mama said Eddie had gallstone surgery. I'm delivering a paper in Arkansas on women's video art in March. Pam had a baby, a boy. I still miss you. Gerrie's dating a guy named Eric. The sun is shining. Madonna has the number one song. I'm wearing your red shirt and hippo tie. Elisa moved to her own apartment. Garth Brooks and Reba McEntire are playing at the rodeo. I'm dating someone. He's taking me to Dallas in two weeks. Adele is in love. Malcolm is in lust. Dr. Yongue is lecturing on Emily Dickinson at two o'clock. I'm going to have pizza for lunch. Arthur Ashe died. Tria graduated last semester. Prince Charles and Lady Diana split. The bus was late this morning. My last test was negative. This guy behind me is talking about Jesus. You will never know any of this.

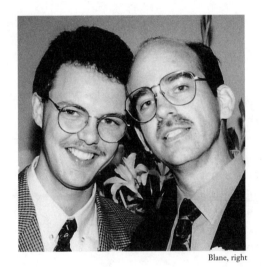

Blane, right

For Blane F. Feulner
April 12, 1954–July 12, 1992

PARTING COURSES

PAUL E. HOFFMAN

Eighteen years of my life
   Have passed in the loving of him.

A model, a lifeguard, an artist—
   Above all a naturalist.
He finds pleasure in a flower, an eagle
   Or a small tiny kitten.
Glowing health, vitality and youthfulness
   Had always been his.

A blond, green-eyed Italian "God."
   We built a secure life
And believed we could do anything—together.
   A house, a garden, dogs & cats,
Vacations, cars, problems & plans—
   Two lives intertwined into one.

Now comes along a new battle
   The doctors say he may not win.
A battle in which I can only assist.

I watch the barrage of attacks,
　　Helpless to stem the tide,
As a muscular, athletic body
　　Wastes away daily,
All I can do is hold him
　　And encourage and forestall.

The future scares me to hell—
　　My life has been his life—
Which has been mine.

A world without him is impossible
　　To comprehend.
Love will have passed out of my life forever.

Lord show me the way to face
　　That dark day when our courses part.
When my friends become my family
　　And a new way must be forged.

Eighteen years of my life
　　Have passed in the loving of him.

————

*To all my friends who have supported me
through a transitional period in my life.*

Our Lives Expire as a Sigh

Evelyn Horowitz

Jeff is waiting for me at the gate. "How is he?" I ask.
"Fine, fine," Jeff answers with a nervous laugh, but his face is
unsmiling. "He's been very quiet. He didn't moan or groan when I
bathed him today. I think he's getting tired of baths."

We go straight to the car. Jeff seems surprised that I have no luggage. "I just couldn't get it together enough to pack anything. Are
Gloria and Eddie still at the house?"

Gloria and Eddie are English friends of Mark's who had arrived
on August 28th for a visit in the Florida sunshine. Instead, they had
been dealing with hurricane season and helping Mother and Jeff take
care of Mark.

I had never met them. When Mark told me they were coming to
visit I'd suggested that perhaps it would be better if they postponed
their trip. "Aren't they very elderly, and haven't you told me that
Eddie isn't well?"

Mark wouldn't hear of their not coming. "They paid twenty-two-
hundred dollars for their tickets, and they can't get the money back.
Besides, I want to see them, and Mother will be here to help me entertain. I've rented one of those scooters, so I'll be able to get around."

I'd spoken with Jeff. "Perhaps you should tell them not to come?"

"No, no, it'll be fine. Eddie's aware of the situation. I've talked
with my boss, and she understands that I'll need some extra time off.

She's very active in Pediatric AIDS charity work and has been very supportive. Don't worry about it; your mother and I will handle it."

It had amazed me that they continued to stay while Mark had gotten progressively worse. I wanted to go to Florida but there was no room for me. "I'm too old to sleep on a couch for any longer than a night or two," I said to Mike.

"Well, you could stay at a hotel," Mike offered.

"No, that'll make everybody uncomfortable. They'll feel obligated to stay at the hotel instead and I gather they really don't have the money. Jeff says they're good company for my mother. I'll stick to the original plans and go down on October seventh after they leave."

"Do what you want," Mike said.

But that was the problem: I didn't really know what I wanted. My moods changed hourly. One moment I was afraid of going. Afraid that my appearance would reignite Mark's rage over our father. The next moment I would feel guilty that I was enjoying life when I should be with Mark because I was his sister and he might need me to be there. Other moments I would be angry with my mother for not telling me what to do. Sometimes I'd be silly and vacuous and sing, "Should I Stay or Should I Go." I somehow believed there was still plenty of time. I had also believed that eight years before when our father had called me and told me he was dying. "Ask anything you want," he'd said.

"Are you afraid?"

"When they were taking me into intensive care and told me I probably had an hour to live, I was. Because there were still things I had to do, arrangements to make. A nurse wouldn't let me make a phone call. I've filed a formal complaint against her; she is a cold-hearted bitch. Now they tell me I've got a year, and it feels like infinity."

"I love you, Dad," I said, realizing how few times I'd told him that since I'd become an adult.

"I love you, too," he said. "I always have from the moment you were born. Come see me soon."

I hadn't gone to see him soon; I'd taken a month, and by the time I did see him, he'd decided to die. He'd refused all medication except for Methadone. I'd stayed for four days, and then he asked me to leave.

"Go home. Please forgive me; I'm tired."

I'd gone back to New York telling myself I'd return to Boston in a week but he'd died two days after I left. Experience does not always teach. Obviously it hadn't taught me how short time is when someone is dying.

I'd been fighting with Mother about getting a nurse or aide to help in Florida. She'd say things to me like, "You have to be careful with help; they'll steal you blind," or "We're going to make an appointment with CAPS (Combined AIDS Program Services) to come in and evaluate him, then they decide what's needed and send either a nurse or an aide in for a few hours a day."

Whenever I asked if she'd made the appointment, she'd tell me, "I called but they're changing locations and can't do anything until next week."

"You told me that the other day."

"Well, it's still true. Besides, Gloria, Eddie, Jeff, and I are handling him. And he's a handful, let me tell you. He's also very funny. The other day he said to me, 'Mother, what's your last name?' I got annoyed and said to him, 'Horowitz, the same as yours.' Now he calls me Mrs. Horowitz. He says, 'Mrs. Horowitz, will you please turn up the air conditioning? Mrs. Horowitz, is your lover sitting in the living room?' He remembers Gloria and Eddie; they make him laugh."

I said to Mike, "She just doesn't want to admit how bad he is, or maybe he isn't. After all, when she called me in July, when Mark was visiting, she told me I'd better get to Boston, as it would be the last time I'd see him and to be prepared for a shock at how he looks. I got there and he wasn't that bad, he looked pretty much the same as he had when he was visiting us in April. He and I had a nice day together playing Rummy Cube. I made him a pork roast for supper because he kept calling Mother the queen of the microwave. My mother likes to be melodramatic. She couldn't just say to me, 'Come visit. I need some relief.' "

As he drives, at what seems to me ten miles an hour, JEff tells me what has been happening the last week. CAPS had come in and referred Mark to Hospice by the Sea. Hospice by the Sea had come in with a hospital bed and restraints. It seemed that Mark would insist on sitting on the toilet, and he was on such heavy medication that he'd fall off and bang his head on the tile floor. "He just doesn't accept that he has no bowel movements, and even if he did, he could make in his diaper. The first two days he struggled with the restraints, but that's stopped; I had to promise he could go to the bathroom on his birthday," Jeff says.

I remembered when my grandmother had been dying. The first time she made in the bed she'd cried almost to the point of howling.

"He takes after his grandmother," I say.

Of course this was the extra kick of cruelty that Mark was getting from the disease. The more common syndrome was to waste, to have constant uncontrollable diarrhea; but because of the liver damage done by the new experimental AIDS drug, D-4T, Mark was constipated but still had the constant desire to relieve himself. The doctor had tried to explain to him the pressure he felt was from the liver and a bowel movement every other day was all his body could handle but it didn't change his behavior. AIDS is a disease where the final months are spent in the bathroom.

"He's stopped eating," Jeff says.

"Do they have him on intravenous?"

"No, nothing. They say the body will take care of itself."

"What they mean is the body will feed on itself," I say before I can stop myself. I look at Jeff; he seems pale despite his tan. He also seems thinner but I won't think the thought.

Jeff is driving very slowly. I don't want to tell him to speed up. I know he needs to talk but I have this feeling that I should get to the house as soon as possible and because of the weather I am already hours late. "Last week at four in the morning he turned on the bedside light, got out of bed, and fell on the floor in the middle of the room. When I picked him up and asked what he was doing, he told me it was 1954 and he was getting dressed for school. I told him it wasn't 1954 but he insisted and fought with me till I had to shake him. I shook him so hard, I became afraid I would hurt him. He can be very strong all of a sudden, and he forgets and tries to go outside."

"From everything I've heard it sounds a lot like Alzheimer's," I say.

"Exactly," Jeff says. "Another time he asked me, 'How will I recognize my father when I see him?' I said what do you mean how will you recognize him? He said, 'How will I know who he is?' We went in that circle for a few minutes until I told him God would take care of identities. That seemed to satisfy him."

As many times as I've made this drive from the airport over the last three years, it has never seemed to take this long, maybe because Mark always picked me up. To describe Mark's driving as heavy-footed would be to understate. He drives like he's a contender in the Indy 500. Jeff is as slow and methodical driving as he is about everything.

Finally we are at the house. We go in through the kitchen. My mother bearhugs me, "He's been waiting for you. All day we've been telling him your sister's on her way. Gloria, Eddie, this is my daughter. Who do you think she looks like?"

"I look like Mark; there's no need for you to say it," I say as I shake hands with a very small, thin blond woman who's wearing very thick glasses, almost bottlenecks.

"I'll take a kiss, please," says a heavy man who looks like a grey gnome.

I'm aware that Gloria is studying me with a look that seems to say it's about time you got here.

I go into the bedroom with Mother and Jeff. The hospital bed has been placed so that Mark can look out a small window, but the sky is overcast with impending rain. In this moment I know: it's almost over. The radio is tuned to one of those almost muzak stations that plays oldies, but not by the original artists; mufake I call it. I don't listen long enough to remember the song that's playing. I almost say, Couldn't you have found a better station?

Mark is covered with an ugly green sheet; the pattern seems to be ivy vines. He doesn't look skeletal, just narrow and bony and yellow. KS lesions have broken out on his cheek and neck. Mother says, "Mark, Evelyn's here. Your sister's here."

I say, "Hello, Markie."

"Hold his hand on top of the sheet."

I take his hand. Then realize and say, "Let me give you a kiss."

"On his forehead, and if you touch him, use rubber gloves."

I kiss his forehead. (I do not remember if I said I love you; I hope I did.) His breathing is gasps but regular, as if he's on an invisible respirator.

"I shaved him for you," Jeff says. "Shouldn't have him see his Evelyn without being shaved."

"Mark, we're all here now," Mother says. But of course, we aren't. Geoff, Mark's twin, is missing. "You can let go now. We're all here and we love you," Mother soothes. "Evelyn, tell him to let go."

"Let go, Markie; it's okay. It's time to go."

"Come on, Jeff, let's leave them alone for a while. Talk to him, Evelyn; he can hear what you're saying."

I sit down by the bed, place my hand over his, and begin to talk.

I talk about how he looks, the music station, the ivy sheets and then, "Don't be afraid. Uncle Austin" (who died three weeks before) "will be there to greet you, and Topper. And all the other old dogs we used to have. Remember: Rex, and Peppy, the poodle nobody ever really liked, and Mandy, what a sweet dog she was, and Greta, what a wonderful dog. Remember she was your dog. You rescued her from the pound. Remember how small she was when you first brought her home, and then she grew and grew and she had those blue almost white eyes. She was the gentlest dog we ever had but everyone who came to the house was scared of her because of that huge collie-shepherd body and blue-white eyes. They'll all be there to greet you, all the dogs and relatives and Dad, too. He'll be there."

I'd run out of things to say and looked around the room. "You did a nice job redecorating the room. What's that print on the wall behind you? I never noticed it; was it always there?"

I heard him sigh and knew, without conscious thought, that he was gone. He'd had his last breath. Being me, I didn't want to think it and make it true. I didn't want him to die with just me in the room.

So I talked on and on and on. I talked about the flight down, about the weather, about Gloria and Eddie sitting in the kitchen with Mother and Jeff. I know I'll never be sure of exactly what I talked about because I'd become a little girl; a little girl sitting there hoping what I was thinking wasn't true, wouldn't come true, yet knowing it was true; at the same time being very aware that I wasn't scared. I was sitting there with the dead body of my brother, and it felt comforting.

Dead bodies had always frightened me. I had not looked at the bodies of either of my grandparents or my father's body. In this room, at this time of day/evening it seemed so peaceful and warm that, strangely, I thought about my birth as I looked at Mark and I was calm, not scared, as if outside of myself looking down on this scene. He had waited for me; he wanted me to see this; he wanted me to know death. I was glad he wasn't alone. I was glad I was there.

After twenty-five minutes when he hadn't gasped or anything I put my hand over his heart to see if I could feel anything. I went to the door, opened it, and called my mother.

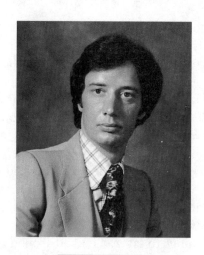

For my beloved brother,
Mark David Horowitz
May 3, 1948–Sept. 27, 1993
Nothing's the same without you.

INCOMPLETE

KATHRYN UDEVITZ HULINGS

I would have poured you water
   when the glass was empty
   and your mouth so dry
Kissed your feverish brow
   when others hid
   behind stiff blue masks
Helped you to the piano
   when the music
   couldn't wait

If only you had called me

I would have lain down right beside you
   when your lover
   couldn't come
Softly swathed my arms around you
   when the pain
   shook down your soul
Let you feel my steady rhythm
   when your head
   sunk to my heart

If only someone could have found me

I would have baked a batch of cookies
　　when the smell
　　brought you back home
Sung a perfect lullaby
　　when you know
　　of my tin ear
Made you smile for a moment
　　remembering "As You Like It"
　　performed in drag

If only I had been there

I would have waited and witnessed
　　when you wept
　　the night away
Whispered good-bye
　　when my hand cradled yours
Sighed in anguish
　　when your breath was still
　　and face serene

If only we had an ending

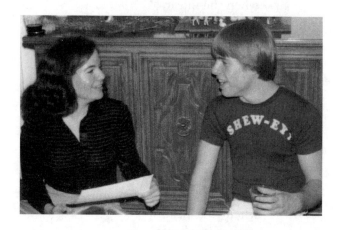

For my dear friend, Scott Caldwell,
with love and respect

FEEDING EACH OTHER

TERENCE K. HUWE

The experience of AIDS in the gay community has been expressed in many ways, ranging from films and novels to the Names Project's AIDS Memorial Quilt. The quilt stands out among artistic expressions, because of its impact on the people who see it. It is impossible to stuff down one's own feelings when faced with the vast acreage of lovingly produced panels, each unique. The quilt bears witness: naming and blessing the dead.

Here is one remembrance from the many acres of the quilt. As with all personal stories told throughout the world, this one reflects both the storyteller and the subject. As with love stories in the lives of ordinary people, it is rich in the fabric of joy and sorrow. As with all stories, the telling is as much for those who are still alive as for those who have died.

Steve

I met Stephen John Risch in 1986. Like so many men under thirty, I was not really looking for love, focusing more on my career, friendships, and my work as a volunteer counselor for people with AIDS in Berkeley, California. I met Steve at a shoreline park that was noteworthy for its cruising potential. We were both old hands in that game, but in contrast to the broad public definition of cruising—an anonymous, unfulfilling obsession—we both brought personality and presence to the ramblings, finding humor and lightness along the way. We both liked to share and talk; this made cruising more fun, similar to other ways of meeting people, such as in bookstores, or at meetings of any sort.

I followed him home to his apartment where we made love and talked for hours. Later that evening, as I thought back to the fun we had had, I felt that I had stumbled upon a jewel of a man. I was drawn to his personality and his life experience instinctively. He was an entomology professor at the University of California at Berkeley, a collector of antique rugs, a world traveller, and not least, an energetic and playful lover.

By any standard, he was a luminous person. His smile invited confidence. His hair was brown and his skin glowed with a general vitality that bestowed good looks on unremarkable features. That he in turn was attracted to me was flattering. I was in the midst of career changes and a stormy breakup; naturally, I thrived on the attention.

After some weeks had passed it dawned on me that I was being pursued. Steve would sometimes meet me for lunch in downtown San Francisco. Romance is a wonderful thing; I recall going to taquerias near Golden Gate University where I worked, and having burritos while we entwined our legs underneath the table; or sipping huge steaming bowls of soup at B&M Mei Sing, a popular lunch spot on Second Street.

One day I got a letter from him saying he needed to stop seeing me because I wasn't available for a serious relationship. Ironically, he agreed to a date with me after the letter was posted. I received the letter on the day of our date, and it was a source of laughter for both of us.

Later that week, I spent most of a Saturday afternoon with Steve, making love and talking while the sun played across the redwood-paneled room. It was a warm autumn day, of the sort that Berkeley is famous for. The light was filtered through bamboo leaves outside the window. A slight crispness hung in the air, and the smell of wood smoke drifted in, suggesting an impending winter that would never arrive. I realized, to my surprise, that I was in love.

We were together for the next several days, talking mouth to mouth, sharing poems I had written or liked, looking at books about Caucasian tribal rugs, meeting his friends. Loving has a way of awakening a new depth of awareness; I remember my skin tingling, and my senses being especially sharp. Life seemed dynamic. I gave in to the feelings. Friends in my volunteer counselors' support group still joke about the way I was behaving.

Steve had already told me that he was HIV-positive, I suppose to spare me from any unwanted entanglement with AIDS. But I had learned through my volunteer work that life is precious, that every moment of conscious living is potentially transformative. Of all the possible worlds I could choose to live in, the world based on loving honestly was surely the most spacious, the most empowering. Despite Steve's HIV status, I could not overrule my love for him. I wanted to be with him always.

I recall standing in the bathroom one day, knowing that I had found my life partner. My inner self churned. HIV had placed a strange and unfathomable challenge at my feet. *"Live now, live in the moment, or run,"* it seemed to say. *"But no sitting on the fence, not in the presence of such joy."*

I could feel the inner architecture of my spirit shifting, correcting and adapting to the currents of the river I was riding upon. Love was now, it was present, a raft on the muddy stream of life during this epidemic. I was vitally alive; my eyes and skin seemed to radiate light outward. This was no time to be asleep at the wheel, evaluating life fearfully by forecasting life and death. To love Steve I needed to be awake, drinking deep, and ready for the possibility that our time would be short.

It is a tall task to summarize the richness of your time together, the qualities of light and laughter, and the overarching presence of HIV. But I want to remember the details because they tell a story of two men, changed by love. I want to remember our story because it stands as a testament to the largeness, the *spaciousness*, of men loving. I want to remember because gay men have a story to tell during this epidemic, because the larger world thinks that it knows us but it does not. I want to tell the story of our caring community of friends, whose love and courage is so great that those who would call gay and lesbian people shameful would themselves be shamed to stand in their presence. I want the world to know how love triumphs when we connect in our hearts, which know no judgment. I offer the following snapshots from our story, as panels in a quilt.

Getting Used to It

Our life together was ordinary in the way of partnerships: nights at movies, a circle of friends who cooked well and dined together frequently, cross-country skiing trips, hikes at the Golden Gate Headlands and Point Reyes. Our sexual relationship was rich and rewarding, and seemed to belie the tortuous psychological gymnastics of sex across the viral barrier, as reported by the gay press. The barriers of fear I saw around me, while understandable, seemed tedious, and irrelevant to loving another human being, safely and sanely.

Of course, there were unwitting trespasses of emotional boundaries, hard limits between togetherness and independence—all this, and more. Yet I felt that this was a time of silent wonder. Writing now, I can see that describing a deep love is a lot like describing a concert to someone; in the end you end up saying, "You had to be there."

I wrote this poem to Steve on his birthday, January 10, 1987.

You are the first sight
I see in the morning—

silver of dawn
shining on your face

I can smell dreams walking
in the air above the bed

touching shoulders, mouths,
tips of hair

Your skin is like the curve of a
mountainside, the sheet is cast aside

I enfold you to me
while bamboo and ferns rustle

You are a hillside to
climb upon

I can smell the life
of the land in your pores

The smell of two men loving
covers us in the morning

Every day I am born,
muscles and hair and heft
in your arms

When we were living in this fashion, Steve's health underwent changes, which we tracked carefully. During the spring of 1989, his T-cell count went down radically. I noticed that his libido had also subtly dropped, but I could remember when it started. A certain fire I had come to treasure was missing; my first thought was "Uh-oh, this is the part where the honeymoon is over." The honeymoon had lasted since 1986, so it seemed reasonable. But a month later, I noticed that he had lost color and muscle mass. A new dynamic arose for us: he could feel himself getting weaker, and he didn't want to talk about it. Dwelling on his health seemed to make his deterioration more real; for Steve, it was better not to give it a name. He became taciturn about his meetings with his doctor.

I tried to stay off the subject, but finally I confronted him and demanded a fuller, less evasive report on this health. It turned out that he had developed a high toxicity of AZT. In effect, he was being killed slowly by drug therapy. Between January and May of 1989, his color and vitality vanished. We hoped for continued stability, for time.

Steve developed Kaposi's Sarcoma lesions in May, and the diagnosis was confirmed in June. I was away on a business trip when he got the news. Returning home, we tried to plan for ongoing changes, marshalling our collective courage. My goal was to be "present," following the Shanti Project's theories about death and dying. Being present became increasingly difficult as he continued to lose vitality.

We proceeded with the plans we had already devised for ourselves. He wanted to buy a house and we followed through on this goal. When our landlord sought to evict us under Berkeley's rigorous rent control laws, we had an incentive to move fast. About the same time, I was recruited for a wonderful position as a research library director at the University of California at Berkeley. All of these events seemed to converge, blending together the promise of forward movement, but HIV was dogging every step. The richness of our time gained a new color and feel. I felt this physically in the region of my heart; I realized that it was breaking.

Family

Steve's family was delightful. He was raised in Minneapolis, and had five sisters. He was loved and admired by his family; he had always encouraged his sisters in all their deeds. His two youngest sisters, Monique and Joanna, lived in the Bay Area, and the other three were married and lived in Minnesota. It was time to tell his family about his diagnosis.

As with everything else, the light and the shadow would be intermingled. His sisters in Minneapolis had looked forward to meeting me since 1986, sensing from afar how happy we were; now they must hear about Steve's AIDS diagnosis just as our friendship began. Towards the end of the visit, Steve gathered the three sisters together to tell them. He wanted to do this privately, so I walked to the nearby health food cooperative in the Seward district of Minneapolis and waited.

Upon returning I first saw how intense the reactions of loved ones were to the news. Having made our collective adjustments, Steve and I were at that moment nursing hopes of longevity. But the impact of the news on Ann, Mary and Martha was devastating.

We did a lot of crying together. This was important and good, but it had a secondary effect on us. The intensity of the reaction—it was as though Steve were already gone—was overwhelming. It restimulated my own pain at his diagnosis, dashed my fragile hopes. My lover was suffering; I was helpless. Revisiting others' pain later on invariably awakens my deep grief and sorrow. Steve's family, whom I adored, triggered this awareness for the first time.

This pain is immediate, and awakens even now. It is sometimes an empowering force, making me more compassionate and tender, and it is sometimes a scythe set against the new seeds I plant. Yet I was not upset with his sisters, who were particularly fond of us. This was our truth now; we were in it together. Ann came to California to visit us as often as she could.

Salt and Bitter Herbs

In the spring of 1989, our friends Rob and Paul held a Passover *seder* and invited many people. The guests included our circle of friends who often cooked for one another, making marvelous feasts. This rollicking group included Steve and me, his ex-partner Steve Cattano and his new partner Cliff Adam and several others. Typically our nights were loud and irreverent; Rob and Steve Cattano had caustic and hilarious senses of humor, and everyone loved sparring verbally.

This was a different night for all of us. As Rob began to start the ancient liturgy of the *seder*, the power of the words brought a depth and majesty to our gathering. The language of the Jews, exiled but reaching forward on the strength of their faith, seemed very relevant to a group of gay men and their friends on that night in West Berkeley. So often we think of our sorrows and grief as moments of weakness—something to be ashamed of, feelings we wish we could avoid. Yet here we were, confronted with a centuries-old history of love and reconciliation in the face of suffering. It was a story to draw strength from.

As the liturgy progressed, Steve put his head on my chest, as though to be close to me. I saw that he was crying, and this caused me to cry. Although I was very much with my own pain, I began to notice that others were crying, too. Of the twelve people present, four were HIV-positive; the others included heterosexual couples and their children, who loved their gay friends fiercely. We were a family, and we were in pain together. It was both miraculous and ordinary: light and shadow. This was not a sorrow that was indulgent, fouled with self pity. Our tears were like those of many other people throughout history, based in truth, cleansing and renewing.

It was a struggle to finish the liturgy. Rob on several occasions had to stop, himself in tears. By then we had drunk lots of wine, downing glass after glass as we followed the *seder*. When Rob completed the service, we laughed a bit, looking around the table. How human we were, how stripped of our artifice, in the face of AIDS. How necessary it was to love the whole person in the face of death.

A friend of mine later said, "With love there is no reward or payback. *Being there is the entire gift.*" On the night of that *seder*, I was richly blessed by the love around the table.

Being Real

I would like to say that all of Steve's journey was like this *seder*, but it was not. It was often hard for both of us to understand what to do. Steve did not want to die, and it was difficult for him to talk about it. As a trained "volunteer counselor," I tried to let him lead in the way he wished to go. I sometimes succeeded in setting aside my own agenda—I am by nature more emotional and expressive than Steve was—but I failed just as frequently. Although he was the one dying, I had needs, too. I was not able to be selfless; my own experience of this process took much of my time and energy.

To meet our combined needs, we organized our friends into a support group, so that we could have some people to call on for basic help and emotional support. We did this outside of the official AIDS support services; we had enough friends and experience to build our network among ourselves. Our meetings were wonderful, full of laughter, tears, and good food. But I learned early on that other people had clear expectations of how the partner should behave, and that I often fell short of these expectations. Some people thought that my frequent tears and sorrow were a burden to Steve (he did not agree); others wanted to see more of us, but Steve wasn't strong enough and asked me to be the gatekeeper. Many felt (inaccurately) that I was instigator of this withdrawal. One friend, his lover diagnosed as well, thought our group was unnecessary and would not come. He said he was a group of one for his partner, and this was good enough. It was very hard for me to navigate through everyone's pain, because it was all valid. It sometimes seemed that I disappointed everyone in one way or another. Looking back, I can see we did the best we could.

There were moments of incredible unity between Steve and me. One day he learned that he would have to have chemotherapy for his lesions. Being a scientist, he loved to talk about the nuances of drugs and therapies; like many scientists, he also believed that science could provide solutions to most problems, such as untimely death. But that night, as he described the poisonous medicines that would be used on his body, he spoke slowly, hesitantly.

I had had my usual day, juggling my distress and clinging to my work for emotional balance. His tone said that something was up. I, too, was frightened by the prospect of yet another treatment. But somehow I remembered to say what I had often said to my counseling clients, when they faced similar news: *"It must have been so scary for you to hear this."*

It was as though a dam burst. Steve cried and talked about how frightened he was of what was happening to him. He was bearing the unbearable. Facing this time and walking straight through it was the only thing he could do. We held each other for a long time.

Later that night he told me that one of the hardest things about dying was not being able to be with me. We had been happy in the way that ordinary people are happy: sharing our hopes and fears, connecting in honesty and compassion, setting aside the endless examination of what is right and wrong about relationships. It was enough; it was the finest thing I had known. My chest was tight: *salt and bitter herbs.* I had wanted more time. Our love, begun in 1986, had brought us to this moment. Our unity was the principal means of bearing these moments.

HIV wrests our fantasies of control and action from us. We are just part of the process, not its director. I wanted to stop the process, to protect my love from his death. But it was his death, and all I could do was be present. We were very close in that time; words were not very important.

Common Threads

Steve died without struggle a few months after that. In August he started to cough and have nausea; three weeks later, he was dead. On the night of his death, after days of laborious breathing and lots of morphine, everything seemed calm. His labored breath had subsided; he could not speak, but he looked at me with calm eyes. The hospital room was darkened, and the San Francisco skyline sparkled through the windows. Things felt complete in that mysterious way that invites much thought and embellishment in literature; he seemed to be at peace.

This story is one thread among many that is captured in the AIDS Memorial Quilt. It gives witness to the care and feeding between gay men. Although our time together was short, we gave of our substance to one another. We were both changed, healed, by the power of love.

I call this story "Feeding Each Other" because of something Steve once told me about parrots. He was an expert about parrots, having raised several while he performed field work in the rain forests of Costa Rica. Once we were in Key West on a short holiday, having dinner at a restaurant with a large atrium. There were two macaw parrots in the cage, sitting two feet tall on their perch. They were feeding each other with great fanfare and screeching. Each partner took a mouthful of food, and gave it to the other from his own mouth. This was the way of parrots, Steve said. They feed each other from their own mouths, and they mate for life. Steve and I were like that, feeding each other from our mouths and hearts, during our time together.

Later, in March of 1994, I read a short tale that was attributed to a Vietnamese monk, who had been asked to describe heaven and hell. The monk said, *"Hell is where there is plenty of food for everyone, but the chopsticks are three feet long, and you cannot bring food to your mouth. Heaven is where there is plenty of food for everyone, the chopsticks are three feet long, but the people feed each other."*

I wondered, upon reading this, at how in 1986 I had stumbled upon heaven in a shoreline park in Berkeley, California, and how my life had been changed. And then I thought about a couple of parrots in Key West, and wondered how they were, two bright spots under the shade of the palms, overlooking a restaurant atrium.

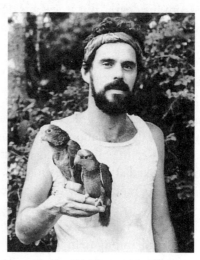

For Steve
Jan. 10, 1950-Sept. 17, 1990

AIDS: Notes of a Survivor

David Israels

When my friend Jeffrey D. Byers died, 434 days after they gave him his AIDS diagnosis in the gray, quiet corridor outside the CAT Scan room at San Francisco General, I began to think of myself as one of the walking wounded.

I joined uncounted thousands of others: we are the friends, lovers, family and caretakers of those who die a horrible death from a senseless microbe called the Human Immunodeficiency Virus. We are witnesses to and survivors of a meaningless viral war. Some of us survive better than others. But all of us, I suspect, feel some affinity with the sentiments John F. Kennedy expressed when he said that after another kind of total war, "the living will envy the dead."

Not every night, but many still, I close my eyes to sleep and unbidden it appears: Jeffrey has come out of his coma. Just a few hours earlier, he began to die and then stopped. That's the way it often is with AIDS patients, the attendant tells me. It's almost as though he's practicing, the attendant explains.

I am sitting by the side of Jeffrey's hospital bed. We are in the living room of my one-bedroom apartment. I have been by Jeffrey's bedside in this dying room for the last seven months.

Kaposi's sarcoma covers his cheeks. The skin cancer forms a mask of purple lesions, bloating his once-handsome, thin face. Jeffrey, who always took such impish delight in his appearance, would be appalled at the sight of himself. But he has no real idea of what he looks like. For the last two and one-half months he has been blind, the retinas of his eyes detached by CMV retinitis.

He gives me his hand. I hold it, gingerly. Painful herpes lesions have run riot over this emaciated body. A large festering sore sits squarely on the top of his right hand.

I can smell the delicious scent from his recently shampooed hair. Ever since another strain of herpes left the nerves of his scalp jangling with pain, we have washed his hair with gentle baby shampoo. I love its sweet fragrance. And I often find myself nuzzling his head, telling him how beautiful his hair smells—telling him over and over again how much I love him.

He tries to speak to me. The words will not form. This is Monday. On Friday sometime between 5:00 p.m. and 8:00 p.m., Jeffrey had a stroke. His left side is paralyzed. His speech is garbled. Most times it sounds as though he's speaking with his tongue clamped between his teeth.

He turns his head toward me, his eyelids shut hard over his sightless brown eyes.

"I'm scared," he tells me. "I don't want to die."

His words are clear and distinct. They echo from that moment to the moment seventeen hours and fifteen minutes later when Jeffrey did die, to the many other moments when this scene plays and replays in my mind.

I open my eyes. They're filled with tears. I will go to the medicine cabinet to get another dose of sleeping pills. I measure my grief in quarter milligrams of Ativan. During Jeffrey's fourteen months of illness, one milligram a night was sufficient. The first few weeks after he died, two milligrams were needed. Now, on a good night one and a quarter will do. On a bad one, the ante is upped to one and a half.

I take these sleeping pills to stop the relentless memories of physical pain and emotional agony that Jeffrey endured. As well as the many moments of unexpected humor and unfathomable bravery. I want instead to enter a state of dreamless unconsciousness—as close, I suppose, as I can get to Jeffrey, who now lies beneath the cold ground in St. Helena, without actually joining him.

My therapist tells me that the process of grief is really all about coming to terms with the fact that I am living. I tell her I think it's more about deciding whether or not I can be in a world that has no Jeffrey.

The awful truth of this matter is made real for me in the third session of my weekly grief group. One of the participants attempted suicide only a few days earlier. It was serious, requiring hospitalization.

When I again discuss this subject with my therapist, Mari's demeanor changes from analytic to worried. She begins to probe gently for suicidal ideas. I assure her that for me suicide is not a choice. "But there are other ways to simply lie down and die," I say. I'm not sure what I mean.

I am, however, struck by the paradox of my emotions. Here I am, healthy and alive, indulging in these questions, while Jeffrey, who wanted nothing so much as to keep his life, lies dead. Yet all I know is that for now I cannot reside in the land of the living. I am too full of the dead to care much about those who possess life.

One lazy afternoon a quiet sadness had descended over Jeffrey. He tells me that he feels as though he were alone on a great ship about to embark. From the ship's railing he can see everyone he knows down on the dock. We huddle there, he says, waiting for him to go.

Shortly after Jeffrey died I made a list that I titled, "The Bare Facts." When I take it out of a file marked "Byers Inactive," here's what it tells me:

I met Jeffrey on April 7th, 1984.

I remember it seemed like the usual pickup at the Midnight Sun, a Castro neighborhood gay bar. We went home to my apartment. We became lovers, I believe, that first morning as we sat curled on my couch, nursing hangovers, eating hard-boiled eggs—the only eatable food in the place—while giggling over a daytime broadcast of *Plaza Suite*.

He moved in with me on a forgotten day in June of 1984. I got him to move out thirteen months later. The reason was simple.

Jeffrey was a garden-variety alcoholic: perfectly capable of holding a job, fine to be around when sober but completely unable to control his disease. I knew he was an alcoholic when he moved in. But I had no idea what that meant. He told me he would stop drinking. It wasn't until much later that I learned how to live with the fact that promises and alcohol don't mix.

Jeffrey was diagnosed with AIDS on November 14th, 1987.

He moved back into my apartment on June 27th, 1988, when he no longer could care for himself. We stuffed my living room with hospital bed, bedside table, wheelchair and enough medicine and other medical supplies to fill a chest. We were allowed an attendant every weekday for seven hours.

Jeffrey's death came on January 17th, 1989. He was thirty-five years old. We buried him on January 20th.

These bare facts, of course, can't begin to explain the bond between us. They don't tell you that he showed me how to give life to the mischievous child tucked away inside of me. How he called me "the little guy" and I called him "the creature." And how, years after our honeymoon period was over, we still spoke to each other in our own silly language— cold weather meant he could call the day chwilly, in the morning he drank cauf and when I remembered the word keister for buttocks, keisters sailed back and forth between us like a ping-pong ball.

It's embarrassing to unearth such personal artifacts but they shed some light on why Jeffrey and I came together and formed a family of sorts and why it was as good and bad as any of the heterosexual varieties I have seen.

After a long day of work, I would feel such a rush of joy when he would call to ask if we were going to be "guys together" that evening. The night would consist of nothing more than dinner, television, the usual silliness and maybe, if we had both had a bad day, a cranky argument.

By then our love was unshakable, though we didn't share the same house or bed. But we were an odd couple even for the innovative world of gay relationships. We weren't lovers—in fact I had a boyfriend—but we were, as Jeffrey's AIDS attendant Caryl Dehlan later said, "like an old married couple."

Later, when Jeffrey became so sick he had to give up his place and come live with me, we spent every night together. But most of them were devoted to just coaxing a little food into him or controlling his pains with multiple doses of morphine or talking him down from rushes of terror brought on by the blindness.

Still, there were occasional times when we seemed to be just guys together.

Times when I switched to one of the music channels on the tube and a song would catch Jeffrey's spirit. He would sit up in bed and begin to move and sway to the beat, swinging his torso, raising his arms and dipping his head. And I would sit up on the couch, watching and clapping and laughing. But I never laughed too hard. I didn't want to start crying because Jeffrey was dancing. Dancing in a hospital bed. Dancing in his hospital bed, blind. Dancing in that hospital bed, blind and dying. So I just clapped and laughed and watched. I watched my little dying guy, dancing.

I force myself to attend a social gathering of gay journalists. It is one of my first forays back into the media world I left behind almost a year ago. I stopped going to these stimulating get-togethers after Jeffrey got so sick. A short while later I stopped writing in order to have more time to take care of him.

About fifteen minutes after I get to the party an acquaintance pulls me aside, "so can I talk to you," he says. He gives me the dewy-eyed look and mumbles something about "I read...your lover." I nod with what I hope is an appropriate mixture of distress and appreciation.

"So how are you?" he asks me, in a voice raw with concern. Though we dip into a few seconds of hushed conversation, he quickly segues into a report on his latest professional exploits.

As I watch his mouth flap I grow angry, thinking that in our death denying culture, few people want to hear how the grieving really feel. I want to scream at him that on this particular day I'm fine—except I'm obsessed with trying to imagine the exact state of Jeffrey's decomposing body.

When I tell this story at my grief group, we erupt into laughter. Of course, we all agree, what else should I have been thinking about? Such thoughts are a natural part of what we're going through. They're also too scary for most people, not because they're morbid, but because they remind people of their own grief.

I make myself turn to the grisly news in each day's newspaper. I am trying to get some sense of proportion, I tell my boyfriend William. I insist on reading about the Salcido murders and watching the broadcasts of the English soccer stadium deaths. I'm hoping they'll help me put my loss in perspective.

But these stories of horror only make me feel numb and a little nauseous. I can't comprehend them, I tell my grief group. The best I can do is try and take in my horror, the one I lived through and seem to own.

To Mari I confess what I really fear—that I will end up holding on to the grief, loving it in a way, because there is no Jeffrey to love anymore. She gives me the same old unsatisfactory answer. I will hold on to the grief as long as I need it. At that moment I feel a huge emptiness beneath my chest. "I miss him so much," I whisper.

To prepare for this story I review Jeffrey's hospital records. For four-and-a-half hours I sit hunched over a two-volume, 800-page thick account of his illness. As I jot notes, I seem to move out of time. I get through some of the pages in what I think is a few seconds and then look up to see that an hour has passed on the clock over the doorway. This happens more than once.

Memories rise to greet me from the turgid prose of doctor's notes, lab reports and nurses' records. They aren't the fuzzy memories of an indistinct time past, but hard-edged, almost like the experience itself. They're reminders of many bad times, but for a bit they do seem to bring Jeffrey back. I feel almost happy.

The price for this visit is high, though. By the next day I find myself thrust back into the deep, weeping sadness that materializes right after a death. My grief group counselor says it's *meshsuggeneh* (crazy) to stir up the past as I did. In her eternal optimism, Mari speculates that I'm trying to "speed up my grief process."

In the grief world, they advise you it will take a year, sometimes two, to "get through a major loss." I've only put in three months on Jeffrey. But if practice counts, I'm well prepared. My father died when I was twelve. My mother died almost three years ago. And then there are all the AIDS deaths: Neil, my friend since college, too many acquaintances to keep count and, worst of all, so many yet to come.

When friends urge me to take time and get away, I start to wonder half-seriously if I should put an ad in the paper that says, "Have sadness, will travel."

I shop, eat, redecorate my apartment, read, make love, watch TV and try to work. But through it all I carry the weight of my dead. And in a year or two, when I "get through my grief," the ghosts will be with me in old pictures and inherited furniture and sharply remembered snatches of conversation.

There is no ending for this story because I'm still in the middle of it. In lieu of one, I offer this experience.

It's morning and as I lie in bed in that half-state between sleeping and waking I have a dream that's more like a daydream.

Jeffrey is on that ship he talked about. But this time I'm on the dock alone, sitting in his blue wheelchair. Though he's a small and distant figure standing far above me at the ship's railing, I can hear him as if he's right in front of me.

"I don't want to die," he says. A long moment passes as though I need time to remember something. "I wish I didn't have to live here without you," I say to him.

As the ship, in slow motion, starts to leave, I turn my wheelchair away. I begin to roll myself, slowly, towards a dark cavernous pier through which I can see the harsh glare of sunlight framed in a mammoth doorway.

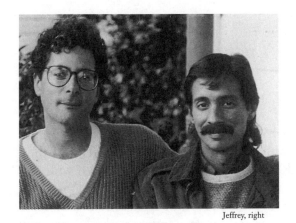

Jeffrey, right

To Jeffrey D. Byers, my little guy.
Always.
July 13, 1953–Jan. 17, 1989

KEN

DONNA JENSON

Journaling has been my private place of seclusion as Ken drifted
from being a vibrant, robust man through all those debilitating
stages as a PWA (funny, I always mix up PWA with POW—but then
a Person With AIDS is sort of a Prisoner Of War).

I'll never forget the first time I laid eyes on him. I knock, the apartment door opens and I'm face to face with a Cary Grant. That smile,
those eyes. Under my skin and into my heart in a New York minute.

"Heard of your peer counseling class through the activist
grapevine." I started a student. Six months later we were buddies. In
two years best friends.

We stayed that way for fifteen years. Colleagues—doing training
and consulting together. Co-counselors—I can't even begin to count
the hours we took turns raging and crying in each other's arms about
past and present hurts. Co-advisors—pushing each other to reach for
our dreams or clean up our acts. We were always each other's first
phone call when something went right or wrong. Sometimes, out in
the world, people mistook us for spouses. Actually, we'd done much
to help each other become committed to our respective partners: his
lover, Todd, and my husband, Chug.

I have a favorite memory from the first time he took me to New
Hampshire to meet his folks. We met Ken's dad for lunch at the country club after his morning game of golf. A puzzle piece fell into place as

I watched this man talking to his son. He adored Ken. Not in a mushy way, just pure respectful love. This straight, middle-class Yankee executive loved the son who had not followed in his footsteps. His voice was warm, his eyes glowed with pride and Ken basked. So did I.

Few knew he was raised Catholic. He looked like a WASP—loafers, button-down shirts, khaki pants, blue blazers, not to mention that fabulous chiseled jaw. Went to Wesleyan. Ivy league all the way, except at college, Ken formed a group for gays. Boy radical in elite clothing, jumped feet first into the civil rights movement of the sixties, too.

His career track and inherent gift was teaching. In the early seventies he moved to New York City and joined an East Harlem alternative school (his African-American students of those years never forgot him).

After ten years of teaching Ken took a big plunge. Became a Professional Gay Man. He courageously closed the door forever to mainstream teaching opportunities by becoming the Executive Director of SAGE—Senior Action in a Gay Environment. His deliberation process was typically thorough and thoughtful. I'll take my share of credit for not buying his carefully crafted counterargument about why he shouldn't face the past. We had made a pact to stand by each other's hopes, not our fears.

There isn't room here to list all the things he did for the gay and lesbian community. He had a vision for leadership that was profound. He was deeply committed to helping the leaders of his liberation movement lead well. That included giving them moral support, helping them solve their conflicts with each other, building bridges with other groups and movements, and pushing them to identify and actualize their respective visions for a better world. A world that would honor and respect every person from every background.

Ken was Ivy League and I was Rock-n-Roll. He learned in school; I'd learned on the streets. He believed in planning and I loved winging it. Together we taught each other when to think ahead and when to go with the flow. Best of all—we loved each other completely, warts and all.

There's no word in our language for the relationship we had. It haunts me. One of the most important, significant relationships of my life and all I can come up with is "best friend." How inadequate.

Here are some of my journal entries since 1988. Just a small sampling of facts and feelings one woman experienced watching her beloved die of this plague called AIDS.

April 15, 1988: (four years before he dies)

What a great time out from our planning session, going over to the (Brooklyn) Botanical Gardens. I love it there on weekdays—so empty you feel like it's all yours. How tranquil it felt, after walking around, to sit on the stone steps going down into the tulip section.

The place was bursting with color. Quietly you interrupt our flower-gazing. "I've got to get used to saying out loud 'I'm a Person with AIDS'."

I shift my eyes from the yellow tulips to the reds, pleading for strength from them, and I respond, "So start here with me."

I don't remember how many times you methodically repeated that phrase. What I remember is each time you practiced it, the blow of its reality would force my eyes to jump to another cluster of flowers. You needed my silent attention—I needed the tulips.

July 1, 1989 (three years before he dies)

Last night I dreamt of you. We are in a small room. You say to me, "I have something for you. I talked it over with my doctor and he thinks I should give it to you, too." You hand me a greeting card. Large and soft grey. No drawings or pictures or anything on the cover. Inside there are words written on both sides in your own handwriting, done very carefully and artistically. Large spaces between the words and in between the lines. Each word is underlined in a gentle wave of red marker. My eyes go straight to two lines in the middle of the message. "I know everyone is approaching death. But I am dying, now."

September 9, 1991 (seven months before he dies)

Ken, as of yesterday your white pallor has moved from the surface of your skin to the depths of your soul. I know that a part of you has already died. That part was the spirit of connection, the vast ability you had to reach into others and draw them out, no matter how hard they protested.

You would make them be present and fully alive wherever they were at that moment. That part of you was the teacher/consoler/insightful discerner who unequivocally loved whoever was in his sight.

You could love the best of us and the worst. You could reach down under anyone's toughness, anger or hopelessness and make them feel they had come to earth to make a difference.

This part of you would sit on the edge of a chair matching minds with great competitors—win them over not only to your point of view but to the delivery as well.

You were a knight in shining armor throughout the gay community for you had slain the closet dragon with more finesse than Fred Astaire on screen. You loved every brand of queer, no matter how outrageous or hard or soft or conservative or la-la they might be—you showed them gays were to be respected by your glowing self-respect.

And you moved the same way through the straight world—through all their homophobia (known and unknown). Loving the part of them that lay beyond the frozen wall surrounding their hearts. Always standing tall and proud as a gay man.

And this part of you stood up to injustice—global and on the subway—like when a man harassed a young woman and you and the other guy closed in on him.

This part of you that connected you to others, this part I no longer see or feel. It seems as though you have buried it, under all the pain you carry for the illness that is attacking your body. I doubt there is any one thing in your life that has taken as much daily time and energy as the application of your drugs now do, with the possible exception of gay liberation.

Unpacking the cartons, hooking up to the pole, inserting your tube and sitting for two-and-a-half hours every day. Not to mention the dozen doctors you see, consult with, get administered to by. They all take more time and energy. This AIDS really does sap life from its targets—one slow day at a time.

I want to scream at you, "How dare you accuse me of abandonment because Chug and I are getting married? It's you who slipped softly away into isolation. Having lovers never kept us from staying connected before—so don't try to saddle me with this crap. That's all it is—self-pitying crap—and I won't stand for it."

You've got another thing coming from your old pal, Donna. I'm sick and tired of not connecting with you. Sure you can't run a marathon any more. Sure you don't want to go for as many hours as you used to. But it doesn't take a whole lot of energy to sit on your bed and talk to me. Or maybe even let out some feelings or just plain snuggle and listen to some good tunes on the radio, hold hands and watch *Roseanne* on TV. There are lots of things to do that don't take any more energy than opening your mouth and talking about what you think or feel or even dream.

I know you're tired and I'm sorry. But I can't stand it that you are giving up. And, damn it, I won't let you!

November 12, 1991 (five months before he dies)

Standing at your bedside in the hospital emergency room it feels like the one-hundred mile drive from Chug's took about thirty seconds. You are convulsing violently.

Todd found you on the floor whispering for help when he got home from work. God, what would we do without him? He's taken such good care of you through all this. I'm sure they're holding a First Class reservation in heaven for Todd.

The doc puts a wooden tongue depressor in your mouth so you don't bite yourself while you shake. All I see is hands moving around the borders of you—nurses, Todd, now two docs. Your torso bounces a foot high. Fear pours from your eyes. Teeth chatter and threaten the losing of the wooden stick. I reach over and hold it in place. We gaze into each other for an eternal second and a question I have held emerges and is answered. I could be there for you, by your side, at the moment of death.

You begin to turn blue. You're packed in ice, I'm expelled from the emergency room. Another waiting woman takes one look at me and asks, "Is that your brother?" Through tearful muffled spasms I utter the truth, "yes."

Each of these rushed trips to the emergency room leaves all of us completely drained. I don't know what's harder—walking in or out of those electronic doors. A pair of thoughts always emerge as I leave. One, this crisis has passed and you're resting. And, two, how much longer do we have?

November 19, 1991 (one week later)

I finally mustered up the courage to tell you about realizing that I can stand to be with you when you die. With great sincerity you simply answer, "Thanks for telling me."

March 10, 1992 (one month before he dies)

It's an unseasonably warm day out here on the island. In front of me the sparkling water ripples to the shore. It looks and sounds as if the bay is blowing kisses to my breaking heart.

Will I ever get back to just *being* ever again? All the years of worrying, praying and wondering. First, "Does he have, will he get...the virus?" Then, "He's got it but please let the cure be found. The miracle drug, treatment, anything that will bring back his T-cells and make him properly immune." Then the realization that "NO—there will not be a cure in time for him."

And now I find myself in moments of not caring about the rest of the world, the whole epidemic. Only You. And now I'm getting impatient. Because I know you're getting "taken out." I know I'm going to lose you. We've made our peace with each other and we've done everything we can with each other (given this superimposed deadline). So now I just want it to happen and when it does, not to have happened.

April 2, 1992 (one week before he dies)

How will I ever get today's image of you out of my head? Your face so dark and drawn, your eyes, now blind, glazed and bulging. Your words making no sense. Spitting up your blood into the basin. I carry the basin to the bathroom and dump its steamy contents into the toilet. How did I do that? How was I able to deposit the blood of your entrails into the sewer? How was I able to keep standing, put one foot in front of the other and carry my body and soul from your bedside and go to the bathroom with a cup full of liquid that belonged in your veins? How was I able to walk back to your bed and put the basin near you on the windowsill—leave it to dry in the afternoon sunlight until your next upheaval—how did I not wail a scream that could wake up all the patients sleeping four floors below and not take handfuls of my own hair and pull with all my might as I dropped to the floor, my knees buckling from the exhaustion? How did I not simply curl up under your hospital bed and cry myself to sleep?

April 7, 1992 (two days before he dies)

For seven hours I sat close, mostly just held hands. We hardly talked. Todd came by on his way to work. As he was leaving he said, "I'm leaving now, Ken. Donna's here, tell her if you want anything."

Your reply was the only thing you said that day, the last words I heard you utter. You lifted your semiconscious head a micro-inch off the pillow and said, "I want out of here."

For over an hour I stared at you, contemplating what you had said, searching for words. Slowly I spoke, "Ken, look beyond here. There are some very special people waiting for you. All the people who have died. Your beloved grandmother—picture her face looking at you, reaching for you. All the friends you have watched go from AIDS. They're all there waiting for you. Todd will be okay. I'll be okay. You can go now."

I don't know where I found the strength to tell you those things.

April 8, 1992 (one day before he dies)

I'm back out on Shelter Island with Chug. I don't know how to come out of this pain. When I'm not with you it surrounds me completely. An all-encompassing pain which will not lift no matter where I am, whom I'm talking to, what I'm doing. The pain just stays, lingers, remains, fastens itself to my breathing and refuses to let up or let go. Like a bubbling fountain it seems to have no beginning and no end. It just is. And it feels like it will always be there—with me, a part of me, a shell encompassing me which determines my very being in the world. I think very little. I have very little desire to think. I have very little desire to do anything.

I just want to be by your bedside—stroking your arm, massaging your hands with baby powder—telling you I love you—calling to whatever spirits or powers to release you from this place and time, to take you out of this present brittle body. The body that looks more and more like the grey slanting trees in our yard, the ones that barely survived last summer's Hurricane Bob. They just didn't fall down as completely as the others. They lean, they tilt. They will most likely never bear leaves again for their roots are too far out of the earth to get much nourishment from that source. That's why I long to be with you—to give what nourishment I can.

April 10, 1992 (eight hours after he died)

You're gone. Todd called at midnight. It's over. I've wrapped my body in a blanket and laid it down on a lounge chair on Chug's back deck. I'm grateful there is sunshine beating down and that my body doesn't need me in order to breathe.

April 12 (three days after he died)

Earlier this evening Chug came home to find me sobbing on the couch. This tender man of mine knows me so well. He just cuddled up next to me and held me close. No questions asked—just loving patience. At the end of this day's trail of tears I had an awakening. Another question answered. Would my inner spark of love for life die with you? In some unknown way I had gotten a glimpse of the fact that it hadn't and *that's* what the tears had been about. I realized that I have been scared about this for years.

April 13 (four days after he died)

I'm really going to do this? I'm going to New Hampshire today and tomorrow I'm standing up at your funeral and saying a fucking eulogy? Where will the strength come from? Will I break down in the middle? Will I even begin? This is the sort of thing you always helped me with—these challenging, impossible moments. You, cuddled up next to me, or even just on the phone telling me why you knew I had what it takes to triumph.

This shouldn't be happening. This should be another weekend trip where we go and visit your family. A drive out of Brooklyn into the country, looking at the sights. Playing with your three nephews, having dinner with your mom, gossiping with your sibs. That's what this trip used to be about. Instead I'm going up there with Chug and Todd. Without YOU. New Hampshire without you. Shit.

June 19, 1992 (two months after he died)

I hate being an executrix. It's like exhuming you every day. I hate the paperwork. It's like a part of you won't be at rest until I finish up your business. Is that true, Ken? Are you listening to me? Right now? Are you standing there with your arms crossed in front of you and most of your weight on your right leg, the left knee slightly bent and a foot occasionally tapping out your impatience in syncopation? Are you annoyed, are you close to getting angry? Well, forget it, Buddy. I am going as fast as I possibly can.

November 19, 1992 (seven months after he died)

Todd writes that he thinks about you every day. I don't have the strength to do that. Or is it the heart? Maybe the guts. I have to carefully pace the amount of time I think about you—otherwise I go numb. Paralyzed once again with the loss of you. Seven months now —I'm always counting. Counting the time since you died. On my fingers no less—April on the right hand thumb all the way around my hands. Months. What will it be like when it's years? I remember someone telling me on the eve of my divorcing my first husband, "Just wait till you're divorced longer than you were married, that will be wonderful." And it was—though I had to wait ten years for that one. So—with the same equation I have to wait until, let's see...I have to wait until the year 2006.

So in 2006 will I still be unable to forgive President Ronald Reagan for his crime of not recognizing AIDS? Will I still blame your death on his seven years of silence about the epidemic, refusing to even say the word AIDS?

A more important question—in 2006 will I be able to think of you whenever and wherever I feel like it and not experience this pain?

January 20, 1993 (nine months after he died)

Grief. Nine months since you died, grief tends to grab me less often but more by surprise. Like this afternoon, listening to a crooner sing old Broadway tunes on the radio. When he finished the first line of "I'll be Seeing You" the first tear had already reached my chin.

I can't see you in the "old familiar places" because neither of us lives there anymore. I could go visit them and you in my imagination but I don't. But I do see you here, at the lake, in such natural, normal, everyday moments—like the sun piercing through the pine trees in our yard or sparkling on the water at day's end.

And each time I see you—how is it I can feel two so completely different feelings all at once? Joy at the presence of your spirit and sorrow for the absence of your smile.

My sorrow cries out—come back to me, dear Friend. Help me think about what I'm trying to do in this here life of mine. Give me those old reminders that I can do anything I put my mind and heart to. Sit with me. Make me laugh. Hold me while I cry. Wrap that big meaty hand of yours around mine and take me for a nice long quiet walk where we look more than speak.

And my joy reminds me how lucky I was to have you as a close companion on my journey. So close that I can recognize you in some fleeting rays of sunshine.

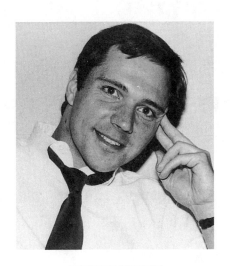

Ken L. Dawson
Oct. 9, 1946–April 9, 1992
Dedication: To all those who loved him
and miss him still.

AIDS Death #54,911

Robert Kaplan

The last time I saw you, Steven, you were huddled in bed,
blankets piled over your body,
you were shaking and shivering so much
there was nothing that could stop it:
your hands bunching the pillows,
your legs thrashing the sheets,
you screaming over and over, Lord, I want to die
please just let me die.

And I sat cupping your head as if that could do anything
as if there was anything I could do
feed you tea hold your hands give you more blankets
crawl into bed and lie on top of you:
my stomach on your back
my arms around your stomach;
anything to give you warmth, just a little bit of warmth.

It was summer; it was New York; I was back in town
and you were dying. I could sit in waiting rooms
I could help you in and out of cabs and up and down stairs
I could cook for you and wash your dishes and
get you shrimp lo mein I could wrap your neck
with towels soaked in warm water
talk with you about our favorite poets and

that little magazine we used to edit and
how you wanted to be back in Indiana and
everything was over, everything we knew was over.

It was summer, it was New York, it had been a year
since I had left; and you had buried your lover
and you had lesions all over your body
and when I sat in bed with you,
pulled up your shirt to give you a massage
and felt your spine between my fingers
you started crying about the last time anyone had touched you
and how your parents were always yelling,
coming to visit and yelling, blaming you for everything,
and all your friends had deserted you except Michael and Anne;
and Anne lived in Boston and Michael never touched you.

Now Michael calls me and I still do not know why I am healthy
and you are dead. Then Michael tells me how you died:
in a hospital, alone, thirty-two. Yes I can picture that.
I can picture that or the night we sat on your fire escape:
it was summer, a different summer; we were smoking a joint and
you were telling me about a man you had just met
whom you really liked, you really liked him a lot.
Was it safe to kiss, that's what you wanted to know. Steven,
isn't that just the most awful question: is it safe to kiss?

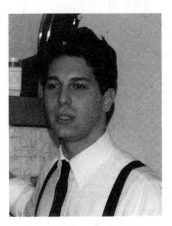

To Steve Cee, dear friend, talented writer.

THE LIVING ROOM

SYLVIA KIMMELMAN

Ring number two, she said,
and wait for the buzz.

I push against the black door
a sort of low church door
at the side of the church.
It sags against the stone floor
and scrapes heavily into a narrow tunnel—
the darkness is a surprise.
    (Later I could read, "Straight is the
    gate, narrow the way," also
    "The best is yet to be.")
After I got used to the darkness
I could read the wall and depend on the light
ahead
at the end. (A preachy wall,
someone wishing to amuse).

In the dark solemn tunnel
opening at last (my first time!)
out. A courtyard under the sky,
like a host at the threshold.

It is winter. A few birds are
restless on a stone garden table
round in the round stone courtyard.

Then—another door and I am in the Living Room, so
unexpected
like entering one of those dreams in another place.
Lamplight and women, voices low
sofas and chairs, dream-like
I blur the faces
I do not speak or wonder how I
    got here. I wait
    Someone asks: Do you belong
    downstairs or upstairs?

I shrug.
Is your child sick?
Has your child died?
Dead, dead, dead, only a word
sticks and stones can
    break my bones...

—Yes, dead.
—Then you belong upstairs.

The downstairs women are quiet now.
Only their hands are stirring.
(Later, I understand. Their hands
    are busy with hope.
Upstairs, the hands have come to rest).

We start at the bottom of the stairs.
She helps me take the turn in the staircase.
Before the last few steps stop
    abruptly
at another door.
I have only to open that door to become
an upstairs mother.

Downstairs, they turn to their work—
The here and now.
How many have vowed, alone,
—Never will I climb those stairs
not all the way—anyway—
maybe one day—if it comes—that day
I will sit on the stairs and listen:
—He said, she said, I can't.
I want, I want, I wish, I must—
Until the words are not needed
        anymore:
Upstairs, those words are useless.

I hear mothers' voices beyond the door
(All speak the mother tongue
downstairs and upstairs, all speak,
        all weep)
All tender, all holding, all telling
        and retelling
Remembering:
All knowing the heart of one another
In this nation of courage and loss.
And sometimes even great laughter
        leaps up
to cool volcanic rage.
We live in scorched earth!

Why? Why? Our young, our beautiful
have left us, have gone before us.
Where is justice? Where is the world?
Where is god?

Here in the Living Room we find no answers.
But hands reach across to share
        the pain.

The mothers' voices are low
there are sofas and chairs
there is lamplight
there is talk in the mother tongue.

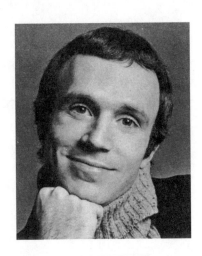

In loving memory of my son,
Seth Kimmelman, died Dec. 5, 1991.
I dedicate this poem to the
courageous mothers of the People with
AIDS Coalition.

SOME NOTES FROM HELL

GABE KRUKS

I
A grown man
but in the moment a child.
Crushed under the weight of reality,
tweed cap covering baldness,
you are totally alone
and very small.

Invisible to all but me,
you are poised like a dandelion
waiting
to have its perfection destroyed
by only the slightest
puff of wind.

II
Waiting for the hour to come and pass
my body is trembling
with the suppressed explosion
of raw pain.
I am counting the minutes
remembering every last detail

of that hell,
knowing that death was close
and in part wanting you to hurry,
yet not believing either.

Lying there in the bed
arms wrapped around you
holding you close to me
and whispering sweet words of love into your ears.
Your body so hot it almost burned me
your feet and hands cold as ice
your breathing labored and erratic.
The endless hiss from the oxygen—
I take the mask off
and wipe your face with a cold cloth.
There is blood coming from your nose
and the tubes coming from your side
have now filled up two containers—
the fluid is dark red.
The phlebotomist comes in to draw blood.
I scream at her to leave you the hell alone—
no more needles or tests.
She leaves.
The nurses all stay away—
they know it is our time only.

I have been here before.
I know that you will fake me out a few times—
and you do.
Your breathing gets harder,
only three or four a minute now.
I hold you closer.
You exhale a last breath—
and I know that this time you won't take another.
Inside me is the urge
to pound on your chest
and make you breathe again.
It takes every ounce of my strength not to do it.
The tears come instead.

I keep touching and talking to you.
I take the mask off for the last time,
wash your face for the last time,
kiss you for the last time.
I shut everything off:
silence at last.
A doctor slips in quietly,
does his thing quickly and leaves.
I am alone with you now.
You look so small
so battered,
a veteran of a bloody war that you lost.
I feel a momentary rage
and I pull all the needles from you.
I want all this equipment gone—but
I am afraid to touch the drain tubes from your chest.

I sit with you
and the tears just keep coming.
Les comes in with a body bag
and asks me if I am ready.
I tell him "no" and that I will do it when I am.
Oh my love—how can this be?
More blood has flowed from your nose
and I wipe it away again.
The girls have gone home,
I am all alone with you.
Everything seems so still and peaceful
in such sharp contrast to the last few days.

It is time.
I wash your body slowly—carefully.
I can't bring myself to pull those damn tubes
I call Les and he does it.
Except they get stuck
and he is forced to cut them off
and push them back into you.
I am screaming inside through my tears.

The bag is white plastic.
Les zips it closed,
but I am not ready yet.
I chase him from the room and
open it again.

It is after one when the funeral home people come.
As they take you away
I have the urge to chase after you.
I can't believe this is happening
as they disappear down the hall with their strange cargo.
If these walls could talk,
what a story they would tell:
there are no happy endings.
It's all done now
and as a final gesture
I walk to the patient census board
and slowly wipe your name from it.
It is indeed
the final act.

III
A five minute wait,
a signature
and
the box handed to me with a knowing nod—
although I am not sure
what it was
that I was supposed to know.

It was much heavier than I thought it would be,
about the size and shape of a shoe box.
I thought about
taking you to the hospital that last time,
and that, now, in this strange way
just a small part of you
was coming home again.

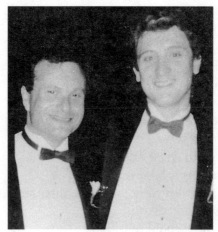

Jurgen, right

For Jurgen, who died July 9, 1988,
dedicated to his courage, his memory,
his loving.

WORDS

STEPHEN KYLE

M aybe we can put some army symbol on it," said Skip. "What's an army symbol?"

"I don't know. A boot? How about a boot kicking someone in the ass?" We both chuckled, which at first seemed sacrilegious to me. But then I pictured Glen with us, like in the old days.

Although Glen was much smaller than me, once he picked me up off the ground with just one arm. He had been out of the army for years, but still stayed in great shape. I had a hard time imagining that I would never see him again. He was always so fit—so *healthy!*

"Glen was a party person," Skip said. "We should show a bunch of people having fun and dancing."

"We could do it with little stick figures, that would be easy. Maybe dancing around something?"

"A mirrored ball."

"That's kind of tacky for a quilt that's a memorial to someone's life, isn't it?"

"He worked at Sears. How about 'Where America Shops'?"

"How would you like a tombstone that says 'Where America Shops'?"

A TV news report had shown the Names Project quilt, which had grown bigger than two football fields. People would make a three-foot by six-foot panel in memory of someone they knew who had died of AIDS. Hundreds of panels were still being added as it toured the country. Some were painted, some were sewn, and others had photos attached. One for a baby had a little pink blanket with small stuffed toys sewn right onto it. There were even panels for Rock Hudson and Liberace. Glen deserved a panel, too.

I didn't know how to sew, but Skip did. He and Glen had been best friends for years.

Skip shrugged. "Well, he was religious at the end, how about people dancing around a cross?"

"You can't be serious."

He grinned.

"I didn't think you could have been serious."

"Well, he was religious only in the last year after he got sick. I don't know if we should make that part of it or not."

Then I remembered something Glen had said once. Somehow, in a crowded bar, our conversation had turned to religion. Glen was saying that Christ was the only "path to salvation" or something. I had never heard him talk about religion before, and was pleased to discover this side of him. But the music was pounding, and people were constantly bumping into us. "Glen, I'd love to pursue this conversation with you, but I don't think this is the right place and time. I can barely hear what you're saying above the din." Glen looked stern, and said "It's *always* the right time to talk about *God.*"

"I don't know," said Skip, "I don't think we should have anything religious."

"Maybe we could have just some vague symbol of all religions. Like a flame. I think that represents the Holy Spirit or something. You're the Buddhist, *you* tell *me*. What's a good universal symbol?"

"I told you. I left that temporarily." Skip had started his own spiritual search, but thankfully was not pushy about it like Glen.

"Maybe we can use the symbol for infinity." I drew it, but Skip showed no reaction. "We can think about it."

Skip was quiet for a while. "It's funny, you think you know someone, but when you try to do something like this...."

I looked at the fresh yellow and red tulips all around Skip's apartment, and at Easter eggs he had painted recently. "It would be easy to pick stuff for you. Like flowers, or teddy bears. Isn't there anything like that we can use for Glen?"

"I can't think of anything. His family gave me stuff of his, but most of it is clothes."

I thought a minute. "Maybe we can use material from his clothes. Is there something we can use? Something you won't be wearing?"

"I don't wear any of his stuff."

"We can cut up something for the letters in his name, maybe."

"That's an idea."

"He liked bright colors. What were his favorite colors?"

"Gee, I don't know. He wore a lot of black and white. Hmm...I just remembered! His parties. At his parties, he always had lots of balloons around."

"Balloons, yeah, I guess I like that. But...I don't know. Something doesn't seem right. I don't want this to end up being silly. I think it's going to look like it was made for a little kid."

Skip was becoming a little cranky. He sneered, "Well, what the hell are we supposed to put on it, a big white mound to show all the coke he snorted?"

By the time Skip had called me with the news, Glen had already been in three hospitals. I was amazed that this had all been going on for the last couple of months; I had assumed Glen hadn't returned my calls because he was too busy getting ready for his big annual party.

Skip said he didn't know the whole story, but it started with a visit from Glen's family. According to Skip, Glen's family was never too accepting of Glen being gay. The only reason Glen entered the army, he said, was because his parents forced him; it was supposed to turn him back into "a man."

Glen's family found out he had recently spent two nights wandering around town carrying his clothes in paper bags because he thought "the church people" were chasing him (which even I admitted when Skip told me about it wouldn't have made me think it was AIDS). And then right in front of them he threatened to slash his wrists, and they put him into a psychiatric ward.

I almost yelled at Skip. If all this had been going on, why didn't he call to let me know Glen was sick? But when Skip said he had been visiting Glen every single afternoon, I understood why I was the last person on Skip's mind.

In a strange way, I was aware that I didn't even want to visit. If I did, I would start wondering about my own death, and I sure didn't want to start thinking about that. But, I thought, if I were in the hospital, how would I feel if people stayed away? So I went. Alone on the hospital elevator, I thought: What am I supposed to say?

I was surprised at how quiet and sunny that part of the hospital was. It was more like a nursing home. When I found the room, at first I thought Glen wasn't there. The man in bed was scrawny and withered, and hooked to an I.V. He turned his head very slowly and looked over at me standing in the doorway. I didn't recognize Glen until he smiled.

He looked like a corpse. The skin on his face was so thin and tight that his cheekbones seemed ready to poke through. Something was wrong with his eyes. They didn't look like Glen's eyes.

I felt awkward; I didn't know what to say. "Are they treating you okay here?"

Glen kept blinking, as if he couldn't focus his eyes. He spoke slowly and softly. "Yes. This is a very nice hotel."

"You mean hospital."

He tried hard to focus his eyes on mine. He looked confused. "Oh. What did I say?"

"You said hotel."

Glen looked a little worried, like he was trying to remember something important. "Hotel...." Then a hint of a smile brightened his face. "Hospital. I said hotel?" He opened his mouth, and I could tell he was about to laugh. Then I noticed a huge silver oxygen tank in the corner. Glen kept smiling, and he wheezed faintly. He didn't have enough breath in him to laugh. "I have fungus in my throat." He sounded like someone else. He didn't sound like Glen. "They keep me on this," and he paused, as if searching for the right word, "medicine, and...I get confused."

He lifted his thin arm and motioned to the nightstand. "Tissue." He craned his neck forward a little as I covered his nose with the tissue. He looked so fragile that I was afraid to squeeze his nose too tight. I wiped his nostrils clean, and dropped the tissue into the trash barrel. I wondered: Can you get AIDS from mucus? I glanced at my hand to see if I had any cuts.

I thought about the movies. In movies, when people were going to die, they just looked a little tired, and people knew how to act and what to say. Glen had cotton stuffed in one ear and gauze wrapped around an elbow. The edges of the gauze looked wet. Veins showed through the translucent skin on his hands. I didn't know what the right thing was to say. I leaned down and put my arms around him, and I could feel tears welling up.

188

Glen wanted to push me off, but was too weak. "I'm a Christian." He was upset. He tried to sit up, as if trying to maintain some dignity. "Christians...I'm a *Christian.*" When he first got sick, he threw out his porno tapes and the phone book with numbers of all his gay friends, some of whom he'd known for fifteen years. He said it was all a sin. Then he started going to Bible study classes.

Where were those Bible study people? I wished they would walk in right then so I could yell at them for messing up Glen's mind. I wanted to say, "Glen, you're *gay!* You're gay, and no amount of praying can change that!"

Instead, I said "But Glen...I just wanted to say good-bye." My voice quivered because I was trying not to cry. "We were really good friends."

Glen stared at the floor like an eighty-year-old man trying to recall something from childhood. He whispered, "Yes...."

I didn't know what to say. We were both quiet for a while.

For Glen, conflict and anger were now unnecessary luxuries—requiring too much strength. He gazed at me peacefully. "Make sure there aren't any Christians around if you do that. Don't let them see."

I smiled and nodded. After a minute I asked, "Glen, is there anything I can get for you? Something outside you can't get in here?"

"Yes." He licked his blistered lips and grinned like a kid about to misbehave. "Chips. Cape Cod Potato Chips."

We gave up on ideas for the quilt.

Skip was doodling on paper, just geometric shapes and patterns. "That's the kind of artsy stuff that Glen liked," I said.

From a box of fabrics, he pulled out a mishmash of felts and cottons, shiny oranges and purples. He cut out a blue triangle, some red circles, and a squiggly green line.

We had been trying to cram everything about Glen on the quilt. But what it needed was simplicity. Just one aspect of him.

I brought a bag of Cape Cod Potato Chips—unsalted ones because of the sores on his lips.

A nurse stopped me in the hall to tell me Glen had been "unresponsive." I wasn't sure what that meant. Maybe Glen realized he was going to die.

When I saw him lying still with his eyes shut, I realized that "unresponsive" meant coma. I felt the bag of chips on the table and stood beside the bed.

Glen hadn't been shaved. One of his hands was curled under the sheets. The other hand lay on top of the blanket. The fingernails were reddish, and white stuff like pus had been seeping out of them.

Sometimes, supposedly, people in comas can still hear everything. Maybe Glen could still hear me.

But words didn't matter anymore. I put my hand on his arm and just stood there.

———————

For Glen and Skip
Glen Holt, died 1987
William "Skip" Alfredson, died 1990

———————

ONE OF THEM

JAY LADIN

"Johnny's got the plague," you say.
They find him barefoot in pajamas flagging down a cab.
You share a cot with his mother
beside the oxygen tent, each of you promising
to wake the other

if he opens his eyes again—Two years:

Robert, body builder, optimist,
a widower too (everyone
was, by then), goes blind;
meningitis grabs him by the spine;
the marbled muscles

that easily pressed a quarter ton

melt overnight. You take over
feeding him, sponging his body, stroking his head.
By the end
he's lost his eyes, his tongue, his mind,
but he smiles as long as he can.

You're next.

You sleep at the office under your desk.
Five-foot-eleven, 110 pounds,
at forty-three, you retire
to a stint in your liver.
You put your affairs in order,

sell your piano, settle your debts. Ten pounds lighter

You visit a volcano with Jim,
dying too (everyone was, by then).
Then you grow too tired for plans.
You nod off, talking
about taking an overdose of morphine.

Jim dies while you're dreaming
you and he are driving
east through needles of rain;
pieces of the car keep falling
until it's nothing
but strands of metal and glass. God-

God-speed you say, hiccupping,

with sores in your mouth and growths on your hands,
clutching a gown to your 88 pounds
while fog spills through the harpstrings of the bridge,
blotting out waves, tankers,
the tourist ferry to Alcatraz. The nurse

who doesn't know why your eyes stay open

gives up closing them. Saline and morphine flow,
and cold pure oxygen.
Your room is filling with men. They arrive
by the thousands and the tens of thousands,
and no matter how stubborn or lovely you were

now you're one of them.

To Daniel Lynn Stimmerman,
Musician, Poet, Gardener, Friend
1947-1992

IN MY HEART YOU'LL STAY

LAURA RIVERO MARCY

I

And as he lay on his hospital bed in our living room of the house we bought together three years before, I told him, "It'll be okay—God loves you. I love you. It's a long, hard road we've gone down together and now you must go ahead and I must stay here. It's okay to go." Within three days he did pass on. On a beautiful, sunny, warm day with the forsythia bushes bursting with their radiance demonstrating God's magnificence at hand.

I will never be the same person who in 1989 stood in the middle of a hospital room gripping my husband's hand anxiously waiting for the doctor to come in to give us the final diagnosis—HIV or not.

I felt I was living someone else's life in a tragic movie of two happily married, thirty-five-year-olds waiting for the family doctor to deliver his death sentence. It felt like we were on a ship sinking so swiftly we couldn't get our life vests on—in fact, our life vests were being taken away from us.

The doctor's words were clear, precise and ringing, "Mr. Marcy, you are HIV-positive and, Mrs. Marcy, you should be tested immediately." How's that for a swift kick over the railing of our sinking ship? The doctor left the room within minutes and my dear husband and I looked at each other. In his hazelnut brown eyes I saw his life. I saw regret, shame, fear and an incredible pool of love for me. We grabbed each other and I felt my tears finally leaving my eyes settling on his shoulder. He softly whispered in my ear, "Laura, if you want a divorce, I'll understand." Ah! With those words, all the love and hope and strength of our bond became clearer. I could never leave my best friend, my love, my teacher. Little did I know that for the next three years he would be teaching me volumes on living, treatises on respect and consideration, synopses on compassion and integrity, theses on suffering and dignity, and finally, doctorates on love, letting go and dying.

This would be the beginning of a journey neither one of us wanted to take. A path through hospitals and in-home infusions, hard-to-keep secrets and dramatic lies, unbearable pain and hopelessness—to our final goodbye and physical separation.

I can never regret our passage together because I am stronger and more confident for it now. But I have cried a thousand tears over the death of my husband. Over the world's loss of such a good soul who tried his hardest and loved his fullest. I wish he didn't have to suffer but my love is not suffering any longer.

After his passing, a momentary calm came over me. I was alone once again in a world made for pairs. At thirty-seven years old I was a widow. All my life when I heard the word 'widow' I thought of an eighty-year-old frail woman dressed all in black. But when I saw my reflection in the store window as I was buying a new outfit for my husband's memorial service, I saw myself as barely a grownup struggling not to feel that life was over for me. My love affair with my husband had made me the happiest, most contented woman in the world. Then his illness appeared accompanied by a slow change in myself. Learning to fight for him when he couldn't raise his head from his pillow, learning to demand for him when he couldn't speak any longer and summoning up the patience to educate those who chose not to touch PWAs for fear of the virus.

Within a period of a few years my metamorphosis was taking place. I knew with his passing that I could work any hospital system to its fullest, that if I had to I could become an aggressive bitch advocating for my loved one in bed "A" of hospital room 370. I know with all my being I will be there again, to hold a hand and wipe a brow next time for one of my children.

When my husband was diagnosed, our hopes and dreams of having and raising a family of our own came crashing down around us. I knew my focus would clearly be my husband, keeping him as healthy as possible for as long as possible. On the day of his fatal diagnosis, a part of me died. The part of me that took life for granted; that bitched and moaned over a rainy day or too cool a cup of coffee served to me. I would never again question how boring the day was or why there were too many dark clouds in the sky. Life and nature took over and made a guessing game for us to play—when would he get so sick he'd be hospitalized? When did death plan to make its face known? Will he suffer so? Will I be able to handle all that will come to me? Would the burden be too heavy? Was I HIV-positive too? Would his illness be the first and mine the second act of this horrific play we were acting out? The doctors have told me how lucky I am. I do not carry the AIDS virus. Shortly before my husband's death, we became mommy and daddy to an HIV-positive baby boy—as of today I have adopted two HIV-positive sons and I'm a foster parent to an HIV-positive baby girl.

II

Together we sat in the front seat
With our two matching medium
Soft chocolate cones.
Licking and loving the sweetness,
The richness, the coolness.
In unison, barely talking
Just letting our tongues
Linger and lap
The way we used to do it
To each other.
My, my, what gratification.
Once when the flesh was strong
And powerful and majestic.
Here we are now —
You're forty pounds lighter
I'm forty pounds heavier
And we're licking our cones
In loving one another.

III

Believe me when I pray to you that I did the best I could and when you cried out—I was there for you. And when your eyes never closed for the last time, I was there for you.

After you went into your coma, believe me, I shaved your face as slowly neatly and as if you were my newborn babe. I guided the razor carefully over every indentation and laugh line. I brushed your teeth. Did you feel me gently tugging at your lips to part them?

The night before you died, did you feel me kiss you all over? In every spot on your body where I had played there before, I had to touch and memorize for the very last time.

But in my mind I play there constantly. You are my playground and the equipment is shiny and new.

IV

Was that you, that tiny
Gust of wind that blew
So sweetly past my face?

Or was that you, the white
Speckled blue butterfly that
Danced in the air around
Our lilacs?

I know it was you at the top of
The stairs that one night
I could never forget your cologne
A favorite fragrance from two
Birthdays past.

If given the chance again
I'd lick it off you ever so slowly
Like a grape popsicle on a cool day.

V

If you were still alive
I'd wrap my arms and legs
Around you so tight
Like the best birthday ribbon
On the greatest package at
The party.

If you were still alive
I'd kiss your incredible mouth
Til we shared the same breath

So the gods couldn't tell
Us apart to take you away
Again.

If you were still alive
I'd tell you over and over and over

Again about my love for you
About my lust for you
About my life for you.
I'd tell you about the moon
And stars and how they can't
Compare to nature's perfect

Bounty in You.
And if you were still alive
Your light would still be burning
In my window
There would be no more dark days
And darker nights
And you would not be but ashes
On my mantle.

VI

When we were married we hoped our lives would run together always growing stronger and older like the knotted, twisted, turning roots of the old sugar maple out in front of the house. I could see us together seventy-five years old walking hand in hand on the weather-worn aged wooden slats of the boardwalk. But alas, we only walked hand in hand, heart to heart, for seven years of married life. Those two-thousand-five-hundred-fifty-five days and nights drew up a blueprint for the remaining days and nights of my life once I became a widow.

If only I had told him once or twice or fifty times more that I loved him. If only I held him closer than I ever had in the past, to press his lifeless body against my living flesh, to try to magically bring back his breath so we could rejoice in a waltz of our loving one another.

AIDS had ravaged his once delectable body—he was my Adonis, so fine, so beautiful. And at his passing, he was like my grandfather. Aged beyond his thirty-seven years, withered and worn, his bones created new angles and lines I had never seen in human form. His face was a

fine translucent sheet of flesh forming over an ever prominent skull —
but in his eyes, oh, those magnificent eyes, there was an eternity.

VII

I send you heavenly hopes wrapped up in butterfly wings with
boughs of forsythia branches.

I send you thoughts of happier times when ours was a lifetime of
giggles, an eternity of hugs.

I send you dreams of you and me when we meet again. I'll know
you—I pray you'll know me. When we meet soul to soul I won't let
you go ever again. Only once, dear love, in an eternity—only once
shall you leave me crying.

VIII

That's it. I picked up your remains today. A tidy brown paper
wrapped package; I've never known you to look so dull. Ha! Ha! I
held you, my love, in my palms and my heart shuddered as deep down
within my soul came a screaming wail that I wouldn't let out, that I
couldn't let out. Not here. Not alone in the middle parlor of the
funeral home. Thank God the funeral director stepped out for a
moment because, my love, I want to jump in that box with you now. I
want to smear your dust all over my body and scream: "My husband
in the palms of my hands!"

IX

Beyond the mountains and in the dunes
There is my love for you.
Beyond the seas and the clouds
There is your memory.
You live in each beat that my heart makes
In every step of the day you are with me.
You have died of this earth
But not of my cosmos.
I will love you till the end of time.
Till we meet again
Face to face
Heart to heart
Love to love
I will love you.

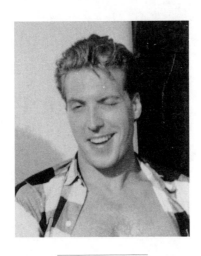

To my husband, my love, Wayne Marcy
May 4, 1954– April 8, 1992

Angels On Your Pillow

William L. McBride

For he shall give his angels charge over thee,
to keep thee in all thy ways." Psalms 91:11

As a child I never believed in angels. Angels were just another myth—right up there with Apollo and Icarus. Whether I saw them in Bibles or on cathedral ceilings, angels were always pictured the same. They wore silly robes. They hovered about with looks of perfect rapture on their faces, and they had ridiculously large wings protruding from their backs. I just couldn't believe that a messenger from God would look like Icarus in drag with the wingspan of a pterodactyl.

The only angel I've ever remotely believed in was conceived in our own Mt. Olympus of myth—Hollywood. I'm referring to the sweet old guy who helps out Jimmy Stewart in the movie, *It's a Wonderful Life*. Clarence is his name. Clarence seems believable as an angel because he's believable as a person. He doesn't wear those silly robes. He doesn't hover about on ridiculous wings. And most importantly, he's not perfect. I guess if you're going to define an angel as a messenger from God, then Clarence would fit the bill. After all, he does convince a human being that his life has value and a purpose, and that's a pretty divine message.

You probably think I'm being sacrilegious about angels. I'm not, though. I'm just trying to explain why I never believed in them. Because you see, I do now. I met one the other night. I really did.

Bart's my ex-boyfriend. He became my best friend. Now anyone who's ever ended a relationship knows that there is something close to Faustian alchemy when a boyfriend turns into a best friend. Such chemistry doesn't happen easily. When we first broke up, I ranted and raved about why Bard wasn't the lover I wanted him to be. I kept this pity party up for a few months before I realized Bart was not going to be who I wanted Bart to be, and I couldn't change him. But I could love him for who he was. That was when the strange alchemy began to work. As I began to accept Bart for Bart, loss became gain. Tears stopped and a treasured friendship began.

On Bart's twenty-ninth birthday we promised to go out for a nice dinner—something different, money no object (within reason). Bart wanted to try one of the latest marketing scams in eating out. Everything on the menu is served as tapas, or snacks. It's a great idea. The menu sounds like one continuous buffet of appetizers. For example:

- Lightly breaded artichokes and capers wrapped in prosciutto and baked with a sprinkling of freshly-grated Parmesan cheese.
- King-size prawns grilled in a fresh lemon vinaigrette on a bed of home-made basil fettucine and sun-dried tomatoes.

Naturally you want to order all two-hundred-and-fifty items on the menu, which is conveniently left on your table throughout the meal. And since the written descriptions are twice as large as the actual dishes, it takes about two-hundred-forty-nine of them to fill you up. But the real genius of this idea is the pricing. Each of these little snacks costs you more than half of what a full entree could cost. Well, fourteen tapas later, you do the math.

Ordering so many dishes takes time. Three hours later Bart and I had downed a couple of cocktails and four dishes each. It had been quite an evening. We laughed over silly self-confessions. We shared important and intimate information.

"Who have you loved the most?"

"What was the kinkiest sex you ever had?"

"If anything ever happens to me, please be sure to..."

Perhaps it was the wine, perhaps it was reality, but by 10:30 we had become somber and reflective. We sat, staring in different directions, lost in our dreams, holding in our despair.

We paid our bill and crossed the street where we waited for a taxi. In the distance a cab came at high speed, but heading in the opposite direction of our neighborhood. Half-heartedly I raised my hand at the cab. Instantly the shriek of tires on pavement snapped our heads up. We began a slow turn as the taxi skidded past about twenty yards, came to a halt only for an instant, then slammed into reverse at the same high rate of speed. As the car neared, the rear end suddenly spun across both lanes, tires squealed on pavement, and the taxi-from-hell headed right for us. Bart and I grabbed each other's arms and sprang back simultaneously. By the time our feet hit the ground, a large yellow car pressed against the curb, the engine rumbling ominously. Neither one of us moved. The car sat vibrating to its engine. Finally, I reached for the back door, opened it, and cautiously stuck my head in.

"Hey, you're some driver," I said meekly.

"Shut up and get in the car," came a voice laden with a deep Spanish accent.

I straightened up and looked at Bart. He stood there wide-eyed and smiling. Something about that resonant voice sent a tingle through me, and I guess through him. It suggested adventure rather than danger. Without hesitation we answered the call and jumped in the back seat. I guess we needed a laugh, a story to tell, if we survived to tell it.

Up front, the driver swung around to face us once we got in. Bart and I drew a sharp breath. Before us was a young man, perhaps in his early thirties, whose handsomeness swept over the front seat like a wave catching you off guard. His mop of disheveled black hair fell in thick curls over his ears and eyes. His high cheek bones, copper complexion, and sharp nose commanded that you focus on his eyes. His eyes were large malted milk balls. In each shone a sharp point of light—like a star reaching out from deep space. He smiled. Every part of his face seemed to glow. The taxi snapped with his energy. I smiled. Bart smiled. He laughed. Bart and I laughed. His message was clear, "It's okay. You're safe now. Let's have some fun." He swung around and peeled away from the curb, never asking where we were going. We watched mesmerized from the back seat. As he drove he kept fiddling with something next to him on the seat.

"Hey, you guys want to hear some good music? I play you the best music, if I can get this thing to work."

Curious as to what he was playing with, I leaned over the front seat. Like a plate of spilled spaghetti, a Medusa-like entanglement of wires covered his lap. Wires lay across the seat, hung on to the floorboard, and disappeared into a dark hole in the dash. He glanced over his shoulder at me and smiled.

"Hey, you want to drive?"

Bart laughed. I ignored the question, then felt a sudden panic. How was he driving? I looked up to see a traffic light ahead changing to yellow. Rear lights from the car a few yards ahead flashed red. Our driver glanced up from his electronic spaghetti, accelerated, steered right, and squeezed between the braking car ahead and three pedestrians who backpedaled over the curb as we sailed past. I let out a breath I didn't even know I was holding.

Maybe he should know we're not in a hurry, I thought. "Excuse me, we're only going a little ways, just past Irving Park. You can let my friend off on Bittersweet, and..."

"Hey, you want to drive?" he interrupted, this time in a tone that was more a challenge than a request.

There are moments in life, rare moments, when you allow someone's energy to consume you, when you let go of your need for control and follow your heart. I looked at Bart. He was beaming from ear to ear. Does he mean it, I wondered? Then I heard myself say, "Sure, pull over."

Instantly the tires froze against pavement. He steered us towards the curb. We bounced off it like a billiard ball kissing the cushion. I leaped out of the car, ran around the back and up to the driver's door. The driver slid over to the middle of the seat.

"I can't believe this," I heard Bart yelling in the back. "In all my years in Chicago this has never happened. Do you realize the trouble you could get into?"

I wasn't sure whom Bart was warning. Do I get in trouble or does the taxi driver?

The taxi driver was fiddling with a tape player, which now lay in his lap. He looked up at me. "Yeah, that's right," he said. "You drive careful."

I put the car in drive. Looking in my rearview mirror twice and over my shoulder three times, I pulled slowly away from the curb. Could I really get in trouble? Plausible alibis for the police began to enter my head.

"Look officer, this guy's really crazy. We just tried to get him from behind the wheel before he killed somebody. It was like a citizen's arrest. You see, what's his name here…" What is his name?

"Hey, uh, what's your name?"

The driver looked up from his tangle of wires. "My stage name is Tony, Tony Barcelona. My real name is William. I got some great music here, man, but I don't understand why it won't work now." He began opening and shutting the cover of the player.

"Nice to meet you, Tony. My name's Willie. That's Bart in the back."

Tony looked up smiling and reached for my hand. I let go of my death grip on the wheel and shook his hand. Then he swung around to meet Bart.

"Hey Mark!" he called out.

"No, Bart," Bart replied.

"Yeah, hey Mark."

"No, Bart," I insisted.

"Okay, Mark," Tony said laughing. I glanced over at him and he winked and flashed that fabulous smile.

I realized I needed to pay attention to my driving, but I couldn't stop glancing down at his fiddling with the stereo. He had rigged a Walkman to two cube-like speakers—each about the size of a package of Graham crackers. From this makeshift boom box he had run more wires into the dash where the radio had once been. Pretty soon I felt like one of those toy birds that sits beside a glass of water and bobs its head up and down until it finally makes contact.

"Where you from, Tony?"

"Colombia," he said without looking up.

"Tony, take the tape out and try the radio by itself. I had one once and…"

"You shut up and drive," he cut me off. Then he and Bart laughed loudly. Tony took the tape out, and sure enough, the radio blared.

"Not bad," he said. "I got some great music. You got to hear it. If I can find it somewheres."

He reached down to the floorboard and pulled out a shoebox full of cassettes, none in cases. Unable to find what he wanted, he swung around to face me and Bart. I tried to concentrate on my driving.

Taxis have a special feel about them. Unlike compacts that jam your tailbone up your spine every time you hit a bump or pothole, taxis seem to float. You feel like you're riding on a cushion of air. You still feel the bumps, but it's more like the turbulence bombardiers must feel as they drop their payload. With each drop you seem to rise higher.

Tony talked the whole way home. Lulled by the rhythm of his Spanish accent, yet buoyed by the energy of his words, we let him lead us into his world. He talked about driving a cab—its hardships, the lousy food on the road. Then he smiled and told us of his girlfriend and the healthy dinners she made him at home. He told us how he had struggled to make a living for himself in a strange country, how he knew he'd be a success. Then he began to share his dreams with us — to be on stage, to be a star. His eyes glowed as he talked about his love of acting. He laughed at almost everything he said. So did we. I found myself relaxing, letting go of judgments, letting go of my own fears of the potholes ahead. Time and distance vanished. This moment with Tony was everything.

Suddenly I realized I was at Bart's street. A little voice inside said keep driving, hold onto this man's energy a bit longer. Another voice reminded me it was my fare I would be running up. I pulled up in front of Bart's building and got out to help him out of the car. Bart gave me a big hug.

"I just can't believe you drove a taxi in Chicago," Bart said in my ear. "This has been great!"

"Bye, Mark," came a voice from the car. We both laughed.

"Bye, Tony," Bart answered. He turned to me before going inside.

"Wait till I tell everybody. This is so funny." He walked up to the door still laughing.

I turned back to the car. Tony leaned over from the center of the front seat.

"I drive now?" he asked.

I hesitated. It sure had been fun, but then, I best not press my luck.

"I drive now?" he repeated.

"Sure, shut up and drive." I answered and climbed in the back seat. I slid over so that I would watch him in the rearview mirror.

"Where you going?"

"Just around the corner. Go down the block and make a left."

"Now you gonna hear the best music!" Tony yelled over his shoulder.

"Is it in Spanish?"

"No," he said as he pulled away. "French."

"Do you speak French, too?" I asked in disbelief.

Tony laughed. "No, I don't speak French."

I heard him plop a tape into the Walkman. The music began softly. Turning the volume up, Tony began to sing along. His deep, rich voice filled the car. He knew every word, in French. He swayed to the music as he wheeled the car around the corner.

I sat in the back entranced that at this precise moment in my life he had appeared. Right now I needed his message. I needed to be reminded to love life.

"IT'S HERE, TONY!" I yelled as we drove past my apartment.

The taxi tires squealed. The rear end sashayed, and the engine slowed to an idle rumbling. Tony turned the music down and looked through the mirror to me. He smiled. "Fare is $5.40."

I reached over the front seat with a ten and then started to get out of the car.

"Hey, wait a minute. I give change." Tony swung around to face me.

"No, Tony. Keep it. You made my friend and me laugh tonight. That was very important."

"But I give change." He put the car in park and began searching for dollar bills.

Never had I dreamed I would fight with a Chicago taxi driver about taking a good tip. Then suddenly I knew I could tell him why.

"No, Tony. You keep the change." I pushed his hand holding the money back over the seat. "You see, Tony, my friend is dying, and you showed us a good time tonight. We needed that."

Tony stared at me. The stars in his eyes flickered and that gorgeous smile disappeared.

"Why? What's the matter with him?"

"He has AIDS, Tony."

Tony immediately leaped at me over the front seat. Instinctively I shoved my feet into the floorboard, unsure of what he was going to do. Two powerful arms reached out and pulled me across the back of the seat enveloping me in a womb-like hug. He kissed me on the cheek.

"Oh, God bless you. God bless you," he whispered.

I couldn't answer. I felt myself go limp in his arms.

"God bless you," he said again. "I'm straight, but we are all human. God bless you and your friend."

I began to feel a deep tremor growing inside me. "No, God bless you, Tony." I pulled away fast, fumbled for the door handle and walked quickly to my apartment door. Tony leaned out of his window.

"God bless you, my friend," he yelled one more time as he drove slowly off.

I waved without turning around. For two-and-a-half years I had stood strong by Bart. I had watched him withstand eleven spinal taps, four sinus operations with only a local anesthetic, catheters attached to his chest, swelling and sickness from experimental drugs, diarrhea for weeks on end, and the slow spread of skin cancer relentlessly stealing away his youthful beauty. I had watched the body of a twenty-eight-year-old champion swimmer slowly waste away into that of a refugee from Auschwitz. And I had stood strong. If he could go through so much without complaining, I could at least hold myself together.

But an unexpected and simple act of kindness can topple the most steadfast resolve. Tony's unquestioning love, his willingness to reach out rather than to run away, had totally taken me off guard. It had undermined my own wall of fear. My fear to feel what I was going through, to feel the pain and loss as I watched my best friend die. I finally began to cry.

When I got upstairs my phone was ringing. I was in no condition to answer it, but something told me to pick it up. It was Bart. He was still laughing.

On the night of August 30th, 1990, the nurse told me that Bart was restless because his brain was no longer getting enough oxygen. He seemed to be struggling for every breath. I remembered Bart's words in the restaurant the night we met Tony, "If anything ever happens, if it ever gets really close, don't let there be any more pain." I asked the nurse to give him a dose of liquid morphine.

Before he went to sleep, he rolled over on his right side. I saw his eyes focus on me for a second. I smiled.

"Hey buddy," I said. "I love you."

He gave me that big grin of his, that grin that said "I love you, too." A few hours later I realized he would never open those eyes again. I reached over and held his hand in mine and repeated the words we often shared instead of goodbyes.

"Angels on your pillow, buddy. Angels on your pillow."

Bart lasted for seventeen more hours. Though he was unconscious, I think he held on until he knew his family had made it into town and to the hospital to say goodbye. Then he finally let go.

A few years and a few more friends have passed since Bart's death. I often find myself wondering what I'm learning from losing people I love so much. I know I try to enjoy life more, especially the people I've chosen to share this existence with. And I don't question and analyze everything so much. I don't always need to see to believe. I accept some things I didn't use to, like angels.

I know now in my heart they exist. Sometimes they appear as real people, out of nowhere like Tony, bringing you love and happiness when all else seems to be falling apart. And sometimes you just feel them, like Bart, watching over you, whispering that you are surrounded by love if you but open your heart to it.

If someday you hail a cab in Chicago and a mad Colombian tells you to shut up and drive, don't be afraid. Climb behind the wheel. It's pure love that's steering you. Listen to it. There's a message from God there.

And if you see a handsome blond in the back seat with larger-than-life angel wings, reach out in love like Tony, and tell him that Willie still loves him and knows he's nearby.

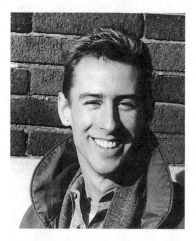

Dedicated to those who choose love
rather than fear.
Bart: June 26, 1961–Aug. 31, 1990

CRAIG

JOHN MCFARLAND

Craig was very good at dealing with other people's crises. At the law firm where we worked, this talent came in very handy. Whenever a person who was white-knuckled with panic stood before him, Craig would grab whatever that person was holding, ask a few key questions and then just do it. No matter if the crisis involved finding a missing page in a mountain of paper or reinventing the wheel, he would get it done. No problem.

In the aftermath of one of these crises, he would sit at his desk, his deep-set blue eyes focused on a framed still from *The Wizard of Oz*. A sly grin on his face seemed to ask, "Like, who *are* these people?" Sometimes, when one of the worst potential disasters had passed, I would hear him give out a fierce chuckle that was half delight and half mockery. He both loved and hated those crises.

One day after he had performed another of his miracles, I went into the men's room to wash off some ink so cheap and hideous that it clearly had to be deadly. Craig was staring in the mirror. He was fingering a huge zit down near his jawline. He'd turn to examine it in profile and scowl at what he saw.

"Blame it on someone here. Blame it on the stress they passed on to you," I said.

"He's the one to blame." He pointed a finger at his reflection in the mirror. "He wolfed down a chocolate cake last night. And here I am the day after. Going to visit his folks, looking like a mess."

"Your mother will say, 'I should have never let my beautiful baby boy go out into a world that covers him with zits.' And you will say, 'Money would help,' and that will be the end of that."

We laughed, as we usually did when we met on the run like this. We'd developed our own snappy little routine in the course of working together. It started when some maniac threw a mass of paper at us, ordering us around, yelling, "This has to make sense in seventeen minutes." In his customary way, Craig asked him what color labels the person who had neglected to anticipate his life-or-death deadline would prefer. "Fuck if I know," the panicked person screamed, "You choose," and ran off. Craig turned to me, that sly smile spreading out from the corners of his eyes and said, "Blue. Blue for BOYS!" The rest came easy.

The decisiveness and humor that Craig gave away by the truck-load to coworkers and friends didn't have a way of getting applied to his own concerns, though. As we became close, I saw him waffle obsessively about the most minor detail although true personal chaos was always about ten paces behind him. The IRS had him on speed-dial. He had two DWI's, but was still sneaking around town in a poisonous, uninsured beater. And his checkbook, for what that was worth, was under lock and key with a CPA. Saving a little bit for himself seemed to be his biggest challenge.

Our folk wisdom claims that gay men can't maintain friendships after sex has ended between them, whereas lesbians hang on to ex-lovers forever, expanding their affectional network to infinity. Craig's life contradicts that bit of folk wisdom. At a party one of his ex-room-mates threw, Craig surveyed the surging sea of men and said with a rueful laugh, "I look around and I can't believe I've slept with almost everybody here. What a slut!"

"And they are all still your friends," I added. "You're like a lesbian."

"Right," he said. "It's my deepest, darkest secret. Keep it to yourself."

The women at work were the first to remark on Craig's not looking so good. It was the flu season when everybody looks dragged out, and I thought nothing more about it. Then one day as he was going by my desk, I glanced up. He averted his eyes quickly, but I couldn't miss the frightened look in eyes that usually carried messages of devilish glee. A few days later, he sat down at my desk and said his flu had been so bad that he went to the doctor. The doctor had given him some weird prescription to help stop a fungal infection in his mouth.

I said, "The crowd you travel with!" His laughter set off a hacking cough left over from the flu. It was May 1985, and we were all going to get an education.

Craig's flu hung on, and during his vacation in June, he got so sick he went into the hospital. He called me from there one day and got right down to it. "It's not the flu anymore. I've got AIDS," he said. I tried to talk over my tears, and hoped I did a pretty good job of covering them. He didn't care about tears, one way or another. He went on. "I'm relieved. I've been living in dread until I knew for sure." This was his deepest, darkest secret, not any "lesbian" proclivities when it came to ex-lovers. Now the crisis was personal and unavoidable. He had to learn to devote his energy to himself.

We continued to have long raucous conversations and long solemn ones, but all over phone lines. He loved the phone with a passion, I found out. Our regular contact was only interrupted when he got the bug to move. From month to month, I never knew whether he was in Seattle or Oregon until he called. Whenever he moved back to Seattle we'd arrange to meet.

By then Craig had become a regular feature in *The Seattle Post-Intelligencer* with a reporter covering his treatment and status as a way to put a human face on what was then in the Pacific Northwest a new and frightening disease. The media coverage was another example of his drive, his path, to be of service to others. The frightened look was now gone from his eyes. I was proud, too, to see that the fight he was waging, the personal one and for all PWAs, brought him to a new level of comfort with himself as a gay man.

When we did manage to get together, we were always in a large group. I remember a picnic we went to when he got out of the hospital after one of his bouts. At first everyone was uncharacteristically subdued. Gradually, we eased our way into teasing and terrible jokes. I caught a glimpse of Craig laughing at one of the worst, falling back on the ground with his dog Casey jumping all over him. He looked the same as he did before he got sick for the first time. He was dressed in shorts and was simply in the moment. The only evidence of his illness was the patch on his leg where the I.V. tube had been a few days earlier.

The last time I saw him was just before Christmas 1986 when he moved down to Oregon to be near his folks. Five of us had lunch in a restaurant we often went to when we worked together two years before. He looked fine and his spirits were high. His divided chuckle and full-throttle laugh were in good repair. On the sidewalk outside the restaurant, we embraced. What others thought of his expressing affection openly to another man was finally not a concern of his. He was tending to his own crisis first. He was beautiful and weary. I could see he was slowing down. This, I knew, was our goodbye.

He moved back to Seattle again a month or so later. I read about him in the paper, and I'd get updates from mutual friends that his condition seemed stabilized. The obituary in the paper, then, came as a tremendous shock. His face looking out at me, smiling and averting his eyes. I was at work when I read it and had to go outside into the rain. You can see it coming, you can plan for it, think you have adjusted to it, know you have said goodbye, and yet the actual loss is absolutely overwhelming.

At the Names Project's stop in Seattle one year, I walked the hall looking down at the heartfelt memorials laid out on the floor. I wondered how anybody selects the key items to summarize friend and lover. It seemed impossible to choose among memories, to call one more important than the next. I looked up and saw more quilts hanging from the rafters. One high up had a white silhouette of a dog standing on its hind legs, and a quote, "I want them all to go to Italy." These were Craig's last words as he died in his mother's arms, but the quote was attributed to Bruce. Who was this Bruce person, I asked myself, looking at the quilt that was on a field of deep blue. Spelled out in large white letters was *Bruce Craig Anderson, 1952-1987.* Bruce, I realized, had been the name he'd been given at birth, and the quilt panel was made by his mother. The dog was his beloved Casey.

I flashed back on our 1985 conversation in front of the men's room mirror, and my words, "Your mother will say, 'I should have never let my beautiful baby boy go out into a world that covers him with zits.' And you will say, 'Money would help,' and that will be the end of that." I know now that there are no neat ends to anything. This is just one of the lessons I learned.

He was the first friend I lost to AIDS. The way the men in Craig's life banded together to help him taught me about the value of true friends. It also made me look closely at my own friends. "Will this person stand by me in crisis?" I am driven to ask now of every one of them. I've found that after you've asked and answered this question about a friend, it is the only one that really matters. And if you can't put yourself at the head of your own list of friends, you're in for real trouble. Every day I see that lesson from Craig before me. It is as vital to me as the laughter, joy and sorrow we shared.

For Craig Anderson, in celebration
of his genius for friendship.
Jan. 19, 1952–Early Spring, 1987

PROMISES SPOKEN,
PROMISES KEPT

STEPHEN W. McINNIS

R oom #626 of St. Joe's Memorial was calm now, except for the low,
almost imperceptible banter from a neglected television set. It
was after 9:00 p.m. and visiting hours were now officially over, though
there were those, such as myself, who chose to ignore hospital rules
when the concern for a patient held more importance. Chris Angeles
was the object of my concern, lying quietly in his bed and fully aware
that this was his biggest battle since he was diagnosed with AIDS over
four years ago. As lymphoma spread through his now fragile body, he
also knew it was probably his last.

Chris and I had been close friends for a little over three years. At
twenty-seven, he was much younger than I or any of my other friends.
But my admiration for Chris was not based on a measure of his age.
In my eyes, I saw him as an old man of wisdom who could wake up to
the face of his own mortality each day and challenge it with the innocence of a second childhood. My admiration for him unfolded with
each passing year as I witnessed him climb out onto many a fragile
limb just to see what was there. I saw him patronize his doctors who
insisted that he take it easier. "The quality of my life is not nego-
tiable," he would reprimand them. So far, he had far outlived all of
their calculated predictions.

For this past week, I came to his bedside every night to spend
what we both knew, deep down, to be his remaining time. As each

214

night lingered, as each visit presented a paler, weaker friend, our silence became longer. Words weren't always necessary between the two of us for we had already said what was important. He would, however, sense when my mood became dark, or possibly selfish in grief, as it had become this particular night. He would try to shock me back to the moment because he, of all people, knew that it was too important and precious.

"I decided to go ahead and be burned," Chris said in a strained, whispery voice, breaking the silence while studying my face.

"What made you change your mind?" I asked, trying to hide my obvious shock.

"Oh, I don't know. Even though it's against the Greek Orthodox Church, I guess I don't particularly relish the thought of having my mother come to the graveyard every week to cry over a plot of earth. It's too morbid for me. I also kinda came up with this idea of giving everybody at the service a tulip bulb with some of my ashes sprinkled over each one. Whad'dya think? You don't think people will think it's too...you know...icky...holding a part of me in their hands?"

"Returning life for death," I responded. "It's got a nice touch to it. As long as you're packaged in cellophane or something, where we don't have to actually fondle your remains. With my luck, I'd probably be standing there at the service, holding a part of you I'd rather not have to think about at the time."

A smile came over his face and his pallid, green eyes regained for a brief moment the richness that had faded as quickly as his health over the past week. At that moment Claire, the night nurse, came in with a tray full of pills; of no real purpose to Chris. Like the other nurses and attendants, she seemed to have taken a special interest in Chris, always checking in on him after her shifts and sending him notes and flowers. He had almost a magical effect on people, the ability to make you feel like you were the only person in a crowded room.

"How's it going, Chris?" she asked in a bright and cheerful voice, a sign that she had just begun her shift.

"Oh, it's going about every twenty minutes," he nodded with a smirk down to the bulging yellow bag that hung off the side of his bed. "It's growing bigger and bigger. Pretty soon it will be walking and talking...like a son I never had."

Claire let out a laugh as she checked his oxygen level and adjusted the percentage a little higher to ninety percent. "Dr. Amison said to give you just a little more air so you'd be comfortable. I'll be back in a little while to change your bag."

I saw Claire's smile quickly disappear as she turned from him and caught my eye for a moment. She walked out and Chris returned the oxygen mask back to his face to gain a few deep breaths, coughing violently between takes to bring up whatever sputum he could manage. He showed a big glob to me as if he were proud. I feigned disgust and slumped back in my visitor's chair.

Only once during our friendship had Chris ever expressed fear. That was five months ago when during a visit to his doctor it was discovered that the cancer had spread dramatically in spite of the chemotherapy he had been receiving. It was his final boarding call. Chris called me as soon as he got home and we simply cried together over the phone. "I'm not so scared about dying," he said. "It's mostly the fear of dying alone."

"As long as I'm around, you'll never have to be scared of that," I pledged. "I just don't want you to give up quite yet." We cried a little more and after a few moments, he changed the subject. He never again expressed that fear, but began an even faster-paced schedule over the next few months that crammed unfinished plans, sorting out his belongings and writing farewell notes to close friends and relatives.

"So how's your new writing class going?" Chris asked. He had again removed his mask and was making an effort to concentrate his interest in my life.

"Oh, it sounds pretty interesting. After each class, the teacher gives us an assignment to write about and the theme this week is pink."

"Pink? As in old ladies' hair and dyed poodles?"

"Yeah. But I'm drawing a blank. The only thing I can think about is that my mother's favorite color is pink. But who cares?"

"Well, why don't you write about…hmmm…why don't you write about pink angel dust?"

"Pink angel dust?" I asked. "What is that, a gay party drug?"

"No. You know. When you die and receive your angel wings? You go up to heaven and the pink dust from your new wings falls to the ground."

"Never heard of it," I replied.

Chris was trying to laugh. "I guess not. I just made it up!"

"Maybe you should be in this class," I said, admiring his ability to still be creative even though he was in a lot of pain.

"One thing I want you to think about," he asked slowly, as if feeling me out. "I'd like you to consider writing a piece about me. You know, to sort of make me immortal." He was shyly smiling, almost embarrassed that he had asked such a favor.

I returned his smile and with sincerity I quietly said: "I promise."

The expression on his face changed suddenly, almost as if overtaken by fear, his eyes stretching to the ceiling followed by a spasm of coughing too weak to be productive. He was gasping in between heaves and shoving the oxygen mask so hard against his face as if to swallow it down his lungs. In a panic, I ran out and brought Claire back to his bedside. She immediately gave him an intravenous injection of morphine to relax Chris' anxiety. I watched her, partially in fear and partially in awe as her expert hands arranged tubes and machines, and all the while taking time to stroke her patient's forehead and whispering calmly in his ear.

I relaxed as Claire continued to soothe Chris, taking his hand and stroking it with gentle care. I sat back down in my chair and took a deep breath. The reality of what was happening had finally taken hold of my shoulders and shaken out any traces of denial. Chris was dying. It had been apparent for some time, but I kept hoping for an outside miracle that would make all this pain go away. I had heard that the caregivers are often the last not only to accept the passage of someone they love but also to anticipate the impact it will have on their personal lives. They become so immersed in providing comfort and support, they lose perspective on what it is doing to them. All of that hit me in that one moment of his spasms and coughing...one moment that told me that I would soon be without a part of my heart.

"You okay, hon?" Claire was standing over me, turning her attention to my own pain. I looked over to Chris who was quiet, in what appeared to be a disturbed sleep. His chin was pointed to the ceiling, mouth open and taking tiny breaths of what was now pure oxygen. "He'll be all right for the evening," she said comfortingly. "Why don't you go on home and get some sleep? You look like you could use it."

"I can't. I promised him that I would be here for him."

"You do what you think you have to do." Claire sat on the edge of my chair and put a hand on my shoulder. "Let me give you some advice from my own personal experience. He could go on like this for days, even weeks. Now I know the two of you are just friends, but your relationship is very special. You made a promise to be with him.

From what I can tell, you'll always be with him one way or another, and he'll be with you. It's something that just doesn't die but will live on long past this lifetime."

"I guess you're right. Thanks, Claire. Will you be here all night?" I asked, wanting the security of knowing that someone who cared for Chris would be there in case he needed help.

"I'll be here the whole time," she said with an assuring pat on my back as she got up and began to walk out the door.

"Claire?"

She stopped at the threshold and turned around. "Yes, hon?"

"How do you do it? How do all of you who work up here do this day in and day out? Where do you draw that line from becoming too involved?"

With a pause, her eyes turned back to Chris and she said: "You don't."

She walked out the door which closed behind her.

I remained sitting in my chair and began to wonder whether Chris was dreaming. What could he possibly be feeling, if anything at all? I closed my eyes and tried to imagine myself in his place but my imagination kept running into a wall. All I could sense was that Chris had arrived in his space with a quiet dignity. It was as if he had cultivated a new friendship different from our own. It was a friendship that I could not be a part of, not now. But through this experience, I knew that one day I would hear that same gentle, whispering voice that Chris was now hearing, and I would embrace it with the same silent strength. That was his gift to me, and one that I would always cherish. I got up from the chair and walked over to his bed. Kneeling down, I picked up his hand with the utmost delicacy, trying not to strain the I.V., and pulled it to my cheek. "Sweet dreams, my dear friend," I said softly and laid his hand back beside his body. I turned to gather my things together quietly when I heard a shuffling of bed linen and a weak, muffled voice behind me.

"Don't worry," Chris said. "I'll say goodbye when it's time." He closed his eyes again as I stood there with the deepest sense of love I believe I have ever felt.

As I left the emergency room entrance of St. Joe's into the cold night air, I felt a quietness that suggested that everyone was frozen in time except me. A fog had crept in, like a predator under the protection of night, only presenting itself when caught in the presence of a streetlamp and the faint glow coming from the few remaining lighted windows of the hospital. It gave a sense of depth to my surroundings, almost a sense of peace laden with mystery. The fog beckoned to my subconscious, offering an escape, a place to wander, leaving what was real behind me, a place that could envelop me and smother my conscious pain. But as I walked off into that void, I found the netherworld to be elusive, teasing me with its lap of security that was always fifty or so feet away. I just kept walking and walking.

I lost all sense of time and direction. Damp and cold, I suddenly realized that I was only a few blocks from my apartment, as if a homing device had taken over. There lay my place of security, where everything would be as I had left it, unchanged except by my own hand and will. I yearned for its comfort and ran the rest of the way. When I reached my apartment, I burst into the foyer, gasping for air and startling my cat. Recognizing her master, she circled my leg and then ran into the kitchen, a not so subtle indication that she was hungry. I gave her a large helping of Cat Chow and stroked her back as she picked at her food. After she was done, I opened the back kitchen door and she bolted off into the black void.

"Here I am safe and secure," I thought to myself and stepped out onto the back porch, again staring out into the dark fog. Suddenly, I sensed a swirl of warm air and a light brushing on my face that felt of fine snow. Without an inner warning, I dropped to my knees, crying out, not caring if the neighbors were peering through their blinds with inquisitive eyes. Nothing mattered at that moment, for I realized that Chris, with a final touch of creativity, had kept his promise to me.

To Chris Angeles, a wonderful friend
who taught me so much about how life
should be lived.
Died April 6, 1992 at the age of 27.

THE LAST OF THE ASHES

MARTIN MCKINSEY

I should have guessed when I got the message to call. My wife was at her Greek class on the other side of Athens. I was thinking about seeing a movie, but at the last minute changed my mind. I went down to use the phone at the newsstand across the street. It was night time, raining, the tail end of October. In southern California it would be early morning and sunny.

My mother answered. From the first word, I knew.

"...He felt he was going down so fast. He was worried about his eyes...he'd gotten so weak. So he decided.... He left you kids a short note. Would you like me to read it? 'Dear Lauren, Kate, and Martin: By the time you see this, I will be happily gone....' "

On my way out, the shopkeeper looked up from his soccer bulletin, and froze when he saw my face.

The previous August, a few days before we left for Greece, I had lunch with my father at the cafeteria across from the County AIDS clinic, where I'd gone with him for his weekly checkup. As we undid our shrink-wrapped sandwiches, he said that if he died while I was away, I shouldn't feel obliged to come rushing back. "I won't know the difference," he laughed. I said I wasn't worried about that, he was doing so much better now.

We flew back anyway.

We all sat around my mother's living room, glum and exhausted. He must have realized, my mother was saying, that there was no coming back. His eyes—all but peripheral vision in the right eye gone, and the other one starting to go. There was also the tuberculosis, the thrush, severe intestinal pains. He weighed next to nothing.

For two weeks he'd seemed agitated, she said, then he was calm. Over lunch, he told her he'd made up his mind. He wanted to do it on Sunday. He would follow the Hemlock Society procedure: pills, then a plastic bag over his head.

She went over to his place on Sunday morning, and sat with him on the sofa. She told him how glad she was that they had met, how much fun she'd had. What a good father he had been. Then she left.

Tony, his lover, couldn't handle much more himself. He took their shi-tzu dog for a long walk in the oil fields. When he came back, my father was dead.

Months later, I found out that my younger sister had talked to him on the phone that morning. I felt a twinge of jealousy, regret. Exhausted by the ordeal of settling into Athens amid general strikes and heat waves, I had forgotten his seventieth birthday. I asked my sister to write me about their last conversation:

> I had sensed the week before that it was coming. The
> night before, I went to a party and drank some tequi-
> la (very unusual for me) because I felt so anxious about
> it. I woke up Sunday morning and just knew. I called
> Dad—the machine was on—and left a message. About
> 11:30, Dad called. He told me right off that today was
> the day, how he planned to do it. Mom and Tony were
> there with him to "get him started." He told me he
> felt very calm and peaceful and was looking forward to
> being gone. He sounded very reconciled and at
> peace—and also very distant. He told me he would
> miss me—that he loved me—he asked me to wish him
> luck. I did and said I hoped it was good on the other
> side. My heart was pounding and I felt really scared. I
> told him I loved him and I held myself together
> because I know he needed me to—and then we were
> off the phone. I put on Beethoven's Ninth and lay on
> the floor through it, crying.

My mother saved us a copy of the obituary.

T.W. McKinsey, a retired attorney who was a co-founder of a Long Beach law firm and active with the Long Beach Museum of Art, has died at his home in Signal Hill. He was seventy years old and had been ill for several years.

McKinsey was born in Walnut Creek and attended public schools in San Francisco, Los Angeles and Riverside.

He had been a Navy pilot and flight instructor in World War II.

McKinsey graduated from Stanford University in 1948. He also received his law degree from there. He and fellow student Martha "Marti" Miller were married in 1950.

McKinsey had been active in the Unitarian Church in Long Beach, and president of its board of trustees. He was an avid sailor and tennis player.

McKinsey is survived by two daughters, a son and daughter-in-law, and two brothers.

He is also survived by Martha McKinsey. They had separated in 1980 and were divorced several years later.

There was no mention of how he died, no hint that AIDS had anything to do with it. Nor did Tony's name appear anywhere. Apparently, this was newspaper policy.

The chartered sailboat thumped against the end of the dock. One by one we stepped aboard: Tony with the bouquets, my mother, my older sister from Colorado, my wife, myself, and the mortician. The mortician carried a clear plastic bag filled with what looked like cement mix, only grainier.

I hadn't seen my older sister in years. Feeling ambivalent toward my father and the rest of the family, she had broken off with us, one by one. Even under the circumstances, it was good to see her. She and my wife had never met, and they seemed to hit it off. It looked promising.

It was a gorgeous November day: bright, sunny, with a crisp breeze on the water. My mother made small talk with the boat's owner, Matthew, a lawyer like my father. "The deceased liked to sail, too," she told him. Terns hung on the wind, eyes out for scraps. The breakwater safely behind us, Matthew cut the engine, and we drifted. The mortician handed me the plastic bag. I was surprised by how heavy it was.

We sat in a semicircle at the prow, and I undid the twistie. Some of us said a few words. Tony was quiet, red-eyed. We began taking handfuls of ash and dropping them over the side. It felt gritty, clammy. I wasn't sure my dad, a private man for all his sociability, would have approved. He had been clear about one thing: we were not to keep his ashes. At some point my sister's emotions got the better of her. Tears streaming down her face, she shoveled one handful after another into the pockets of her windbreaker. ("I got greedy," she said later.)

They sank quickly. Once, when the boat turned into the wind, they blew over the deck. I pictured Matthew hosing them off afterwards.

In the end, I just shook the bag out over the side, and stuffed it in my pocket. Then we scattered what was left of the bouquets and turned the boat. When I looked back, the flowers were gone.

"At this moment it is appropriate for each one of us to reflect upon the meaning of life and death...."

Jack, an old family friend and former Unitarian minister, had flown down from British Columbia, where he managed a shopping mall, to deliver the eulogy. The night before, he had told us about the book he was writing, about how the Bible got Jesus all wrong. Then he asked us if there was anything we particularly wanted him to say at the service. With the limited truths of the obituary in mind, I asked him to be sure to mention Tony if he was going to mention us kids. After all, Tony had been my dad's central relationship during the last five years of his life. But Jack said there was no real reason to mention any of us, so the matter was dropped.

Pulling into the mortuary parking lot, we saw one of my father's brothers on his way in. It had been nearly twenty years since I had least seen him. His face looked like something that had been broken to pieces, then glued back together wrong. He greeted us sheepishly, as well he might. Inside was my other uncle, a high school coach with tattooed arms. I wondered what they knew. The rest were old family friends or professional friends, many of whom I barely remembered. Tony sat near the front with his parents, who had flown in from the midwest. A few gay friends were sprinkled through the audience.

After a nod to the spiritual realm, Jack began to reminisce about the old days, the fifties and early sixties. Unfortunately, the gauze of the years had intervened. In his version, my father, a career atheist, became "a religious leader of his community" with whom Jack, during his years as a minister, "spent hundreds of hours discussing religious philosophy." ("God schmod," my sister whispered in my ear.) He had also, Jack went on, been a dedicated husband, and the loving father of three wonderful children. And he named us, one by one.

"When Tom and Marti arrived in Long Beach in the early 1950's," began the next speaker, an attorney whose family's history was intertwined with ours, "they were simply the brightest and handsomest couple we had met." He then gave a decidedly more profane version of those years: parties to rival those of Zelda and Scott Fitzgerald; squalling babies and house payments, intellectual discussions late into the night. He praised my father for his mordant sense of humor, and for a compassion not normally associated with lawyers.

It was all very moving. Still, taken together, the effect was to throw us into a peculiar time warp. It was as if the past twenty years hadn't happened—twenty years that had transformed my family No mention was made of what may have been the central fact of my father's existence, the two selves around which his life had revolved since youth. No mention was made of the cause of death, though most of those present must have known. Maybe this too was part of the etiquette of funerals. Still, it was strange being wafted back to that earlier time. From that perspective, my mother became his bereaved widow, though they'd been divorced for years. We three kids became his orphans. Tony was erased.

Midway through an account of a wild midnight swim in the fifties, there was a small electronic beep. I looked over and saw Tony reach down to switch off his watch alarm. I remembered the watch had belonged to my father. It had been set to tell him when to take his medications.

Last to speak was my father's law partner of forty years, who had to cut short a ski trip to Sun Valley. He talked as best he could of what those years had meant to him. But mostly he took deep breaths and fought back tears. This is my sharpest memory of that day: a man I'd never felt especially comfortable with, who had always seemed a little cold, standing up there with his handkerchief, tears dripping from his walrus mustache.

A few days later, my wife and I flew back to Athens. Tucked away in a suitcase was a plastic bag full of ashes—the ones my sister had pocketed that day on the ocean. I had convinced her to let me take them with me and scatter them in the Aegean, in memory of the trip he and I had been planning before he got sick. Fistful by fistful, she had poured them back into the bag.

They sat in a drawer in our Athens apartment until the following summer. It was strange coming upon them while I rummaged around for something else. In the ten months since he died, I'd barely been able to spare my father a thought. Once or twice I took out the bag and pondered the ashes with the same uneasiness I'd felt that day on the sailboat. I'd heard somewhere they have to grind down the bones.

A week before I returned to the States (my wife was already back), I borrowed a friend's motorbike and sleeping bag, and grabbed a ferryboat for the islands. I picked Milos as one of the farthest from the polluted seas around Athens. I would spend the night on the beach and devote the next day to thinking and writing about my father.

Mid-August is the peak tourist season in the Cyclades. Milos was mobbed, but I staked out a spot on the sandy bay south of the harbor and unloaded my things.

That night, I went to a noisy celebration of the Dormition of the Virgin, a major holiday. I sat on a ledge in the church courtyard and watched people mill around. A fiddler and mandolinist ran through their repertoire of island songs, while locals danced in a cramped circle nearby: generations of them, little girls and their grandfathers, middle-aged brothers and sisters, a great-grandmother or two. People wandered in and out of the church, where the Virgin's ornate bier was on display: lavishly decked with flowers.

I spent the next day on the beach by myself. That evening en route to the harbor to catch the last boat, I stopped at a roadside chapel and lit a candle. It was a habit I'd picked up from my wife, a lapsed Catholic who'd reverted to this custom. The small, simple chapel was dedicated to "St. Alexios, man of God"—someone I'd never heard of. His large icon stood before the sanctuary, its gold leaf gleaming in the light of the oil-candles. He wore a rough animal skin and leaned on a staff, like John the Baptist. His free hand held an unfurled scroll that read, in Byzantine script, "Stammering tongues shall utter peace."

Before leaving Greece, I sent a postcard to my sister:

> I scattered the ashes from aboard the F/B Salamina on its overnight run from Milos to Athens. Not much to it—my main concern was how not to hit people in the face who

were standing farther back in the boat. Given Dad's doubts about the afterlife, it seemed right to be doing it at night: all that blackness churning past. Back in Athens, the streets were wet. It'd rained, unheard of for August. I rode the motorbike into town, at dawn. Over Mt. Pendelis, the clouds were starting to break up....

I haven't heard from her since.

T.W. McKinsey (1920-1990)

WHEN MY FRIEND DIED
OF AIDS

MARGARET MCMULLAN

My friend Ken died of AIDS on a lovely sunny morning three years ago. I wasn't there. Before he was unable to talk, he told me he didn't want me to come. He worried about what I might think of his living conditions. He worried that he might lose control of his kidneys while I was in the room. He wanted me to remember him as he was.

Now I think we both made a mistake.

In college in Grinnell, Iowa, I didn't go anywhere without Ken. We stood in lines together, ate and gossiped together, danced together. He never told me he was gay. He didn't have to. He was a tall, lanky, handsome Black man who didn't date women. And he never spoke of his personal life. He thought it was in bad taste. I can remember once, when we blew off French class to watch Erica give birth on *All My Children*, Ken told me he wanted to get married sooner or later. He wanted children of his own.

That was the year he started seeing more of Randy and less of me. They went out until Randy dumped him for another man and left to join the Navy. I knew Ken was devastated but he never talked about it.

AIDS wasn't even an issue the year Ken and I graduated from college. It never would have occurred to me to tell Ken to be careful when he called to say he had just landed a job as a steward. He was happy and excited. He had never been to Europe before, and the airline was sending him on a non-stop to Germany.

Six years went by, and I didn't see Ken until our college reunion. I had moved to Fayetteville, Arkansas, where I was teaching English at the university. Ken was living in Newark, working as a paralegal. He looked good then. His hair was shorter and he was more muscular. We were among the few who had neither spouse nor pictures of babies to show. We went to the pub. I told him about all the trouble I'd been having with my current boyfriend. He said I had always been too hard on people. After a while, I, too, was blunt. I told him I was worried about him, what with AIDS and all. I was relieved when he didn't get mad. He told me about what he knew and what he read. He told me about Jamie, a man he was seeing, on and off. He told me he was scared.

We danced to Devo and the Stones until two o'clock in the morning. I was the one to give out first. When we left, we swore we would stay in better touch. That was in June. At Christmas we sent each other cards.

It was Jamie who called me from a pay phone in the early spring. He said he had heard a lot about me. He also said that Ken had tested positive for AIDS and already he had lost a lot of weight. The telltale Kaposi sarcoma blotches were beginning to show on his skin. Ken had just quit his job, and Jamie said Ken didn't want anybody to know.

After the first jolt of fear, I felt, I admit, hurt. Ken hadn't made much of an effort in the past to keep our friendship alive, and now, here I was talking with his boyfriend, a man I had never even met.

"What do you want me to do?" I asked.

Jamie paused and I imagined him looking out of the phone booth. Maybe he could see Ken's apartment up the street.

"If he knew I was calling you, he'd kill me," Jamie said. "You know Ken, Mr. Proud. Just call him. Write to him. Let him know you're there."

When I called Ken that afternoon, it took a long time for him to answer. He had dozed off during *Star Trek*, he said. I could hear the TV on in the background. He was surprised to hear from me. "Your social life must be really crummy," he said.

We gossiped about an ex-boyfriend of mine whom I had seen over Easter. Ken remembered him from college.

"He's turned into everything a person hates about the eighties," I said. "Me, me, me. Selfish city. He didn't even say I looked good. All he said was, 'Gee, I never knew your arms were that skinny.'"

"He was always like that," Ken said. "I mean, you could be out there dying and he'd forget to write."

I started sending Ken cards every week then, and poems written by my neighbor's children. One was called, "How to Stop Being Scared to Death." "Get your Mom to read you a story," little Angie Jones wrote. "Turn on a hall light."

"What's gotten into you?" he said when I called again near the end of April.

"You could be writing back, you know," I said.

"I suppose," he said. "But then I'd have to keep on. It's damn difficult corresponding with someone who writes back all the time."

He had been making a sweet potato pie since noon, he said. It was two o'clock. He would peel a potato and then he would have to rest. He needed the calories, he said. He'd been meaning to put on a little weight. Jamie had mentioned that Ken had already discussed funeral arrangements, and it hurt that Ken couldn't be that honest with me. He still needed to pretend, so I pretended back. I spoke to him as though he had the flu.

"Make yourself a toddy," I said. "Read *People.*"

As the weather turned warmer, Ken complained of being cold all the time. We would make bad jokes about all the places he wanted to visit. Venezuela. Mexico. He wanted to be near the ocean but there were either revolutions there or devil worship. "I don't want to be sacrificed," he said, and he laughed so hard he coughed.

"Visit me," I said. "We don't have an ocean, but we've got lakes." He ignored me.

"I've always wanted to move to Virginia," he said. "You know, buy a house of my own. With a garden. Maybe I will in two years. Richmond would be nice."

Ken and I became friends again while he was dying. He asked what I was doing, whom I was seeing. He told me about his travels. He talked about Jamie. And, inevitably, we would reminisce about college. On the phone, he wasn't self-conscious since I couldn't see the way he looked, or how much hair was already gone. By this time I was in touch with Ken's mother about his deteriorating condition, but with Ken I still pretended he had the flu.

On Memorial Day, Ken called me from St. Michael's Hospital. He had had a seizure the night before. Luckily his mother and his sister had been there with him, watching a movie on the VCR. He couldn't remember anything. What really bothered him, he said, was that I wouldn't know where to reach him. He wanted me to know where he was.

I called every day after that, in the evening around seven because, he said, that was the calm time of the day when everyone left him alone. I wondered how long Ken would go on pretending. Finally on a Sunday, when his mother left the room to pray in the hospital chapel, Ken told me.

"I have the AIDS virus lurking," he said.

"Lurking?" I said.

He laughed. "Yeah."

I said I was sorry. I asked him what he wanted to do.

"The doctor says I can go back to work. That I should."

"What do you want to do?"

"Sleep."

"So sleep."

"Yeah."

"Do you want me to come?"

He laughed. "Margaret," he said "I'm not terminal. Not yet."

That was the last time Ken spoke of having AIDS, but it wasn't the last time he told me not to come. He made it clear: he didn't want visitors. "It just kills me to see those people walking through that door—and the look on their faces when they see how thin I've gotten," he told me once.

I baked him cookies. Fattening ones.

The phone calls were difficult because I was never sure if there would be another one after I hung up. Ken would have to force me to say good-bye.

"Okay," I would say. "I'll talk to you again. Tomorrow."

"Okay."

"Okay."

"Okay, Margaret. Get off the phone."

We were running out of things to talk about. Everything I told him about my life seemed extraneous. So he spoke of his ailments, his doctor whom his sister had a crush on, and George, a hospital room-mate who didn't want to go home.

"Can you believe that?" Ken said the night George left. "He didn't want to leave because he'd paid for his TV till Sunday."

Ken wanted desperately to go home, but his doctor said he would need a full-time nurse and neither he nor his family could afford one.

Than late one night, Ken called me. He sounded drugged, his voice soft and dreamy.

"I wanted to tell you something," he said. "Now I forget."

After that night, Ken started having trouble speaking. The words were there, he said, but he couldn't get them out clearly. When a nurse gave him a form to sign, he couldn't remember how to spell his last name. He couldn't eat without throwing up. His kidneys were failing and he had diarrhea. He kept asking me the time, the day of the week, the month. He hadn't been outside since April and already it was June.

I made him a video. Since you won't come here, I said on it, I'll bring me and my life to you. Just press stop when you get bored. I showed him my apartment, my garden, my friends. It was summer solstice, the longest day of the year, and we filmed ourselves telling ghost stories around a bonfire in my neighbor's backyard. We wrote out wishes on scraps of paper and burned them so that they would come true.

I told Ken that one of those wishes had to do with him.

Ken was too weak to watch the video.

I called him on his birthday. His sister answered the phone.

"Ken? Kenny, it's me," I said.

I could hear him whisper something. Then I heard him take a deep breath, and with all the strength he had, he screamed out my name like a question, like an incomprehensible question.

Ken only lived to be thirty for a week.

Sometimes, when I'm lying awake late at night, I think about how it might have been if Ken had let me come see him. We would have stayed up past visiting hours, sipping the wine I sneaked past the nurse we'd have nicknamed Tank. We would have joked and laughed till our eyes watered. Then, maybe, Ken would have remembered what he wanted to tell me the night he called.

When word finally got out about Ken's illness, all his friends wanted to see him for one last visit. And, despite his request for no visitors, a college friend from New Jersey did get to him. She called me to say how much better she felt.

"I fed him a banana," she said. "And when I combed his hair he opened his eyes."

I imagined her with Ken. I assume he had been too weak to refuse her attentions, but I also know that he must have welcomed them. Anybody would. And even though I suspected she made the visit more for herself than for Ken, I was jealous. She had the chance to touch him again. She had the chance to say good-bye.

I tried to remind myself that Ken hadn't wanted me to see him, but if there are any lessons to be learned from this, I know now that when a friend dies, you're only left with what you did for him and what you think you should have done.

For Ken Johnston
July 9, 1959–July 16, 1989

REMEMBERING JAY

DOROTHY MERTON

This spring my godson died of AIDS. I loved him as I love my own sons. My own sons will not die of AIDS. But I want them to remember Jay for the reasons I loved him and mourn him like a mother.

In a sense, I was his mother for seventeen years, and my husband was his father. For seventeen years we knew that he was gay, while his own parents did not know. We welcomed him, listened to him, shielded him, and sometimes entered into deceptions that kept his life in the city a secret in his hometown. And yes, we did warn him. At the end, he came for a visit home to his mother, who had been widowed less than a year. He died in her arms that weekend, of pneumocystis carinii pneumonia. She had known what his illness was for several months, even before his father's death. The nurses told me that she threw herself across his body, screaming, "You come back here! You can't do this to me!"

Now the shame of her secret weighs on her like her grief. Jay had finally told her what we alone knew, that he suffered from Kaposi's Sarcoma. He never told her that we had known of his gay life since 1970. She telephones me often at night to grieve and be reassured of our friendship. "This is our secret," she says hopefully. But it really isn't. Though staff at the hospital and the mortuary have kept professional confidence, people who knew him since his student days at the local high school and college could see the truth through the heavy makeup he taught himself to apply over his facial lesions. Faculty members who have spoken to me have all been compassionate. They know the real loss to the very world they value.

"He was, he was a good boy," his mother says, with defiant sorrow. And he was. "Caring" is a word I've grown to despise as a catchall for anybody showing the least human concern. All ten speakers at his memorial service in his cathedral used it. I'd rather tell just how much Jay cared for people right to the end.

He was taken to the hospital fighting to breathe, just twenty-four hours after flying home, with a load of gifts for his mother. In emergency, he immediately told staff he had AIDS. "He didn't have to tell them," Laurie his nurse says to me. "He was so considerate, letting us know. That was the kind of person he was." She smiles. "I shook all over when they told me what he had. I thought, I can't go in there! He was covered with sweat. I had to say to myself, 'This isn't how you get it, Laurie,' Then I was able to touch him. I think he wanted to be touched."

Out of his mother's hearing, Laurie remembers, "We asked him if he wanted to be put on a respirator, and he said No. His PCO$_2$ level, which indicates his breathing capacity, was forty-one. Ordinarily, when the level is fifty-five, we put a person on a respirator." She thinks he may have known how very bad off he was. But at 11:00 p.m., three hours before he died, he rang for assistance to get up to go to the bathroom. "I think he was trying to protect us, by not using a bedpan." Just before 2:00 a.m., Laurie checked and could hear him breathing. His mother's arm was around him, from the chair where she had fallen asleep. Ten minutes later, Laurie found him making no sound. His mother's rage she understands. "You walk a mile in that lady's shoes," she says. Her voice is firm. "After Jay, now I'll never be afraid of it again."

I had held him and kissed him and said goodbye at five o'clock. We had been given tickets to dinner theater; I didn't return. I didn't believe he was dying. He was rational, his executive self. "I just cannot comprehend the complete reversal of my condition," he said irritably, his exact words. For a year he had been taking AZT, with no severe side effects. He had followed the medical course of his illness with interest. It offended his sense of orderliness and organization, but he dealt with it practically.

As I sat with him while his mother ate in the cafeteria, he groaned twice, softly. "Excuse me if I groan." He turned his head to me. "I just feel I have to groan every few minutes." Restlessly he kicked away his sheet. I saw his feet. The cruelty to his feet, he who loved to run and to walk and to dance: gauze-wrapped, open sores, swollen, black with the lesions. I kissed his feet. The athletic legs were shrunken bone-thin. His trim body heaved for the air that would not come. "Mother will give you the gift I brought you," he whispered.

He showered me with gifts. My magnificent *Illustrated Gospels* is from him. My life subscription to *Bird Watcher's Digest* is from him. There were icons, jewelry, books, imported delicacies from the city like Brazil coffee and Russian tea, imported cigars for my husband, a continual flow of letters, cards (always for Mother's Day), remembrances.

What other gifts? "His listening voice," to use his mother's words. For the office his voice was crisp and commanding, though even there he listened well. For those he loved, the voice was always an invitation to tell him more. There was so much I had saved to tell him that very weekend, that now I cannot. For him I saved my dreams of something larger than the life I live here. He listened. He eased the problems that came in my own marriage and with my own sons.

He loved life. He took his greatest joy in the beauties of nature and art. Artists, writers and dancers came to his services and wrote loving letters to his mother. He loved his work. He had talents for fund-raising. On the job he was rewarded handsomely, but he gave the money freely also to his church. He loved his church with a special devotion to the Mother of God. He was altar server, choir member, youth leader, parochial school trustee, and the chair of years of dinners, conferences, and committees. His faith kept him buoyant. In midwinter as we walked together before his death, he said joyously, "I feel an invincible summer within me." It was the summer sun of his belief in goodness.

There was nothing unnatural about his love. Not for me, not for all the others of whom I was sometimes jealous, because he poured out his gifts for them just as unstintingly. Was his love for Devin unnatural? If it was, I conspired in that, too. His last Christmas before he died, they came to spend the week at his mother's house. I arranged for a service of covenanting between them to be read at my son's home. I asked my son to agree to it for my peace of mind. My son is a licensed lay minister and officiated, while we sat around the dining table: my husband and I, Jay and Devin, and my son's wife. The two of them read together the Baptismal Covenant from the Book of Common Prayer. We used the proper readings for the calendar day, and my son chose some prayers. There was no blessing, no absolution, nothing forbidden. I had my son enter it in the Register of Church Services at our church, as a service of "private Evening Prayer." It is written there for those of us who sat around that table to remember Jay. It gave me, it still gives me, peace of mind.

They lived together over seven years. At the wake, I sat with Devin, alone in the row of chairs furthest back. He huddled in an overcoat he would not take off, staring dry-eyed at the mourners. "I can't be a part of all this," he said dully, though Jay's faith was his own. Without caring one way or another, I wonder if my neighbors speculated about the two of us. He telephones Jay's mother often. She was the one who had to phone him with the news. He writes to me. From a letter of late spring: "I am beginning to climb out of my depression, thanks to my many friends here and the project for adding a third floor onto our house here at Castro Street.... Some things are beginning to come together. I started to do some volunteer work, working for a group called 'Pennies from Heaven.' They collect pennies in jars which are left in stores and bars throughout the city.... The money goes into a fund, and anyone (children, women, as well as men, after being diagnosed with AIDS) simply has to apply and will receive $1,000 for emergencies, or just to catch up because of all the initial outlay of money it takes to get the medicine for AIDS patients."

Wholeheartedly, Jay would have approved. He was an activist, and an advocate. He intended to give his last months, after he could no longer work, wholly to volunteer his management expertise at AIDS centers. But he died just after he had resigned from his position.

Again and again, in my tortured memory, I go with him up to the moment of his final breath; and then I am turned back, and he has gone. I want to talk about him. I want to tell him more, all that I had saved for us together that spring. I can talk to him now only in prayers.

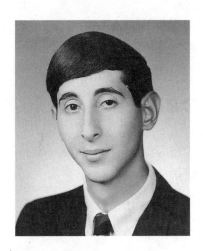

For Jay, this spring and always
June 1, 1950–Feb. 27, 1989

No More Poems For The Dead

Victor Mingovits

no more poems for the dead
no more poems for the dying
no more poems for the brothers
who died too young
to ever use Grecian Formula
restores lost color to grey hair
down cosmetics aisle past
the styling mousse

no more poems for the dead
no more poems for the dying
no more poems for the friends
whose laughter instead has grown grey
& smiles forced through I.V. tubes
cramp through veins
bring little more than grimace
to ashen lips
no more poems for the dead
no more poems for the dying
no more poems for the husbands of men
conducting symphonies of alliteration
bing & beep of hospital emergency

as all visitor faces collage with dementia
and recede

no more poems for the dead
no more poems for the dying
no more poems for the living who endure
our eyes desiccated by grief
tears begin to flow from fingertips,
spine,
throat
o, this desert of the soul,
mirage of echoes and hope
our own dementia
until the promised hum of the EKG
when the dead become our poems
written in misshapen ovals around each cell
in fingertip, spine and throat
and we can finally rejoice in the sound of
no more poems

for Janet, Jay, Jim

Years of Memories Gone in Minutes

Beverly Mire

I watched one of my friends die last Wednesday. When we met five years ago, Eric had just been diagnosed with Kaposi's Sarcoma. Within a year his skin was covered with reddish-purple stains. Within two years, cancer had begun to rot his insides.

When we met five years ago, Eric was a muscular guy who rode his bicycle up and down the hills of San Francisco. When he died, his legs were so swollen with edema he could hardly walk.

Eric's lover Joseph and I have been friends for over ten years. We were once part of a sixsome who couldn't breathe without calling each other, and although the makeup of our group changed, four of us are still tight and Joseph and I have seen each other through births, deaths, broken hearts, a year-and-a-half-long three-thousand mile separation, and the frustration of seeing the Forty Niners blow a chance to go to the Super Bowl for the third year in a row.

Now we have seen Eric die.

For about a month before he died, Eric talked about taking an overdose of morphine, but vacillated between wanting to and not wanting to. One day he'd think he felt better and didn't want to die. Another day, wearing diapers because he'd lost control of his bowels depressed him so, he wanted to die the next day. His indecision took such a toll on Joseph's emotions that Joseph finally took the two of them to a therapist and with her help told him either to do it or not, but to stop playing with his emotions.

Shortly after that session, Eric was mugged as he struggled home after doing errands on Castro Street. He couldn't run, but he could scream a wild scream—he hadn't lost his lungs—so the thief ran away without getting anything, no wallet, no jewelry, no nothing. The thief didn't steal anything tangible, but he did steal Eric's will to live. Shortly after, he set the date.

Eric had a vain kind of strength that wouldn't let him believe he was any less than perfect. Because he refused to let on that his immune system was breaking down, that he was sick, that he was incurable, I for one was able to live in denial. Even when he finally began to complain that he wasn't feeling well, when I'd stop in he'd be in the garden, down on his knees, separating red and purple cosmos to give to his friends. It didn't register for me that he was going to die.

On a late August afternoon my denial was shattered when Joseph followed me down to my car after a visit and told me Eric had decided on a date. He planned on calling me at work next Wednesday, he said, and say it was an emergency. I almost asked him to change from Wednesday to Thursday since Wednesday is my busiest day at work.

Joseph swore me to secrecy. Obviously, by law, the doctor could get into trouble for teaching Joseph how to administer a lethal dose of drugs. And of course Joseph, who it would turn out only had five months to live, could get into trouble, too.

Whether or not I could get into trouble didn't seem to be an issue, and I didn't even consider it a possibility.

Wednesday turned out to be a beautiful day to die. The sun was shining, the air was as snappy-fresh as ginger ale and there wasn't even a stray finger of fog coming over Twin Peaks. By 9:30 a.m. I was standing in a coworker's office explaining that a friend was dying and I had to leave. He looked up, asked if my crucial work was done, barely heard me say yes and put his head back into his computer.

The first thing Joseph said when I got to his apartment was how nice I looked. Eric was taking his time about signing a codicil to his will, and Joseph was getting antsy. "We're late getting started," he said, almost impatiently. The plan was to have Eric die by early afternoon. "We'll have plenty of time to take care of everything else, and then I'll take you to Zuni Cafe for dinner," Joseph said to me. Eric didn't ask what I would order.

The document signed, Eric got up from where he was sitting on the couch and waddled through the kitchen and into the bedroom. As he slid into his newly-made, fresh-sheeted bed, I went over to a comfortable chair in the corner and let it wrap its arms around me. Joseph had stopped in the kitchen and was making scrambled eggs and toast so Eric wouldn't die on an empty stomach. And he would keep the morphine down.

While eating his scrambled eggs, done slightly moist just the way he liked them, Eric told me he decided to die wearing a Sand's Casino t-shirt because in the fifties his mother was a dealer there. When Joseph took the tray away Eric lit up a cigarette as Joseph slid a needle into the shunt in his arm and pushed some buttons on the morphine machine. I noticed then that little conversation had passed between the two. Everything was focused on getting on with death: signing the will, filling the stomach, being sure Joseph really knew how to increase the dosage.

Joseph was sitting on the bed looking like a hospital visitor. By the time the cigarette was three-quarters gone, Eric was already nodding. Joseph slipped the still live butt out of Eric's hand—it was the first time I'd seen Joseph touch a cigarette, never mind let someone smoke in the house—mashed it out and increased the dosage. For a long minute the only thing we heard was the morphine machine half-humming, half-clicking in a low, mournful tone.

Eric looked like he was napping. His head leaned on his shoulder and every once in a while he'd make a face. A few minutes passed after the cigarette was out, and he snapped his head up and opened his eyes. I told him he frowned while he was out and he said that his mother used to call his frowns, "brussels sprouts faces." "It was the face I'd make when she made them for dinner," he said. "I called them little baby heads. I hated them. Now I love them."

Joseph leaned over to the morphine machine and without moving his head, Eric's eyes followed Joseph's actions. His eyes started to droop. A few minutes later his head leaned on his shoulder for what would turn out to be the last time. He told Joseph he wasn't wearing the ring Joseph had given him because he was afraid his hands would swell up and the mortician would have to cut the ring off. He nodded again and I said, "No brussels sprouts faces." He closed his eyes, gave me one, and went to sleep.

That was at about noon. Right in front of Joseph and me, Eric's body and spirit engaged in the ultimate boxing match. As he lay there we could see his face turn ashy white as the essence of Eric tried to fly away. One foot was outside the covers. I looked at the skin on his legs. It was gray and rough like an elephant's. The part below his ankles looked like your skin does when you walk in wet sand on the beach and then the sun dries it.

I looked at the purple lesions on his arms. I still didn't believe he was dying, but I was praying for his spirit to wrench itself free. Joseph increased the dosage, and the morphine machine started to hum with more energy.

Eric seemed to stop breathing and he started to gasp for air, making loud snoring sounds. He did that for five or ten seconds and then relaxed. Joseph moved closer to him and Eric's arms went limp. His hands were balled into loose fists and Joseph stuck his thumb down one of them and held the fist with both hands.

Time became space. I was losing track of where one ended and the other began. Joseph loosened his grip on Eric, got up and walked to the front of the apartment. Eric started gasping for breath, so I walked over to the bed, sat next to him and told him it was all right to die. He calmed down and I put my hand on his heart and felt it racing. It slowed down and then stopped for a few seconds. Then Eric began reaching for breath again, half snoring, half snorting, and his heart, jump-started, began pounding. As I held my hand over Eric's heart, I could feel the blood flowing through his veins like the last sips of soda through your straw.

"Let it go," I thought. "Let it go." But Eric's body wouldn't go easy. He had been a salesman, and during a conversation we had a few days ago, he and I laughed about how he never gave up and how he turned no into yes. Now his body was saying no to death, but his spirit was screaming yes.

Mid-afternoon was passing. Joseph had thought for sure Eric would be dead by then. I was still sitting on the bed and Eric was still struggling while Joseph walked from the kitchen to the bedroom and back again. He was worried the morphine would run out.

Eric started snorting again. I asked his struggling body if he changed his mind, and said it was okay if he wanted to live. "No," Joseph said angrily. "Don't tell him that. Let him go. He'll be mad if he wakes up and is still here."

I got up, went out on the small back porch and sat in the sun for maybe half an hour. When I went back into the bedroom, Joseph rose, went into the kitchen and brought back a bottle of wine. He cracked it open and we both drank some. We sat and watched Eric struggle, then be calm, struggle, then be calm.

The doctor had said that if they started at ten o'clock Eric would be dead by two o'clock at the latest. At seven o'clock, Joseph, though he was holding it together, began to panic. The morphine was gone and there was no one he could call to ask what to do.

I walked into the living room, moved the towels Eric had spread across the couch so he wouldn't stain it when he sat there, lay down and dozed. I woke up not knowing where I was until I heard Joseph's slippers slapping across the kitchen floor. I sat up, he sat down next to me, leaned on my shoulder and said, "He's gone. Finally he's gone."

I got up and walked back to the bedroom, which was now flooded with unnatural light. The reading lamps attached to both sides of the bed were spotlighting Eric. I sat next to him. His eyes were closed and there was a tear in the corner of the left one. His mouth was agape, as if he were about to pull another breath. I put my hand on his arm, being careful not to touch a lesion. His skin was still warm.

A half hour later two nurses came to tell us Eric was dead. An hour after they left, two gentlemen from the Neptune Society drove up in a discreet white van. They put Eric into a plastic bag, strapped him to a stretcher and deftly maneuvered his body down the stairs and drove away. I was careful not to look at Eric's body as they carried it by the small mirror in the living room. I once read in a Russian novel that if you see a dead person in a mirror it's bad luck.

In between phone calls, Joseph and I asked each other how we were. Fine, we said. After he spoke to Eric's sister, who was Eric's only surviving immediate family member and his best friend, Joseph called his own sister-in-law in Ventura who told him she, Sam and the two children would be down next week. Then Joseph pulled out the futon in his front room for me to sleep on and he changed the sheets and went to sleep in the bed his lover died in three hours before.

The next morning was bright and glorious. The sun streamed in the front room and Joseph and I stood gazing across San Francisco, assuring each other we were okay; I drank a cup of strong coffee and got ready for work. Just before I left, Joseph hooked himself up to a funny little bulb that somehow sent a painkiller directly to his heart.

He assured me he wouldn't leave me for a few years. But, as with Eric, I don't believe Joseph will die.

To my favorite Forty Niners fan, with fond memories
June 26, 1955–Jan. 30, 1993

TO PLUTO'S HOUSE:
AN AIDS ODYSSEY

MICHAEL KIESOW MOORE

Accepting the possibility of death—honestly and completely—frees up a whole lot of energy to live.

—Keith Gann

When Keith asked me if I'd be interested in taking him to Iowa to see his family for Thanksgiving, neither one of us realized that we were planning a trip that would radically change the lives of many people, especially ours. For Keith this trip was about healing, healing the rifts between him and his family. It had been some years since he had seen his brothers and sisters and their children; his relationship with his father resembled that of two strangers; and at this time he was having a difficult conflict with his mother; she wanted him to move back home. She could not believe that these friends Keith talked about could take care of him the way she could.

For me, this trip symbolized the reason why I moved to Minnesota from Washington, D.C. I wanted to spend time with Keith, to participate in the very thick of his life. If I had stayed in Washington, Keith's life would have veered far from mine. He would become a specter the way many of my friends had in their last years: because they lived far away, it was often through second sources I heard how they were doing; how they were dying. I could not let that happen with Keith.

As we crossed the Iowa border, Keith's spirits began to sag. He was getting tired. The sun had gone down. It was that time of year when the days grow short but you still expect the sun to operate on its summer schedule. As we approached Ames, Iowa, Keith asked that we stay the night at a motel. Council Bluffs was too far.

After dinner Keith asked me to help him bathe. I thought all he needed me to do was run the water for him. After I got the water going, he instructed me to set towels at the end of the bed and to turn up the heat. Then he took his clothes off and asked me to help him into the tub. Because I had never seen him naked before, I was shocked by the sudden intimacy between us and the sight of his deteriorating body. I was aware that Keith had lost weight but it was only now that I clearly saw the devastation. I could see each rib jutting against his thin, white skin, skin that looked so delicate that these sharp bones would surely tear through. His legs and arms were spindly sticks. This was why Keith needed help into the tub. There was no more muscle in his arms. Without someone to help him out of the tub, he would be trapped by his own weakness. Not only were his legs rickety, but slightly bowed, turned in. It was a miracle that they could even hold him up.

The water turned lukewarm and Keith asked me to help him out. He put his soggy arms around my neck and I lifted him. I then walked him to the edge of the bed where he sat down. With him seated, I dried his shivering body. While rubbing his fragile limbs I realized for the first time that Keith really was going to die.

I remember the first time we met at a gay and lesbian Quaker conference in New York City...the first of many Quaker conferences I would attend. Keith is one of the more colorful characters there. He is a typical carrot top redhead, hair that blazes like Lucille Ball's. His skin is white and freckled, with texture like an albino's. And he uses his uncommon features like a canvas for a showy style: baggy pants, vivid, colorful shirts, dangling earrings and bejeweled brooches. One night, we and a few of our new friends barhop in the Village. We end up at The Monster which has a fabulous dance floor downstairs. And we dance. Keith and I storm the floor. Behind us a huge screen plays film clips of Fred Astaire and Ginger Rogers. The deejay throws the spotlight on us and the New Yorkers stand to the side and give us the floor. That night the spirit of Fred Astaire is alive and well in our dancing feet.

Keith and I slowly walked to his parents' house. For me it was a new place filled with new people. But for Keith, it was his history. Each step to the house was a step backward in time. This was where he played with his sisters. It was on this lawn his brothers chased him. On the porch swing he shucked corn and snapped beans. And behind the shut door, his father watched TV while his mother baked pies and cookies.

We opened the metal gate to the house and slowly walked forward. The front door opened.

"Hi, Ma!" Keith said.

A jumble of voices called out "Keith...Keith's here!" And then there was a hush. Keith leaned on my arms as I led him up a few steps to the screen-enclosed porch. Though Keith walked into his past, everyone else stood fully in the moment. The man whom they once knew as brother, son, had become somebody else. His appearance before them cried out the words, "Your life will no longer be the same." Keith moved in front of me, entering the house first.

I glanced at his mother. Her whole body was shaking with pent-up tears. Keith's sister, Sharon, looked directly into my eyes. Tears were flowing down her cheeks. She didn't want Keith to see that she was crying. We all walked into the dark living room where the TV was turned on to a football game. "Hi, Dad," Keith said.

"Uh...hello, Keith." His father got up and let Keith sit in his chair. Introductions were made and I briefly shook hands with everyone. I was motioned to sit in a chair next to Keith. Looking around the room I saw that beside the TV was a set of shelves. On all the shelves were pictures of the family, the children, the nieces and nephews, the grandchildren. I kept looking for a picture of Keith and at last found one. It was a recent photograph in a lavish porcelain frame on the very top shelf.

"So what's for dinner?" Keith asked.

"Oh, the usual, of course," his mother hastily said. "You know, turkey, dressing, potatoes and a couple pies."

"That sounds so nice, Mom. I'm hungry today for a change. I should be able to eat tonight."

The dinner was a huge production on a David O. Selznick scale. The dining room couldn't hold all the people, so the children ate in the living room, happy to get away from the grownups (AKA "the grumps") and to sit in front of the TV and watch *Bambi*. There were a number of people at the table whom I was never introduced to: Keith's brothers and brothers-in-law. Their conversations centered on sports and hunting. Unlike Keith's sisters, they neither asked who I was nor wanted to know.

The food was passed around. Turkey—carved by Mr. Gann at the head of the table—slices of steaming white and dark meat. Cranberry sauce. Mashed sweet potatoes, orange and buttery. Dressing and gravy. The adults chattered and the children were noisy. And throughout the dinner Keith smiled and kept saying, "This is so wonderful."

Keith and I are at a national Quaker conference being held in Northfield, Minnesota. We are walking along a dirt road. My mind is on the memorial service we had the other day for Jan Sutter, the first of the many gay Quakers our community lost. While attending his service, I missed John Willig's which was being held the same day in Washington. Mitch's memorial service was a couple of weeks ago—a religious service in New Jersey which he would have hated. And next week I will attend Randy Brown's service. It's getting to the point where we who go to these services say to each other, "See you next week," knowing that we are referring to the next ceremony for the dead.

Keith's voice breaks into my wandering mind. "I have AIDS Related Complex." I look at him, aghast. I don't know what to say. "I haven't told many people yet," he continues. "For now I'd appreciate it if you keep it between us."

The plates were cleared and the coffee was poured. We prepared ourselves for the last ritual: the carving of the pie. Keith started shivering. "I'm cold," he said. "I think I'd like to take a bath." Keith's mother showed me where the towels were and how to work all the strange knobs. This time, helping the naked Keith into the water wasn't so jarring. Something had changed since that bath in Ames. I knew how to do this. For the first time in caring for Keith I felt competent.

"The water's getting cold," Keith said, his teeth starting to chatter. I turned the hot water knob. Only cold water came out. "I'll be right back," I said. I went into the kitchen where Mrs. Gann and Keith's sisters were cleaning up and explained the problem to them.

"Well, I suppose we could get some hot water boiling, do you think that would work?" Mrs. Gann said. I thought it a great idea and went back to Keith to tell him what we were going to do. And in a few minutes we had the kettle brigade going. As each pot of water was ready, I took it into the bathroom and poured at the far end of the tub. After five large kettles of water, steam returned to the bathroom and Keith sighed with pleasure.

That night Keith slept in one of the beds and I slept on the floor in the living room. Mrs. Gann seemed disappointed that she didn't have enough beds. I assured her that I liked hard surfaces and the floor was just fine. After all the lights went out, I luxuriated in this break from that long, stress-filled day.

A few hours after I fell asleep, I heard my name being called. "Michael...can you come here?" I threw on a robe and came into the room. Keith's teeth were chattering. "I had night sweats again. The sheets are all wet."

Keith's mother heard our voices and came into the room. As I pulled the sheets off the bed, I explained what was happening. "Oh, I'll get some more sheets," she said and set to work remaking the bed. I led Keith to the bathroom for another of our routine baths.

The time changes to January. A chilly time of the year, though not much snow. The chill comes mostly from the omnipresent dampness that seeps through clothes, skin, even the city's ubiquitous marble. I get the call at work. "I'm in the hospital. Pneumocystis." I am in a fog of disbelief. It can't be happening, I think. Not to Keith.

I mention the phone call to my coworker, Ed. He is clearly shaken, but he says little. Something inside me says, "Him, too." I leave work and go for a walk. When I come back I tell my boss that I am moving to Minnesota.

As I make my preparations for the move, Ed continues acting uneasy. He never tells me what's going on. Feeling his desire to keep himself private, a privacy that he perhaps wants broken, I never ask. A few years later I learn that both he and his partner, Tim, died of AIDS.

My memory of the next thirty hours becomes dim. From that moment on—Keith's waking in the middle of the night—there was constant motion. It was like Keith was the calm center of a hurricane and we were all the intense winds that swirled around him, full of flurry and action. By the next day, Keith's mother and sisters realized that taking care of Keith was more than I could handle by myself. Soon they too were helping with Keith's frequent baths, getting him his glasses of water, pulling out blankets and turning up the thermostat.

His night sweats came on like clockwork and so before going to bed we decided who would have the night shift.

In the midst of all this chaos, Keith's one big dream happened. There were many times when, after talking to Keith's mother in the kitchen over coffee, I would come into the living room to see Keith and his father in deep conversation. I never knew what they talked about, but in the coming months Keith often told me how his dream came true: he had reconnected with his father. The language they now spoke with each other was love.

That same evening, while we were eating the Thanksgiving remains, something strange started to happen. "While I was at the Democratic convention..." he started to say. Then he stopped. He looked into the distance, his eyes slightly glazed. "Uh...what was I saying? I don't remember."

"The Democratic convention," someone prompted.

"Oh yeah. The Democratic convention. I...I..." His eyes again went blank and he stared for a while. "I don't remember. Oh well." He laughed nervously. For the rest of the dinner, he said little, often staring across the table blankly.

After dinner we set him up in the living room covered with a blanket. "Would you like some tea?" his mother asked. "Or maybe some water?"

"Um...let me think a minute." He paused, concentrating deeply, his eyebrows furrowed. "I don't know what I want. Uh...what do you think?"

"Well, I don't know," Dorothy said. "I just want to get you whatever you'd like. What do you want?"

"I don't know. I don't know!" Keith started breathing harder. "Oh, just bring me some water," he said angrily. We all exchanged glances.

"I'm so scared," Keith continued. "I don't understand what's happening to me." He started to cry.

Everyone looked at me. "What should we do?" Dorothy asked. I wanted to yell that I didn't know, that I was tired of having all the answers. "Is there a hospital in Council Bluffs?" I asked.

"Yeah..." Dorothy slowly drawled, "there is ..." She looked at Keith. "I don't suppose they've dealt much with AIDS?"

"Oh no...I doubt if they have ever had anyone there with AIDS."

"I really think Keith needs to go to a hospital, but it doesn't sound like the one here would know what to do."

"No...they probably wouldn't. What should we do?"

I thought really hard and then remembered that I had the phone number of Keith's doctor in my wallet. I told everyone and said I'd call him. We all glanced again at Keith. He was still looking around blankly, his eyes reflecting only a void.

I made the call and had the doctor paged. Once he was on the line I explained what was happening. He agreed with our assessment that Keith should be treated in Minneapolis and he told me to get Keith there as soon as possible.

I went back and told everyone. We now had a plan of action and we all felt some relief.

Our last hour was filled with a final flurry of activity as we prepared for the trip and said our farewells. Once we finished packing and getting Keith dressed, Dorothy gave me a hug and Tom shook my hand. "Thanks for all you've done. I don't know what we would've done without you," Dorothy said.

"Take care. Please call us when you get home," Tom said. He was never one with many words, but it was clear that a lot of emotion bubbled between his words.

I'm Keith Gann from St. Paul, Minnesota. I am a person with AIDS. I rise to speak in support of the Majority plank on the HIV-AIDS epidemic. I am outraged at the immorality of a President who sat idly by, refusing to say the word AIDS publicly for six years while thousands of my brothers and sisters got sick and died...

I am frustrated with those who call me a victim, stripping me of both my personal and political power. I am not a victim. I cannot think of myself as a victim and survive. I am a person with AIDS. I am your brother, son, neighbor, friend, lover. I ask each of you to personally take responsibility for eliminating the word "victim" from your discussion of AIDS...

I want you to know that AIDS is a life-threatening illness, but is not one-hundred percent fatal. There are already many long-term survivors. This is not denial—this is hope. Please join with me in remembering those who have died and loving those who are living. Together we can stop AIDS and live well and live long. Please support this Platform. Thank you.

—Keith Gann, speaking at the 1988 National Democratic Convention

After a long journey, I got Keith to the hospital. But once he met with his doctor, he demanded to be taken home. And so I brought him home. As I got Keith ready for bed, I left him for a moment and made a phone call. It was now one o'clock in the morning. The ordeal at the hospital had lasted over six hours. Our mutual friend John Yoakam answered the phone. I explained that I needed a break and hoped he could spend the night with Keith. He hesitated. I had awakened him and he had guests visiting, but he also heard the urgency in my voice. Not comprehending the long travail encapsulated by my tone, he said he'd come over.

I returned to Keith and gave him some water so he could take his sleeping pill. He swallowed the pill and his eyes suddenly rolled back. He fell back onto the bed and his arms and legs started to flail about.

"Keith!" I kept yelling. I ran to the phone and dialed 911. I yelled something about a seizure and hung up. When I ran back to his room he was lying lifeless. He looked like he was dead. At that moment something inside snapped. Until now I had been the one with the answers. Since that bath in Ames, I had kept my emotions in check and put myself into automatic drive. But now I lost it.

I started crying loudly, my whole body shaking with sobs. Though I tried yelling Keith's name, all that came out was an unintelligible roar. I could no longer speak words. I ran around the apartment. Into his room where his lifeless body lay, into the living room, into the kitchen, back into his bedroom, sobbing and crying out sounds that were not words. It was like my body and everything that went with it—my mind, my conceptions of the world, the boundaries of real and dream—all had been ripped off. I had suddenly plunged into a state of being that was purely insane. I was now at my journey's final destination: the house of Pluto where only madness ruled.

The phone rang. It was someone from 911. "You hung up on us. Please tell us what's going on." I answered with a sob. "Take a deep breath," this person said, "and calmly tell us what's happening." Somehow, the fact that they called back when I didn't give a phone number helped me return to my body. I said he had a seizure. Once it was ascertained that he was no longer in danger of harming himself, I was told to see if he was breathing.

Slowly I returned to his room, afraid to discover the truth. The only way I could do it was because I knew there was someone at the other end of the phone. I stood over Keith. He was so still. I looked at his chest. Yes. He was breathing. He wasn't dead.

I returned to the phone. "Okay...we'll send some paramedics. Stay by him to make sure he doesn't hurt himself."

And so I sat by Keith, watching him breathe. He now seemed at rest, as if he were sleeping. Once the paramedics arrived, I called Keith's doctor again. As I explained what was going on, one of the paramedics came out. "He's regained consciousness." As I went to Keith's room, John Yoakam walked through the open door.

"Who are all these people?" Keith asked me.

I told him that he had a seizure and these paramedics wanted to take him to the hospital. "But I don't want to go to the hospital. I want to stay here. I won't go to the hospital."

The paramedics left after I signed a form that Keith refused to be taken to the hospital. Once gone, I returned to Keith's room. John was getting Keith's coat on. Somehow he had magically done what no one had been able to do. He had talked Keith into getting admitted.

We got him to the hospital. After yet another wait, he was finally wheeled to a room. I went to the end of the hall and lay down on a sofa. John wanted to stay with Keith until he fell asleep. And so, by 3:00 a.m. I finally closed my eyes with a quiet sigh.

This account has been written after a distance of four years. Since Keith's passing in 1990, I have lost many more friends and lovers. It seems like every time I get a break from the storms, a new loved one tells me that he has AIDS. Friends ask me how I bear such loss. My answers vary. One is that I am an emotional catastrophe, full of pent-up emotions; I veer in and out of depression. But in moments of calm, my answer is that I survive by telling the story. I have learned that in the course of any person's life, one of the most powerful things they can ever do in life is to tell their story.

As I look back at this story, I see that my greatest challenge right now is keeping the lessons that Keith gave me in my present moment of living. It is too easy for me to get swept away by the flow of the everyday: paying bills, doing laundry, trudging through snow and minus-twenty-degree temperatures. But Keith's teachings are some of the most profound lessons one could ever come by, teachings that should not be forgotten.

One of Keith's teachings was the meaning of compassion. Compassion doesn't simply mean that you give people whatever they want. Sometimes compassion means being firm and unyielding. Keith also taught me that you shouldn't give up on people. Sometimes all people need for transformation is a loving hand extended to them. Keith also showed me how ephemeral life is, that we do not stay in this plane for very long. While here, we must live with diligence. And Keith also taught me that I am both strong and weak, which is all a part of being human. In the course of caring for Keith, I met myself.

Keith spends the last days of his life at Grace House, a hospice for people with AIDS run by a friar named Brother Paul. One night, around two o'clock in the morning Keith calls out and I come into the room. He looks at me strangely and then says he was just talking about me. Keith explained that he had asked if I could come too, but "the guy at the top shook his head."

Another morning I walk into the room and Keith's eyes get real big and he says, "Who is that with you?" I look to my side and don't see anyone. "That's the most beautiful person I've ever seen."

On the last day of his life, five of us stand around his bed: me, Brother Paul, Dorothy, and his sisters Sharon and Bobbie. We take turns holding his hand. We all know that this is it. And so does Keith. He is awake and cognizant, the most aware he has been in weeks. But he can't talk. He can only mouth words. At first I don't know what he is saying. And then it is obvious. "I love you...I love you...I love you...."

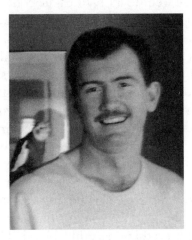

With love to Keith Gann, my friend,
remembering and missing you

Birds

J. Fraser Nelson

I

Love Story was the first movie I saw where someone died and I learned the way you died was this: you were born beautiful and rich or beautiful and talented, you went to an Ivy League college, you fell in love, you got an important job in a big city and an apartment with lots of windows, you got a sudden, faultless, fatal illness, you became even more beautiful, and you faded from view in a sunlit private hospital room, a little pale, but loved and all-knowing and smiling.

Seven years of working on the front lines of AIDS have taught me differently. This is what I know now; this is how you die:

You know it is starting when you look in the mirror and see a bird. Your eyes get bigger, and new nose bones jut out over your lips. You are scared to go to sleep and so you sit up, vigilant in the night, listen for the changes in your body and stare down at anything that comes near. You take thirty pills each day, hoping that one in the lot will make you feel a little better, give you just one normal day. The sores in your throat make everything taste like blood. The diarrhea comes so often, fast and hard you don't want to eat, and if you do, you throw it right back up no matter how nice the restaurant or the company. Your teeth turn black. You get so thin and gray and horrifying no one argues when you say how hideous you have become. Just a few people, some of whom get paid, drop in on you now, so you close the curtains and turn up the heat. You lose your muscles so you can't walk or straighten out your legs, and you wait through each season under winter blankets, your face toward the wall. You can't get up to change your own sheets and you smell bad five minutes after a sponge bath. Your bladder and bowels become willful and you have to wear diapers. You get a skin rash that makes your ear disintegrate into a gray powder that reeks of rotten flesh and your hair falls off in chunks with the scalp attached. You lose your eyesight so you can't see the TV and since most people have long since stopped visiting, you lie in your own infectious waste, alone. Your skin is tight across a face that no one recognizes. You are more hatchling than human, lips stretched across teeth, bony mouth snatching, gaping, hungry for a full breath, helpless, eyes darting, looking at those around you with a horrible need for everything, all of it back, a way out of this stinking dark nest. There is so much pain that you beg to die, beg your last friends to kill you, take overdoses of anything you can get your hands on. But you don't die for a long time yet.

II

My mother stopped believing in God when I was eight. That was the year of phone calls that sent us upstairs to be quiet, or outside to play, a year of calls that brought us home from school early. First her brother Hank, then her favorite Aunt Katherine and then her father, all dead one after the other, with Robert Kennedy in between. Uncle Hank and Robert Kennedy became for me the same fallen hero, frozen in black and white photographs, forever handsome with their short Princeton hair cuts, with their dogs and kids all around, with their blonde widows left behind. I felt linked to the world through a common tragedy. I became political and protested Nixon's bombing of Cambodia on my New Jersey suburban town green. I started talking back to adults.

I repeated the story over and over again to friends. *My Uncle Hank died of a brain tumor when he was only thirty-two. His brain had a tumor the size of an orange. They said he had only six months to live, but he wanted to live so badly he lived for a whole year. He died with a smile on his face.* At night I tried to picture smiling in death.

We went to church because we were a young Episcopalian family on the move, but I no longer prayed. I had given faith my best shot and my mother had given God a chance three times over. There is in my memory her simple statement: There is no God. I was released.

Without a God and without the consequences of a hell or a heaven, death became less heroic and life more frantic. I became a Marxist. I became a secular humanist. I became an existentialist. I became a socialist. I worked for Democratic candidates. I made sense of it all and went out to do good and work for positive social change and justice. I worked in an abortion clinic and never once thought of death. Then came AIDS, and death caught up with me.

Now I begin friendships with people who are already dying. It's easy to say "Well, we are all dying; I could get run over by a truck tomorrow," but I have never known anyone to get run over by a truck. I started to think about things like quick tragic death by truck last winter when I spent a lot of time driving home from my friend Eric's bedside, back across the Mississippi from Minneapolis to St. Paul. Why have I attended more memorial services than baby showers? Why is it that my father called me for advice when his parents were dying? When did I learn to wait quietly for the last breath? This was not the career I had planned; this is not what I imagined life would be like.

III

Ruth, Jimmy and I are on the ferry to Fire Island. It is 1977 and we are spoiled preppies driving the family Vista Cruiser. We are off for a big weekend at their grandmother's cottage, and have wine and pot I bought from the guy who works in the morgue at the hospital where I have my summer job. The ferry is full of gay men, and we stare at them. They all seem to know each other, and stand in loose groups like a floating cocktail party, laughing and sharing a sense of tight anticipation. They are definitely going to have a good time with their tanned terrific legs in short shorts, groomed mustaches, bright tank tops, and nice luggage. Ruth is figuring out she's a lesbian and Jimmy wants to lose his virginity with me. It all seems possible. We feel adventurous, away from the Ethel Walker School and the Phillips Andover Academy and among these handsome New Yorkers.

IV

In 1981 nothing was unsafe. Studio 54, cigarettes, and cocaine were politically correct, and we stayed out late, even on week nights. In those days, you walked down Christopher Street through a wall of gorgeous men, studded and shining black leather men, lumberjacks in tight pants, dancers, body builders, each beautiful. I walked home from the subway alone at night and did not worry. My best girlfriend Nancy and I scored dollar joints in Washington Square on nights we didn't have dates. We were having a lot of then unregretted sex. I could hear it through my walls; it is chronicled in my journals.

When my parents came in from New Jersey they had to turn off the West Side Drive onto Christopher Street at the even then notorious leather bar Badlands. They never failed to say 'Jesus, who *are* these people?' and roll up the Volvo windows. One visit, a tall transvestite rollerskated by and winked at my father and I smiled back, in proud collusion. I loved it when those things happened; those moments that placed me far from New Jersey and prep school and debutante parties and all that had been planned and was anticipated. It was a lot of fun back then; it was my *Breakfast at Tiffany's*; it was exactly like New York was supposed to be. AIDS didn't exist for us yet.

In a different New York the *Village Voice* was printing strange stories of rumors that the CIA was putting a poison into the water to kill off gay men by giving them cancer and weird diseases. We didn't pay much attention. I had my first job working on Mario Cuomo's campaign for Governor but I don't remember writing or reading a policy statement about it. I think the big issue of the campaign was infrastructure.

V

Roanoke, Virginia, gateway to Appalachia, is called the 'Star City of the South' because the world's largest neon star sits on top of Mill Mountain. Roanoke also boasts the world's largest miniature Graceland complex which includes doll-sized replicas of Elvis' birthplace, the Tupelo church where he first sang, the Memphis Civic Center, and a fully landscaped Graceland, down to the pool and horse pasture. The tribute has never been vandalized—that's just the kind of place Roanoke is.

I got to Roanoke at about the same time as AIDS. Several gay men asked me to help start a local AIDS project because I was young, heterosexual, had a background in community organization and sexual politics and could say condom on television with a politic smile. Being marginally employed, new to town, and recently unengaged, I said sure. The state of Virginia gave us $7,500 to stop the spread of AIDS and care for the sick in the twenty-nine counties of southwestern Virginia, a seven-and-one-half hour drive through the Blue Ridge mountains from end to end. Wayne Slusher put a hotline (982-AIDS) in his upstairs bedroom and we were in business. In the morning he would play back the messages. One woman called us 'dirty flies on doo-doo' and said we would burn in hell or be killed. We were dirty faggot queers who deserved to die. There was not much use calling the police to report threats, here in the shadow of Jerry Falwell's Thomas Road Baptist Church. Eventually people with AIDS started to call, and we had clients, right there in Appalachia, just like New York.

VI

I am sitting next to Harry's hospital bed, which is in his living room. Harry was the first official client of the Roanoke AIDS Project. For eighteen months we watched *All My Children* together when I made him lunch. Harry's last words were, "Where are my noodles?" — but that was more than two days ago. Harry is no stranger to death or other adversity. He started doing tricks in the bathrooms of mining town movie theaters when he was ten years old. At seventeen he was shipped off, illiterate and in government shoes, to a New Jersey Job Corps program. "Whoever dreamed that up must have been a real fool, thank you," Harry would say. Eventually he became a nursing home aide and an unsuccessful transvestite prostitute in the Star City. He was a plain man even in makeup and in full health, too unassuming to drive a hard bargain.

Death and funerals are important to Harry. He admires the big Baptist services where they wheel the casket up the aisle and the family follows slowly behind crying, up to the front pew and sits down to face dozens of huge flower arrangements while the preacher talks about the dead and their loving family for at least an hour. His photo album contains pictures of family members and friends in open caskets, a yellowed shot of Harry and his brother as children, kneeling in little suits with hands held before them in prayer, looking down at a child's white casket, and many obituaries and funeral cards. There is only one picture of Harry as an adult—a color polaroid of him dressed as a cheerleader. I have the feeling that the only time in Harry's life that anyone was important was when he or she died.

Harry told a television reporter doing a story about the AIDS project that I was like the daughter he never had. The day I told him I was engaged to be married he told me he could die in peace. My fiance has carried him home from the hospital to this room. I want his death to be perfect for him.

I watch for the signs I was told to watch for. His breath is cautious. His hands are turning lilac, and when I hold them I can feel the effort it takes his heart to keep pumping. I hold his hands as I would a bird, gently so as not to crush him, but strongly so he can't get away. His eyes have stopped darting. He does not turn to look panicky at me any more but stares ahead and up. I look at his urine bag, how dark the liquid is, and how little from the hours before. I don't know what to do because there is nothing to do.

I slip a dropper more of morphine under his tongue, and the bright blue liquid reminds me of "Tidy Bowls," a drink that was popular with preppies one summer. It occurs to me that in other circumstances it would be illegal to have such a big bottle of such a controlled substance. I wonder who placed this bottle in my hands. I wonder who is letting me minister the liquid that keeps the pain away, that keeps the breathing steady, that takes the edge off death and hastens its arrival. I have no idea what I am doing alone, here. I want someone to come by and be with us because I am not sure how much to give, what's enough, what's too much.

At night I lie on the floor listening for the slow chunks of breath to rise up and out of Harry's filling lungs. I wake only when they stop, and in the light from the bathroom, I watch Harry's face and eyes, open and staring up to the narrow light cast across the ceiling, and wait. I hold my breath; his starts again, like a scuba diver, deep below me.

After two more days friends and AIDS Project volunteers come by to wait with me. Harry's younger brother, Jimmy Dean Earls, sits in the front parlor because he cannot bear to watch. Oldest brother John Wayne Earls is driving his truck somewhere in Tennessee. This is my first death, and I've read somewhere that coaxing can help. I speak softly in Harry's ear so that the others cannot hear, "Please die if you can." Our head volunteer John, who was a priest before his homosexuality got in the way, asks Jimmy to sit by his brother's side and tell him it's okay to die. We leave, but after a few seconds Jimmy yells for us to come quick because something's happening and we run from the front room to watch as Harry pulls in one last breath and opens his eyes wide and looks straight up to me and dies. I see Harry's chest fall still below me; his warm breath rises up and enters my lungs. I see the others turn away, putting their faces in their hands, pulling their shoulders down. I hold Harry's breath in my chest and I wait for him to start breathing again.

I did my best with Harry's funeral but five years later I still worry that he was disappointed. I did not have any money for a fancy church tribute and neither did anyone else. Harry told me he had a plot at the Blue Ridge Gardens, but when I showed up it turned out he still owed them for his mother's burial three years before. I negotiated with the limited authority of an AIDS Project Executive Director and got Harry a spot directly on top of his mother at a substantial discount. I went to the richest church in town, St. John's Episcopal, and cried until they gave me enough to pay off the plot. Other friends planned the service, I just said we needed flowers. The county provided a pine box covered with gray fabric. It looked good against the bright green astro turf and the southern red clay. There were lots of flowers and the whole AIDS Project turned out. It was a beautiful clear southern summer afternoon. Two nuns said a few things, and we sang "Amazing Grace." At the end I was handed a red balloon, and I walked away from Harry and the crowd to release it. I wanted to believe that he could see me, the speck of my red balloon, my white dress, all the flowers, my face looking up to him. I told Harry I was sorry his casket wasn't on wheels. I stood there for a long time, looking out at the Blue Ridge Mountains and up to the crows and hawks flying above us, trying to take in steady breaths.

VII

Sean drove limousines, and his mother was a devoted Catholic transplanted from New York to rural Southwestern Virginia. Sean was so tall, good, handsome and funny that Mrs. Hegarty seemed not to mind that he was gay. When she went north to visit and saw how skinny, sick and tired he was she brought him straight home, thinking it must be New York City that was doing this to him. AIDS was a surprise, and we rarely mentioned it by name.

After Sean came out of Roanoke Memorial Hospital for the last time I started coming by as often as I could, but it was right before my wedding and I had a lot of things I needed to get done. We drank iced tea and talked wedding plans, and Sean promised he would be there and drive us away in the white Cadillac. Eventually Sean stopped talking. By the time my big day came Sean was only eating chocolate milkshakes, but so rarely, we fed him from the same one over and over again out of the freezer. He didn't seem to mind.

I tried to remember all my religion when I sat with Sean and his mother, mainly because the priest didn't seem to be coming by as often as she needed, and a lapsed Episcopalian was as close to Catholic as she was going to get in Blue Ridge County. She had a traveling sacrament kit and I would help anoint Sean with oils. I bathed his feet gently so that the pain of his damaged nerves would not bring him up out of his bottomless, blind sleep. The certainty of the ritual had a calming effect on the three of us, but I always worried on the drive home that someone would catch me taking faith.

I remember one June afternoon when all the lilac trees were blooming just in time for the wedding. Mrs. Hegarty and I were sitting in Sean's room and the window was open so that Sean could smell the spring. All the lilac blossoms outside the window were white, but three framed by the sill formed a perfect purple triangle. Mrs. Hegarty asked me what I thought it meant and I said, "It's the Holy Trinity." When I got back from my honeymoon Sean was dead.

VIII

When I met Angela's mother she was working double shifts at the Lynchburg Country Club to pay for Angela's dental bills. When Angela was born at the University of Virginia she had to have transfusions and one of them, Linda explained, was "bad blood." Now when Angela needs to see a dentist she has to go to a special university clinic because no one else will clean the teeth of a five-year-old with AIDS. The university clinic is expensive and since Linda still owes a lot of money for Angela's transfusions, the University has begun garnishing her wages. Linda wants Angela to start kindergarten next year, but the principal, himself a member of the Country Club, said she was not welcome in the public schools. We sit together in big leather chairs in a dark corner of the Men's Lounge between her shifts and try to figure out what to do. People with AIDS didn't sue back then.

Angela's neurological problems made her walk like a drunk, and she was always covered with bruises. She tottered around the paneled walls of our low-budget offices, laughing through the tangle of her long blonde hair with the bangs cut straight across. When Angela became a client of the AIDS Project we went out and bought toys. Because of her we got brave and went mainstream—Toys for Tots, church suppers, holiday gift drives, the Make a Wish Foundation. Other clients started bringing their children to the AIDS Project to play, and we got a paint set donated. Angela was our collective and individual hope, because none of us, sick or well, could imagine that she would die. She was our innocent victim and since nothing could happen to her we reasoned we all stood a chance.

Linda never fought the Lynchburg School Board because before too long she got caught up in other problems, like finding a way to pay back the hospital so Angela could go there for treatment, and finding a loaner children's hospital bed, and finding money for the funeral. In the time I knew Angela she lost her baby teeth and grew replacements, but I can't remember how old she was when she died. I don't remember her last name. This worries me. I wonder if I have gone beyond some human point of care or remembrance. I get angry with myself for not remembering the date of her death, for not honoring it in some way. I say to myself that if I could only remember I could spend a moment on that day in hope that there is a good life after a stupid death for children at the very least, to pray that there is a place of peace for their mothers, to pray for a hell for hospital bill collectors and for the members of the Lynchburg Country Club.

IX

In those days there was no money to care for people and few drugs to keep them from getting infections and dying within months. We kept secret lists of doctors who would treat someone. We stashed the AZT of people who had died in our desks for the next who needed it. We did not have time to do aerobics, find personal space, "journal," reconnect with our spirituality, or take care of ourselves. At national meetings we would talk about who had been hospitalized with what stress-related illness, who was dropping out of the work and who had found out that they, too, had it. We ran a separate body count of who among us had died.

Four months before my wedding I was driving home from Charlotte in a sleet storm, and I lost all the feeling in the right side of my body. I was told to go straight to the emergency room and to bring things for the night. Chris and I sat next to each other on the hospital bed while the doctor routinely asked if there was history of brain tumors in the family. I said that I had an uncle who had died of a brain tumor at age thirty-two. I did not mention that he died with a smile on his face.

The clients of the AIDS Project loved coming to visit because it evened the score. I got so many flowers I was sure I was dying. One doctor told Chris he should not marry me because eventually he would have to feed me strained baby food—so much for *Love Story*. But once I found out it was only Multiple Sclerosis and not a brain tumor or AIDS things were great.

Getting MS is a sure sign of burnout, one that even a burned-out person can recognize. I had been handed an easy excuse to get off the front lines. I told friends I was quitting to sell Isotoner gloves—one size fits all. My husband and I moved to Minnesota, to the promised land of progressive Scandinavian Lutherans, America's socialist state. One of the first people I met was Eric Lerner.

Eric liked movies where people died too, but I would bet he hated *Love Story*. Soon after we met I ran into him and his younger brother David outside of the video store on Snelling Avenue in St. Paul. They both looked sick: Eric gray and shaking; David frightened and pleading. They were renting *Long Time Companion*, a movie in which almost everyone dies of AIDS. I say, "Eric, that is so sick!" and David nods enthusiastically. "I want him to know what it's like," Eric says. "I want him to really know." David and I laughed about that the next summer at Eric's funeral. I am glad that David missed his brother's version of an AIDS movie; it was not made for television.

X

The Democratic Convention is on, we're talking politics and AIDS, Eric is in a good mood. I ask, "Eric, this close to death is there anything you are hoping for?" Eric does not look away from Tipper, Al, Hillary and Bill, and says, "I hope that when I take that morphine and the rest of those Seconals I can keep them down." He has talked about killing himself many times, and there were times when I wished he would do it. Once, he took a handful of pills and ran naked down the hallway of his old folks' apartment in Saint Paul, screaming. During the Halloween blizzard he fled the psych ward of the county hospital and ran barefoot through thirty inches of snow in a flapping hospital gown. One day he called me at work demanding that I bring him a gun, and when I refused he said he was going to order one through the mail. I laughed. "You and Lee Harvey Oswald," I said. Eric invites me to his euthanasia often.

At the Ethel Walker School the seniors took "Situational Ethics" and learned Kubler Ross's "Stages of Death" as though for some foreseen future purpose. We read about life after death experiences. We argued about life after death experiences. We argued about life and death, suicide, life after death— this was heady college-bound stuff, better than religion. Now I see death more like the Myer's Briggs personality indicator test than a road map to some state of all-knowing bliss. I have learned that people die just like they lived, even more so. Shy people die quietly, not wanting any fuss. People who are loved die with a smile on their face. Curious people look at the action around them, ask questions and provide a running commentary on the process. For many, death is just another thing that seems to be going wrong with life.

Eric was pissed off from start to finish; he had gotten tripped up in the anger stage long before any death sentence. His anger kept him alive through years spent in the company of rich lonely men, through years of heroin addiction, years on the street and through six years of AIDS. For months now, all Eric talks about is pain and AIDS. He is down to a few friends: Earl, Elizabeth, Cindy, and Joanne and Mary, who knew him from treatment and took him in when he could no longer be trusted to live alone. He throws things at us, calls his mother who has come all the way from New York a fucking bitch, screams at the nurses, and smokes Marlboros one after the other, truly incessantly. He never says he's sorry. He doesn't say thank you anymore, either, not when you fluff his pillows or change his diaper or come to the hospital with a café latté an hour before work. He tends more toward asking you why the fuck you forgot the sugar. He abuses the drugs his physician has prescribed.

Eric screams on and on: "This sucks, this sucks, why me, why the fuck is this, look at me I am like a fucking pig lying in my own shit, I love you so much, get a gun, this is ridiculous, it won't be long, I can't stand this, I have a plan, keep it quiet, don't tell anyone, this sucks." His constant euthanasia plans are making us crazy; we are on a twenty-four hour call. He hoards his pills like a magpie's silver, secreted away. But we know just where they are because he can only reach so far outside his nest. For Eric, death will come more deliberately than suicide.

Looking back now, I realize we took the drugs away only when we knew he would not kill himself, just stay as high as possible and make our lives even more miserable. But by now Eric is too tired and scared to be nasty. He no longer talks about killing himself, he simply asks to be put to sleep. I am glad he is too blind to see the pills he could use and too weak to reach them. He spends his time drifting in and out of morphine hallucinations. He looks at my husband and says, "I just saw the most beautiful thing. You were holding a little girl in your arms and you loved her so much." Chris, who wants us to have a child, says, "That was a great dream." Chris is having a hard time meeting men in Minnesota, and I think to myself that it is not fair that they can't stay friends.

XI

"This is to certify that Eric Lerner is a member of the Cremation Society of Minnesota and as such has made complete prearrangements for cremation service after death and that the Society is to be notified at the time of death. twenty-four hour Emergency Number (612) 825-2435." The frameable certificate is dated and signed on January 8th, 1992, by Kevin Watiton, president of the society. Earl says the certificate is "good for one redemption." I am sitting by Eric's body looking at the cigarette burns on his fingers and at the last tufts of hair that stand almost apart from his scalp, like the feathers of the old dead birds in the dioramas at the New York Museum of Natural History.

The kids who lived in Eric's house have come in to look, too. They stand in the open door, and the smell of the fried chicken I brought replaces the stale cigarettes and urine. They ask to tie friendship bracelets on Eric's wrists, which curl up under his chin. The bracelets are woven of yellow, purple and orange string, and it is hard to slip them under his stiff arms. Eric's brother David does not want Eric moved until he is cold. This is something he is learning at naturopathic college in Seattle. He says we are to feel over Eric's heart because it is the last place to grow cold. It has been three hours since

Eric's last breaths, a smooth series of three, no gasping. His skin is the color of Minnesota's summer sky at nine o'clock at night, when the northern lights give dusk a greenish hue. Joanne decides he is cold, and calls to redeem our certificate.

I stay to keep company with Eric. Under his bed are neatly lined size thirteen shoes of Italian leather; a folded walker lies against the wall. On a table are the *China Handbook Series on Politics* and Joanne's Kool cigarettes. The toothbrush, the lotion, the diapers, the alcohol, the infectious waste, the saline, the morphine, the dying flowers. Eric's tray, his phone, his Marlboros, his pie pan ashtray, his pills, a glass of water, his world, those objects he could reach.

Joanne comes in to disconnect the morphine drip and the condom catheter. We remark on his urine output, considering he hadn't had anything to drink in two days. Eric is dressed in a tie-dyed t-shirt, and his belly is flat as a plate. He lies on his side, legs curled as tightly as his hands. I sit, remembering the pain in those legs, how they hurt when they touched. I hear him yelling to me to lift his legs and pry them apart when he wanted to turn: "Separate them! Separate them!"

Two members of The Cremation Society of Minnesota arrive in black pants, white short sleeve shirts and matching ties with leafy green patterns. They do not have much to say. Eric is long since too stiff for a gurney so they place him on a canvas hammock and cover him with a burgundy fake fur blanket. His knees jut out as he passes by. Joanne follows him out and stands alone on the front lawn, smoking. We sit quietly and listen to the metallic clunk of Eric being placed in the back of a windowless grey van. We joke that we didn't even ask for credentials.

Earl and I take the cold sheets from the bed, and when we remove the plastic mattress cover, a warm blast of cigarettes and urine hits us. The mattress is hollowed out to cover a water bed, and Earl says, "The state should pay for a waterbed for every smoking AIDS patient on Seconal, so if they set themselves on fire they'll put themselves out." We carry the mattress to the garbage, and I start to cry from the smells. I try to remember if Situational Ethics taught us that the human being does not remember pain.

XII

I have come to regard funerals the way I used to regard weddings. Like Harry, I observe the display, look at the flowers, listen to the music, take in the environment, and decide again what I want mine to be like. When I first moved to Roanoke and was in the midst of complex love problems I went to a Tarot card reader. She saw a lot of men in my future, men whom I would come to know very intimately but love platonically. I explained that they were the AIDS Project. Seven years later, lying on an acupuncturist's cot, I am told that I have built up a lot of unresolved grief. Memorial services are supposed to help with that, but I am always too aware of my surroundings and too unsure of what happens next to grieve properly.

Eric's funeral was held on a Friday at five o'clock, two weeks after Eric died because his parents wanted to save money on air fare from New York. We gather in a semicircle around a red cooler containing Eric's ashes in a wooded glen in a park he loved. The family is seated. Mr. and Mrs. Lerner are hunched in their folding chairs like they are preparing for a crash landing in a plane. To start us off, Earl reads a letter Eric published in a magazine by people with AIDS. Eric sounds hopeful and joyous, talks about going out to dinner with a girlfriend, about sobriety, and about renewing his friendships and his life. I wish I had known that person. A friend sings "Love Will Guide Us" so clear and sad. Mosquitos are biting us all, reminding us of him. David is crying now. One by one Earl, Mary, and Cindy and I speak about this man, his pain, how easy and hard it was to love and care for him, and then we turn the telling of his memory over to the others. There are a lot of people there that I don't know, that I never saw when the drugs took over or the Bird Look came, but it appears that they have known Eric a lot longer than I did. I try to concentrate on the red cooler, on moving my anger through the plastic and into Eric's bones.

Earl, Elizabeth and I keep scratching at our stomachs and legs, but it's not the mosquitos. Eric's physician looks us over and concludes that Eric gave us scabies. We will need to get some special lotion after the refreshments. I am looking up into the trees, looking for the birds that are singing.

XIII

A few weeks later I asked Earl, "I wonder how Eric is doing?" Earl replied, "He's dead, how the hell do you think he's doing?" I knew that, of course, but there are not a lot of people to whom I can ask that question. I would like to make sense of things. I would like life to have a purpose. I would like death to have meaning. I would like my friends to be remembered as heroes. I want them all to be doing fine. I want the dead to hover around me whispering warm breath on my face and neck, I want postcards from the Blue Ridge Parkway, visions of holiness, birds singing to me from a lilac tree. It is not that I want my friends to be alive—I was always so relieved when they died. I just want to know that the dead are doing okay.

To Wayne Slusher, whose love and compassion are there for the long haul.

OCTOBER 20, 1993

LESLÉA NEWMAN

Happy birthday, baby.
Did they throw a big party for you
in heaven?
Were there lavender balloons everywhere
and white roses in tall crystal vases
and a big chocolate cake
with thirty-four candles glowing in your eyes?
Was there a chorus of pretty boys
singing happy birthday to you,
their arms outstretched
wine glasses raised high,
your amber reflection in every one?
Was there laughing and dancing
and drinking and cruising?
Did you pick one special boy
to celebrate with
or were there many?
Two years ago you told me you were dying
to have sex.
"At least I won't need rubbers
in the afterlife," you said,
no bitterness left in your tired voice.

Oh baby, there are no condoms in heaven.
There are no hospital beds, wheelchairs,
or catheters in heaven.
There is no AZT, DDI, KS or PCP in heaven.
Only all those pretty pretty boys like you
who went through hell to get there.

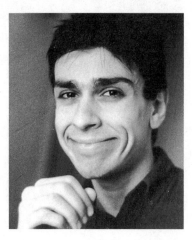

for Gerard Rizza, 1959-1992
"most ordinary boy"

THE CINNAMON GIRLS

ALLISON J. NICHOL

The day John Kennedy was killed, Sister Mary Margaret gave us Hershey bars and holy cards. I cradled Saint Patrick as I crushed the almonds between my baby teeth, taking comfort in the rush of sweetness as I rolled the chocolate over and over on my tongue, making it last as long as I could.

Sister sat slumped in her chair in the front of the room sobbing with the face of a foregone conclusion, the Sacred Heart dripping velvet blood just above her head. We didn't understand what had happened exactly, not even after Father John came in a few minutes later and in the shaking voice of a young man said, "Children, the President has been shot."

All we knew for sure was that Sister Mary Margaret had never cried before, not even when Elizabeth Joan Marie O'Rourke threw up all over the back of Sister's habit during her first communion, so something really terrible must have happened. It took me thirty years to see another face as gripped with grief, confusion and shaken faith as Sister's was on that day. Thirty years to understand that, for Sister Mary Margaret, more was lost that day than our only Catholic President. That day God and the devil ran neck and neck in a dead heat to a photo finish.

John and James died only a few months apart in 1990. John got sick first. We knew right away, although denial is a useful tool and we used it as best we could. We knew that if John had AIDS then James did too. So they coped with AIDS, like everything else that had come their way in the past fifteen years, with courage and dignity and humor and each other.

I'm sure I drove them crazy the first year. In a moment of weakness they had agreed to move into my house. I thought I had used my lawyer wits to outlogic them— Why pay two rents? Why have to climb all those stairs at their third floor walk-up? I have this big house. It's paid for. Don't be ridiculous. And on and on until they finally gave in. I know now that they agreed because I was their best friend, and they knew I wanted to mother them and sister them and love them for whatever time would give us.

We played backgammon and bridge and blew bubbles out the window on Pride day and when they could manage we would invite five friends over so we could square-dance. I sterilized the house, bought a humidifier, a purifier, learned how to make pot roast, real mashed potatoes and other variations of 1950 make-people-fat food, ran endless mineral baths, and, in between, felt guilty that I wasn't dying, too.

We told the story at least fifty times that year to everyone who had heard it before and anyone who hadn't. We were striving to preserve our history in the memory of others. And so we told them how we had all gone to the gay square dance convention in New York five years before and got stuck sharing the same room even though we didn't know each other. They loved to tell the part about how they were apprehensive at first about sharing a hotel room with some lesbian they didn't know because they were afraid I might put some evil curse on their penises making them forever unusable. I loved to tell the part about how I had never even seen a penis before that weekend much less a penis in pantyhose and a penis wired with a black orchid. And we all loved to tell the elevator story.

John was dressed as Amber Waves, head to toe in lavender polyester and orange crinolines. His eyes, the color of blue printer's ink, caked with sparkling silver eye shadow. James chose a more formal look, his broad shoulders almost bursting from his floor length red satin gown. A small tuft of blonde hair peeked through the V-neck, a faux diamond choker set off his beard quite nicely. I wore my black tuxedo and white Stetson and tennis shoes. We got into the elevator on the first floor on our way to the "Honkey Tonk Queen" contest.

We had assumed wrongly that the entire hotel was filled with gay guests. When we reached the third floor the elevator lurched to a stop and the door opened to reveal seven members of the Southern Baptist Revival Convention, who we found out later were unable to secure rooms across the street in the hotel where their own convention was being held.

They were busy talking when they first got on the elevator so they didn't really notice that two of the girls on the elevator were really guys. I heard John and James each suck in a sudden breath. By the time we reached the tenth floor the interlopers had caught on and one said, "God save us all."

The mere mention of the "G word" sent Amber spinning into action. She started to swish and sashay as much as the room allowed. Then she reached into her grey straw purse and pulled out a piece of Brach's cinnamon candy. She unwrapped it slowly and with an exaggerated pucker rolled it over and over on her tongue. Then she bent toward James and grabbing his shoulders placed her mouth over his and slid the candy into his mouth. They slid it back and forth between them a few times. Then James reached over and grabbed me by the waistband and pulled me until I was standing in front, facing both of them. Then he stooped down and put his mouth very close to mine with the piece of candy sticking out from between his teeth. I took the candy in my teeth and transported it back to Amber. This went on for the balance of the ride. And so from such simple beginnings were born the "Cinnamon Girls;" incomparable, inseparable, insatiable.

I worked on the Names Project panel on and off for over a year. It took me a year to begin and a year to finish. I wanted it to be perfect and in the end it was. It was awash in crinolines every color of the rainbow. I sewed our "family photo" from New York in the center and stapled a border of Brach's cinnamon candy around it. Next to the picture, as promised, I glued John's favorite t-shirt, the one with the picture of Pope John Paul II on it in a big red circle with a slash through it with big block letters underneath that reads THE PATRON SAINT OF LIARS. I even lacquered the letter from John's parish priest in which he explains with great regret how unfortunate John was to be a "victim" of AIDS but church rule prevents the possibility of a Catholic funeral. I folded it, blessed it with Evian and scotch and shipped it.

The quilt has become so large now that I knew if I didn't go when I was in Washington for the March, I might never again have the chance. I had gone with Deirdre and David, my two new best friends, and enveloped in their arms I felt safe and strong enough. We had just finished attending the candlelight vigil at the newly opened Holocaust museum.

I thought the vigil had drained all of my emotions. We had stood for two hours partly in the rain listening to the horror stories of gays imprisoned, tortured, killed by the Nazis. We held candles and each other, finding in our small circle enough collective strength not to pass out or run away.

We strolled the short distance from the museum to the quilt in silence. Deirdre and David each held one of my hands as we inched our way through the crowd of mourners searching for the panel. And then just like that, there they were, my cinnamon girls. I let go hands and reached down, patted the panel, smoothed out the crinolines that had bunched together a bit, and then bent all the way down to the picture and kissed one, then the other. I caught my reflection in James' favorite compact mirror. There was that face again, drawn, sunken, unforgiving, and I wept. For myself, for John, for James, and for Sister Mary Margaret.

For the boys: If love could have kept them
alive, we'd still be dancing.

DENNIS

NINA

December 6th, 1993, was my fortieth birthday, a day I thought to celebrate, to have a huge surprise party with all my friends to marvel at "How did we get so old, so fast!" Instead I was in New York Hospital making the hardest decision I shall ever have to face. It was the day I decided to stop all treatments for my husband, Dennis, who was dying of AIDS-related brain lymphoma. Most specifically, I had to stop his TPN (Total Parenteral Nutrition), which as his "food" was keeping him alive—barely. As I stared at this man I loved, who had come into my life less than nine years ago, all I could think of was "How did this happen?" How did this happen to someone who loved life more than anyone I knew—how did this happen to the vibrant, funny, most caring and handsome man I knew? Yes, we were too young to be so old, too young to have this happening to us.

Dennis was born on December 18th, 1954 and grew up in a broken home. His father left with his younger brother when he was only five. This started his lifelong fear of being abandoned and "not loved enough" by his ever-elusive father. He credited his mother, Eileen, for many things—his optimism, his caring of others, his sense of righteousness. He grew up under the worst of circumstances in the best of times—the sixties, a decade that most of us have romanticized as part of our youth—the decade of the Beatles, Vietnam, free love and, of course, drugs. Dennis did them with abandon. It all started innocently enough, pot, hash, acid—and eventually heroin. He smoked it throughout the seventies. Unfortunately, his "only smoking" changed one day in the early eighties and he used a needle only once. I don't think (and neither did he) that it's important to know how a person got AIDS. You can't differentiate it. When you do, you fall into "good" AIDS and "bad" AIDS. It's all bad, no one deserves it and everyone suffers just the same. I just felt it was so ironic that it was the only time he used a needle. But as Dennis used to say, "It takes only one time."

Dennis finally got clean in early 1984 and I met him later that year. I was so attracted to this beautiful man with the brilliant blue eyes, dazzling smile, incredible style, and childlike wonder.

He was so happy to finally overcome his addiction and all of the adversities that had affected him all his life. He felt as if he was given another chance. He embraced life like no one else I knew. It didn't matter to him that he had had such a hard life, he was never angry, bitter or blameful. He accepted everything—as he later did his illness—with dignity, grace, humor and courage. He seemed unstoppable.

We were married in June of 1987. Not only were we lovers but best friends and remained that way throughout our lives together.

He found out he was HIV-positive on October 26th, 1987. Both of us were totally shocked. Were we in denial? We knew he had used a needle, but we really never considered the consequences. Were we stupid? We used to watch TV and every time there was something on about AIDS, we'd remark on how lucky we were to have found each other in these very scary times.

I remember that day well. I was working and felt so lucky that I had finally met someone like him, and when I spoke to him that day I told him how much I loved him. He told me he had something very important to tell me. I didn't think anything of it—until I saw him. As soon as he started to speak, I knew. As he tried to console me (which was often) the first thing I thought of was how we'd have no children—then I asked about me (my test did come back negative and to this day I haven't the nerve to go back again) and then asked about him. I knew he would die—there are no words to describe how I felt. He felt he could beat it and we'd try together. We just held each other as I cried. I know he tried to be strong for me as usual. But that night I heard him cry out "Ma" in his sleep. He later told my mother that the train ride home was the longest in his life, knowing that he'd have to tell me the news.

How do you get up the next day and continue on with your life? We did—okay, we took two days off from work—but we did. We decided to become macrobiotic, totally holistic and spiritual. Truthfully, I have lost most of my faith in God. He never did, he felt that there was something after this lifetime. We continued on with our lives as best we could. We went to the gym every day, we went to work, we went out to great dinners and took great vacations. Very few people knew that Dennis was HIV-positive. That was more my fault—he felt no shame and he wanted everyone to know. I felt that people would think it a "newsworthy" event and gossip. Wrong? Yes, I know that now and perhaps I made it harder on him and everyone around us.

Den thought that I'd leave him when I found out. We had only been married four-and-a-half months. I remember when I later told someone, her response was, "Well, why don't you leave him?" And I asked her if she would leave her husband if he had cancer. That wasn't something I would have considered. I took my marriage vows very seriously and I would never do that to this person I loved so much.

Of course, our lives changed. At times the tension and stress were unbearable. I had all the anger and rage he didn't have. Our lives did change, but they were as normal as could possibly be, given the circumstances. Dennis and I were both incredibly strong people and we weren't going to let this stop us. Not that everything was sweetness and light—we had some very dark moments. He was so special, so uplifting, so positive about everything. I handled it a lot worse than he did. I often screamed, at times I blamed him for ruining my life, but underneath it all I was just so scared, so angry I was going to lose him. I tried to be more like him, I'd look at him in awe. After all, he was the one with the fatal diagnosis. If you knew Dennis before and after his diagnosis, I don't think you'd see much of a change. Many people didn't. He'd still have that very open quality and wonder about him. He wanted to soak everything in—he'd talk to everyone about everything and anything. He still spent tons of money on his very serious fashion habit (Giorgio Armani clothes were a favorite). He'd even spend twenty dollars on a mushroom! And all the time I'd be screeching about money. His reply was always "Don't worry about it—it'll work itself out." I admit I became very indulgent—I knew beautiful clothes and good food gave him great pleasure, how could I deny him anything? But underneath it all, he did have his moments and doubts. He was such a free spirit—he felt his illness hindered him, he always had to worry about what he ate, what he drank, knowing that the wrong food or water could ultimately kill him. What bothered him most was how he felt he couldn't dream anymore.

Dennis was in pretty good health until the summer of 1990. We were going to Italy and France the end of August and he had gotten a little thin. He really didn't feel well—his chest was "tight," and he worried about PCP. I told him we could cancel our trip, but never wanting to disappoint me, we went. He was sick that whole trip. I remember listening to his labored breathing at night and feeling such a sense of gloom. By the time we got to Paris he was very sick. We did leave Paris early and he was diagnosed with PCP. He said that was the worst day of his life because that was the day he had full-blown AIDS. And he cried. He spent forty-five days in the hospital and made a miraculous comeback. He went back to the gym and looked better than ever.

We did many things during the last three years. We skied out west, summered in Montauk and went to Germany seeking a holistic cure. He catered elaborate feasts for a Buddhist Zendo. It gave him such pleasure to plan those menus and go shopping around town. Even when he became sicker and weaker, he'd still do it. At those times, my mother would take him shopping and my parents would make the three hour trip with him and spend the weekend. I always had to work and felt I missed something very special. He always got a standing ovation at the end of each meal.

The year 1993 was a bleak one for Dennis. He was diagnosed with a parasite that causes chronic diarrhea or "wasting syndrome" so prevalent in AIDS patients. He was weak most of the time and had lost a great deal of weight. He'd go to the gym in baggy clothes and take yoga. He'd look in the mirror and say, "Just look at me—what happened to me?" We did go skiing at the end of March. He did it for me, I did it for him. He could only ski a few hours a day and slept the rest of the time. I'd just sit there and cry. It was so hard to see him like this. His days now consisted of going to doctors, taking more meds, sleeping and trying to stay alive.

We went to Montauk on Memorial Day weekend with my parents. We managed to take walks, but he didn't have the strength to do much more. On the way home he just slept in my lap as my mother cried. He wanted to see San Francisco and Northern California. We went at the beginning of June and stayed with friends. I noticed such a decline then—I was always afraid he'd die when we were away.

One of Den's biggest fears was getting dementia or toxo—he complained that he thought he was losing his mind and I'd just try to reassure him he wasn't. He had lost a great deal of weight by the July fourth weekend. He looked like my grandfather did when he was dying. I was convinced he wouldn't make it past the summer.

His doctor didn't recognize him on his next visit and wanted to put Dennis in the hospital. His worst fears were confirmed there—he had brain lymphoma. Dennis kept saying, "I have cancer, I have cancer *and* AIDS," over and over like a mantra.

He started radiation when he got out of the hospital. He now needed his mother to stay with him while I was at work. This bothered him so much. We were so protective of him. He felt he had lost his freedom and we were telling him what to do. It was just out of concern that he would fall or lose his way. Radiation made him weak and tired. He lost all his hair and looked like a little Buddha. He would rub cream into his burnt head all day, and could barely keep anything down.

He knew he was dying and felt such despair. He felt he had ruined his life when he had so much to offer. He still had his spirit—he wanted to get everything in. Every time he passed flowers, he would stick his whole head into them, just smelling them for a few minutes. He still gave to others. When he was finished with his radiation treatments, he gave flowers to all his technicians, and sent a delicious breakfast to his doctor and his staff. Shortly before he died he asked me if he'd be remembered as a lover of children.

When Dennis and I went to his doctor on November 16th, his condition had deteriorated so much that his doctor told me he didn't think he'd make it 'till Christmas. All I did was cry. Dennis went right to sleep when we got home. I tried to light some candles by his bed and couldn't. Dennis woke and asked why I was crying. I told him I couldn't light the candles and he said, "Tell me the truth," and went back to sleep. Dennis went into the hospital the next morning. His Total Parenteral Nutrition had infiltrated the port in his chest and I took him to the emergency room. At times he wasn't conscious and was in much pain. We spent Thanksgiving in the hospital. He slept most of the time, had stopped talking and eating. They removed his port and wanted to put in another. "Why?" I asked his doctor.

"What's the point?" That's when I decided to stop everything. Even though Dennis had a living will and made the decision for me (as his doctor pointed out), I still have doubts. I remember when "he came back to life" and spoke and said I was beautiful and that he loved me. But I knew and know I did the right thing.

Dennis wanted to die at home and we took him to my parents on Friday, December 17th. I know he knew we were there. He slept all day. The next day was his 39th birthday—we gave him chocolate ice cream and he said "Umm." His mother and two of his dearest friends came over. He opened his eyes so wide when he saw them and fell back to sleep. The next morning his breathing became very labored and he didn't moan when we turned him. When his hospice nurse came, she said he was in a coma and actively dying. It seems even when you know the inevitable, you are never prepared for it. He died that day, December 19th, at 10:26 p.m. I was with him the whole day holding his hand, talking to him, soothing him. His mother left the room for just a few minutes and I knew he would die then. He did. I felt he knew he was home, he had his birthday and died when his mother left the room. He knew when she left—he knew it would be too painful for her to watch. I felt his spirit leave and when I looked at him, I realized his body was just his earthly shell. In addition to myself, he left a loving mother and stepfather, my parents who loved him like their own son, my sister, brother and their spouses who also loved him like their brother. And many, many others who loved him deeply. Even his doctor told me that all doctors wish for patients like him. He touched everyone that he met.

How do I go on? I don't know. How have I gotten through these past two-and-a-half months? I don't know. I have never felt such sadness, such emptiness, such overwhelming grief. I slept with his ashes the first day I got them. I skied half a day at the mountain he learned to ski on and cried all the way up and all the way down. I listen to music. I saw *Philadelphia* and play the soundtrack over and over. I wear his clothes all the time. I bury my face in his closet. I watch our wedding video and wear his wedding rings under my own. I walk around with tears always behind my eyes. I don't answer my phone that much. I try to make risotto like his and fail. I usually cry from the time I walk into my door until the time I go to sleep. I talk to him as if he were still here. I try to understand all this, and feel like a Vietnam Vet or a Holocaust survivor. I try never to forget his deep, wonderful laugh and the way he would kiss my nose. I remember his courage and strength and how he would console me and say, "You poor dear, I'm sorry this happened to you," when in fact it was happening to him. I try to remember all of this, his touch, his smell, his voice, his kindness, his gentleness. Above all I remember how lucky I was to have known and loved him.

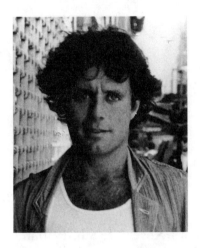

For Dennis Janis...I thought we'd have forever...
Dec. 18, 1954–Dec. 19, 1993

Ginkgo Trees, Eureka Street

David O'Steinberg

Prologue

Marty Selim, born November 8th, 1950 in Glendale, California, grown up in an L.A. he once said "no longer exists" except in his treasured childhood memories. He graduated from the University of California at Irvine with a degree in Social Ecology and later received a teaching credential. Marty worked as a substitute teacher in Ukiah, California, before going to teach in a private school in New York City. He returned to San Francisco in 1977 and, among other jobs, worked for several years as High Coffee Priestess of the Meat Market Café. He shared his last job as a typesetter with his best friend, the late Fraser McBeth, at the Bank of California.

Marty, who stood at six-feet-five-inches, founded the Tall Men's Dance/Theater Group in the seventies, bringing together tall gay men who finally had somebody their own size to pick on. He kept a journal for nineteen years, and loved writing, literature (especially Dorothy Parker), family gatherings, clean windows, and traveling. Marty's playful wit attracted many friends, and his true art was the coffee klatch where his coffee-making rituals rivaled the Japanese tea ceremony. In a journal, he wrote that he loved to have friends over, get everyone buzzed on coffee, and blab.

Marty was diagnosed with AIDS in March of 1989. His final days were full of humor, *kvetching*, gratitude for friends and family, simple weariness of being sick, and love. Marty was a real *mensch*, never a gilded saint. I miss him.

December 17, 1991

I make a left onto Eureka Street just to see them: seven ginkgo trees evenly spaced along the downhill sidewalk. In the bone-chilling morning mist, their yellow leaps out in contrast to the milky winter sky overhead. Only a scatter of yellow leaves lies beneath each tree. Ginkgoes hold most of their leaves until a certain moment—a week?—tomorrow?—when suddenly, all the leaves fall, leaving the tree bare, the sidewalk carpeted yellow. I drift slowly past the ginkgoes, then release the brake.

I've just left Marty's house for work, after spending the night there. His roommate Terry is away for the holidays so Marty's arranged a schedule of friends to take care of him. I was to take the first watch and last night was my second consecutive night with him.

Marty and I have been friends since 1979. I first met him through my roommate Gerry whom he'd just started dating. When I asked Gerry where they met, he said, "I went to the Stud on Punk Night and this big, wild thing was pogo-ing up and down like mad on the dance floor, and then he slam-danced into me, so I slammed back and that's how we met." They were perfectly matched: Gerry's six-foot-six-inch stature gave him only a slight edge over Marty's six-foot-five.

Twelve years later: Gerry has been dead two years, Fraser for over a year, and Marty's in his third year of full-blown AIDS. I yearn for Gerry and Fraser more keenly after each visit with Marty. Too many friends are gone and so before I left work last night, reluctant as I am to ask for help, I ask my lover Ruven to bring dinner over to Marty's place. I'm relieved, arriving at Marty's, to know Ruven will bring burritos soon and I won't have to fix dinner.

As soon as I say hello to Marty, he starts telling me, "Someone's coming from Pacific Bell tonight, my phone went dead today, it threw me into a panic. I tried Terry's phone, but that's dead too. Michelle just happened to stop by this afternoon, she went right out to call the phone company." Uh oh, partly my fault.

"Marty, I unplugged Terry's phone last night when I was meditating and forgot to plug it in when I was done. Shit! I'm sorry."

"Oh, God, really, Terry's phone just needs to be plugged in? But mine's still dead, listen, I felt so cut off, I couldn't call anyone all day. I needed to call the night nurse to see if she could come earlier tonight." The night nurse, one of three who administer antibiotic infusions daily to treat a blood infection that in turn has caused another infection.

I try to calm Marty down by telling him I'd call the night nurse from the corner phone, but Michelle did that, too. After seven hectic hours of word processing legal documents, I want to meditate, as I usually do after work. I'd even settle for changing out of my work clothes first before I have to deal with anything. I'm too tired to think clearly, though, and I start doing things for Marty. Then Ruven arrives. I tell them to eat, I'll join them in half an hour, but no, they'll wait for me.

In the other bedroom, I sit on Terry's bed, covered with dog hair from Annie, who's used to sleeping there every night. I repeat the mantra, hoping calm will enfold me quickly, but after seconds the doorbell rings. Annie explodes into ragged snarls of barking, and Ruven clatters after her down the stairs. I realize it's a phone repair-*man*, wonder if he's cute, and wish I wasn't meditating. I try to continue, but Ruven and the repairman clatter down the hall and back, clomp downstairs, then back up, then down the hall again and then...and then...it's quiet.

I'm hardly breathing, a thousand thoughts flood my mind, the switchboard on overload. Have I repeated the mantra? I think: "Maybe I'll skip this, I don't feel the least bit calm, I'm completely tense, why bother doing this, no, I need these twenty minutes..." When I'm done, the repairman's checking something outside, the burritos are in the oven.

"Why are the burritos in the oven?" Because Marty told Ruven to put them in the oven to keep them warm.

"But they're veggie burritos, the lettuce will get all soggy!" I go yank the burritos out of the oven and as I'm gathering dinner dishes, I wonder what drugs Marty might be on now—did he take what he was supposed to? How much morphine, which he doesn't like to take unless that hard lump in his gut really hurts—and did he break down and take a Xanex when he was panicked this afternoon? I'll have to check the daily medications log he keeps obsessively.

The burritos are good, but Marty eats less than a third before setting his plate down. Ruven finishes his quickly, then leans back in his chair, and bangs the floor lamp behind him with his head. The cramped bedroom seems too crowded, I want Ruven to go home, and suddenly I realize—only nine days till Christmas—no cards, no gifts, no tree, no holiday anything in the room. Marty's brother is going to Hawaii with his family for somebody's wedding, and their father's decided to stay in L.A. Do they think there'll be Christmas with Marty next year? I want them to come help us, we don't have it in us much longer to see Marty through to an end which does and doesn't seem far away.

But there's no family to scream at, there's only Marty, who's sick, and sick of being sick, and Ruven, who brought dinner, who becomes the lightning rod for my frustrations. I really want to crawl in bed with him and stay cuddled up for the next twenty-four hours.

After we finish eating, Marty feels a wave of anxiety and restlessness. The bedroom seems claustrophobic again, full of too many objects. I think: "I want control of this situation, I want all the clutter out of here, a dying man—I mean sick—a sick man ought to have a neat, clean, simple, tidy, organized, orderly room to be in. I'll send Ruven home, then do the dishes, they're all over the place—glasses, coffee mugs, our plates with mostly eaten burritos, lost my appetite too, halfway through mine, hard to look at Marty when I eat, terrible though true, don't ever say a word. Do I want Ruven to leave, yes, concentrate on Marty, I want to go home, I don't want to deal with this anymore, I don't want to take care of another friend with AIDS, only one more night after this, I'll do the dishes right *now*, that's it, hands in hot water will calm me."

I ask Ruven to help me gather the dishes. Marty says he's feeling more fidgety from anxiety and asks if I'll massage his feet, the only thing that calms him. "Why doesn't he take the Xanex like his doctor told him?" I think. "Maybe he hasn't taken morphine for a while; when it wears off he really feels that pain in his gut, the anxiety intensifies too, but he doesn't want to take the morphine because he's afraid he'll get hooked. For crissakes, his doctor prescribed it for him, it says right on the label for every four hours, or as often as needed!" Before I say anything, Ruven says "I'll massage your feet, Marty, after I take these dishes to the kitchen."

"Let me have those dishes," I tell him, quivering tensely. My head feels like it's going to pop off.

I'm filling the sink with hot water when the repairman comes up the back stairs into the kitchen. He's friendly, but not as cute as I'd imagined. "Everything's working, let me call his room on the kitchen phone," he says. Marty's phone rings at the other end of the flat, and I hear Ruven ask if he should answer it. I yell, "It's the repairman calling from the kitchen to see if Marty's phone's working," then the doorbell rings, the dog barks and romps downstairs again, followed by Ruven. It's the night nurse, here earlier than usual for the third infusion. Nothing's ready, and I zip into Marty's room to push chairs against walls, then roll the I.V. stand in from the next room, thin plastic tubes dangling, empty veins. Ruven and the nurse enter as I'm settling Marty closer to the edge of the bed, along with a certain configuration of pillows he likes just so, to prop him up: "I need another one, that big one on the floor over there, bring it over here, okay, now turn it sideways on top of the other pillows so I can lean back against it." And would Ruven massage his feet some more? Ruven would. I carry away the last stack of dishes, brushing past the repairman in the hall, who's on his way out. "See ya!" he chirps, clumps down the stairs, and the front door *slams!*

I pause in front of the sink, hands full of dishes. I can't get my breath to go below my sternum, so I plunge my hands full of dishes in the hot water, shut my eyes, force a slow, deep breath, another, then another. "This is an impossible life," I think. It's all I think, over and over, as I try to relax one small notch. Except for a few people, friends visit less than they intend to. His roommate can't take it anymore. My breathing deepens a bit as I soap the first glass. I wonder who's going to get Marty a Christmas tree, and what will he do Christmas eve, Christmas day? "This is an impossible..."

Ruven comes in the kitchen. Marty fell asleep during his foot massage, the infusion will take another half hour. I tell Ruven I need time alone before Marty wakes, and ask him to leave. As I walk him to the door, feeling guilty, I apologize for being so tense and irritable. Kiss, long hug, then I watch Ruven walk down Douglass Street. He looks back and waves before getting in his car. The night air is raw though the empty street's quiet is inviting, but a walk right now isn't possible.

I finish the dishes, scour the sink, put on tea water, and turn off all the lights except the one above the stove; its low level light seems soothing. The water boils, but I want decaf instead of tea because I've just noticed, as I cleared the cluttered kitchen table to wipe down, a plate of Christmas cookies someone brought today, probably Michelle. I decide I'll only have two, but devour a half dozen.

When it's time to get Marty settled for the night I'm exhausted, and at 11:45, I'm thinking about work tomorrow. Marty and I start haggling about what medications he should take. He cuts me off: "First I have to double-check my medications chart." After careful evaluation he says, "I guess I could take more morphine now, and I only took a quarter of a Xanex this afternoon when I was in a panic about the phone going dead."

"A quarter of a Xanex? Why didn't you take a whole one? Your doctor said you can take four every day!"

"I didn't want to fall asleep when I was home by myself without the phone working." That's a reason? If it was me...

"Well, why don't you take the morphine and a Xanex and maybe you'll sleep through the night for a change," I say, realizing as the words come out that *I* want to sleep through the night.

"Well...I don't know...I don't think I'll take anything, well, maybe, I'll think about it. Right now I want to brush my teeth."

Right now I want to strangle him.

"You're kind of pushy tonight," he says before shuffling down the hall.

When I hear the bathroom door close, I root around in his medicine basket till I find it, then take half a Xanex. After a second, I swallow the other half, too.

I sleep well and in the morning feel surprisingly calm. Then, while I'm fixing breakfast I remember taking the Xanex. Marty's bright and chatty this morning, how wonderful. After I went to bed, he settled on one dropperful of morphine and half a Xanex, and only woke once, around 5:00 a.m. He felt anxious and wanted to crawl into bed with me. Anxious—the word he uses repeatedly, that skates over the thin ice of his real fear, the unmentionable "x" of anxious.

"Well, why didn't you? I told you to, if you woke up like that."

"I didn't want to wake you, you have to work today."

"Oh, just get in bed with me if you wake up again feeling that way." This morning I'll skate over the "x" too.

"Okay," he says grinning, "Next time I will. These eggs are delicious, I think I'll even have another half cup of coffee." I'm suddenly so happy Marty wants more coffee. He's nearly given it up lately, for health reasons, claims the coffee connoisseur, who's drunk lattés, cappuccinos, French roast, Colombian, dark roast, light roast, coffee, coffee, coffee for years. Marty, who taught me to disdain the use of low-fat milk in coffee: "It makes it the wrong color, it doesn't taste right and, besides, what's wrong with fat?" Cholesterol's the least of Marty's problems. I pass him the half-and-half.

At nine o'clock, the morning nurse arrives for the day's first infusion. Marty looks more gaunt in the morning light, cheekbones more prominent every day, but he's so cheerful this morning, so gracious with his nurse. Now I don't want to go to work, and think about calling in sick. Marty would love to have me with him all day, but I think of how much I wouldn't earn, how much I owe, expenses for the week, the holidays ahead—I'm going to buy that Christmas tree after work, today, and decide not to call in sick.

I turn left onto Eureka Street, to see the yellow blaze of ginkgoes again. Sadness—with no resolution for it this morning—wells up in me, and I linger longer than usual, finally stopping the car in the middle of the street. I think of the ginkgoes all the way downtown, forgetting them only after the rush of work comes at me.

January 7, 1992

10:00 a.m. I'm at work when I call Marty's hospital room to check on him. David answers: "Marty got up last night to go to the bathroom and tried walking to the toilet, but he collapsed halfway there, the nurses found him on the floor and got him back into bed. He's not responding to anything, his doctor's not sure if he'll snap out of it, like he did a few days ago after they brought him to the hospital after he fainted at home, maybe this is it, I can't tell..."

I arrange to leave work, call Ruven in his office, then wait on the corner of Battery and Sacramento where he picks me up ten long minutes later.

The too familiar scene in the hospital room: David and his lover Reggie, Marty's father and stepmother are grouped around the bed. Shortly after Ruven and I arrive, Terry comes in. Marty's breathing is labored, his long neck stretched out from the exertion, like a horse's neck, I keep thinking. After half an hour David, Ruven and I go to the cafeteria for coffee and lunch. David's been at the hospital since 8:00 a.m. and wonders aloud again, "Is this it? Or will Marty go on like this for hours, for days? What if he dies while we eat lunch?" We're all like rubber bands stretched to their limit, ready to snap.

We return to Marty's room. He's the same. This could go on for a long time. Everyone quietly settles into something: quiet chatter, reading newspapers, gazing out the window, pacing. Then Terry goes up to Marty and says, "Marty, I'm going to massage your feet for a while, okay?" Hearing is supposed to be the last thing to go. She takes his right foot and gently kneads it. After a few minutes I decide to massage his other foot, but first I have to pee. When I stand, David looks up from reading *The Chronicle* and glances at Marty. "Is he breathing?" David asks quietly. Everyone looks at Marty's chest, waiting for it to rise. But the eyes play tricks, so used to seeing the chest inflate...A certain moment, January 7th, 1992, 1:38 p.m. All the leaves fall.

In memory of Marty Selim,
and all we have lost to AIDS.
And for all surviving these losses,
and for Ruven, love.

MY CHILDHOOD FRIEND

FELICE PICANO

James was my childhood friend. I don't mean that I knew him for decades or that we played together back in the fifties in Arizona. I met James only last year, a little more than a year ago in fact. It was an all-day writing/publishing seminar hosted by the Publishing Triangle and I was a panelist. Afterwards, as I helped fold up chairs and put them away, I said hello to an acquaintance. James was with him and introduced himself to me in that most startlingly forthright way of his. He asked, "Are you seeing anyone?"

It took me half a minute to figure out that I'd been asked out on a date. I fudged a little, then said I didn't date. James said that was okay, he didn't mean *that* kind of a date anyway. He got my phone number and phoned a few days later. It took only one dinner at a local restaurant for me to discover James hadn't been lying. This wasn't an ordinary date and James wasn't an ordinary person. Although he said he was attracted to me, he also told me he was HIV-positive and symptomatic, and although he played it down I already knew from experience what that meant: a fine romance, with no kisses.

That first evening James made his pitch: what he wanted in me, his new friend, he said, was not a lover, not a boyfriend, not a sex-buddy: what he wanted was someone to go out with occasionally, to talk with about books and writing, current events, nature and science. James had recently developed a foot infection and he couldn't get around that well until it slowly healed. So he was bicycling. He wanted me to get a bike and bicycle with him. He promised to teach me how to play chess, which oddly enough I'd never learned. He promised me we'd see interesting new places and have fun.

And so it was. I got a bike from a friend who'd had an accident with it and whose father had fixed it—not at all well. I dragged the bike home on the subway and together James and I fixed it in my living room. Then, pleased with our labor, we went bike riding. It had been years since I'd biked in Manhattan, but James knew all the short cuts, all the untrafficked routes, all the choice little off-ways and by-streets. He showed me lower Manhattan by day—and even more interesting—by night. One of us would hear of a fireworks display or unusual 19th Century clipper ship berthed at the South Street Seaport or a jazz concert at Battery Park or a Dominican gala at some East River Park and we'd jump on our bikes and take off. And he did teach me chess. Not that I play brilliantly, but I sometimes win and I know when I'm losing and can generally make even that interesting for my opponent.

Sometimes a friend would join us in our bike jaunts, and several times James and I found ourselves bicycling right into the middle of hot spots: the Democratic Convention where we'd snuck behind police lines to get a better look; Chinatown and Little Italy on the night of the Fourth of July with people tossing wrapped tenpack sticks of firecrackers under our bicycle wheels as we tried to speed away before they exploded. More often we found ourselves exploring areas we barely knew or had only heard of—an amazing residential suburb hidden deep in Harlem uptown, a tiny craftspersons' colony behind the smokestacks of industrial Brooklyn. James would call me up at ten o'clock or even later on a summer night and tell me to meet him downstairs: he wanted to go bike riding. And as with any childhood friend, I would hesitate only a minute then sacrifice my TV, movie or book to meet him. When I'd arrive downstairs, he'd be in the lobby, sitting on the stone bench opposite the doorman, his lame foot sticking out, looking pensive. But he'd stand up and greet me with his leprechaun smile. "This is what I thought we'd do tonight," he would begin, breathlessly as though already in the middle of doing it. Or "I've been thinking about this article I read today in the *Times* Science Section." And we'd be off.

For me, the last few years have been a sort of second childhood. Not because suddenly I'm rollerskating and bike riding and playing backgammon, chess, checkers—all childhood activities. But because with the death of my last close friends and especially with the death of my companion of sixteen years, I've found myself suddenly at sea, unsure where I'm going and why, where I've been and what it could possibly signify, confused as to what I'm still doing here when so many are gone. Loss unmoors us. Twelve years of constant devastating loss have snapped my guide lines, cut my guy wires. I exist in a child's world again: fearful, uncomprehending, not knowing what to do next.

James was fascinated by this aspect of my life. For him, it was only with the arrival of his positive—fatal—HIV test results that his own childhood really ended, only then that James found himself a journal-writer, a poet, a book-craftsman, a computer aficionado, as a grownup. James' views of gay life were by no means entirely positive when I first met him. Because of his background and especially his ultraconservative mother who'd raised him alone, James had fought his homosexuality much of his life. He'd been married, had a son, divorced, entered destructive relationships with men involving drugs. While I'd existed for decades within a large, creative, sophisticated, beneficent gay environment—an environment now obliterated by death, James seemed barely to touch gay life. And when he did, he'd found it exotic, and after all not very consequential. Now, it thrilled him to suddenly have new male friends, like myself and several others, with whom he could be fully himself: gay friends with whom he could talk and argue and discuss and discover and grow.

Once he came to know me better, James also found a task: to reconcile me to life. Although I was healthy, I'd grown sick of living. With everyone I'd ever loved dead, I was repulsed and disgusted by the teeming throngs of the unheeding who were alive. Although he was often sick and in pain, James loved life, not with the desperate grasp of the ill, but with the sane curiosity of the healthy. He simply wanted more of it. We would bike ride late at night downtown through the immense, empty, echoing lighted-at-midnight buildings of Wall Street and the Financial Center, then back home past the Clinton Street Housing Projects and we'd stop for hot bialys just made that minute at Yonah Shimmel's Knishes Bakery and as we chewed our fresh-baked bread from astride our ten-speeds, James would wonder about the life of every family in those immense projects, every person behind those scores of windows and tiny balconies.

We argued of course. We'd bicycle a while, then he would tire and we'd stop for a rest at that circular park in the heart of Stuyvesant Town, or at the little blue-lighted wooded-over harbor area at the end of Battery Park City on the Hudson with Miss Liberty in full view, the lights of the Verazzano Bridge dancing in the distance, or that miles-long bike path that runs along the East River, where we'd stop to face a spectacular view of the Williamsburg and Brooklyn Bridges, the Domino Sugar sign behind them. Once in these perfect settings, we'd attack each other's most cherished beliefs.

James couldn't understand my intense misery, my sense of loss of the world I'd lived in so long. When, as he would point out gesturing around us, there was so much still to have. What was the difference how much there was around us, I would argue, when I didn't want any of it, while what I did want I could never again have. I was being foolish, sentimental, wasteful, James would counter. He'd clearly never loved as well as I had, nor had he ever had friends and lovers as worthwhile as mine, I'd say, or he would realize the immensity of the loss. James used his optimism, his cheerfulness to cudgel me into thinking his way. I'd use my bitterness and cynicism and his own health condition against him, cruelly as a stiletto. All this, James would say, and I wouldn't even grasp at it. All this, I'd respond, and it would all be taken from his grasp so very soon.

Then we'd get on our bikes and ride again, and all the frightful things we'd said to each other would vanish. We'd point out details as we rode past them, signs, people out late, like childhood pals who'd fought hard and gotten dirty, then got up, brushed themselves off and were pals again. We'd arrive at his building or mine and hug and shake hands and make a tentative date for our next outing. James never managed to eliminate my depression. I never managed to dent his optimism, his belief in the future.

Even during his one, mercifully short, final stay in the hospital, James was always finding something new to learn and discover. When he could do so, he'd be upstairs in the Sloan-Kettering library and whenever I would visit I'd be told to bring only serious magazines, *Natural History*, *Discovery*, *Scientific American*, *The Atlantic*. As James' body weakened, it seemed paradoxically that his spirits rose, his cheerfulness grew, his mind lifted free to range farther and farther.

Once or twice, when I visited, James even said he hoped to get well soon so we could go bike riding again. He thought it would be a really good summer for bike riding. So far, it has been. I bicycle to some of the same places we went to, along the East River around the lower tip of Manhattan to the Staten Island Ferry, across the Brooklyn Bridge to Cobble Hill and of course down to the Hudson River parks. But I bring my Walkman or a book now. And even if I do miss James, I'm seldom alone. For while it's unclear whether or not James succeeded in reconciling me to life, it is clear what he gave me—himself and those parts of my own city I'd not seen or had forgotten. Both are gifts of inestimable value.

James kept me distracted and interested and intrigued and sometimes irritated every moment we were together. He did so selfishly and selflessly, as a child would: James was my childhood friend.

For James Turcotte, childhood friend,
Nov. 30, 1945–May 11, 1993

A Travel Back

Darrell A. Pittman

A few years ago, I traveled back to Los Angeles for the death of my best friend, David Trujillo. I had relocated back to Detroit one year previously to that April. I missed David terribly through that first year. When I left L.A. due to personal illness, I didn't think that I would ever see David again. He had already been diagnosed with Pneumocystis pneumonia. I knew I had to leave the big city to get back to my family, but it was extremely difficult. How do you say goodbye, when it may be the last?

When David's lover Gary called me in Detroit that April evening, I could hear the coming event in his tired voice. He said that David wanted to see me before he died. I now remember crying and telling him that I just didn't have the money. I was embroiled in a battle to get my social security benefits. Money was nonexistent.

I was then living with my other best friend Kevin. He said that he would pay for both of us to go to L.A. with his income tax refund. I couldn't thank him enough for such a gift. I would be able to spend what became the last month of David's life by his side. I would never have thought that such a thing would be happening to me at twenty-eight years old. I didn't think that I myself would be living with AIDS. I didn't know that by my late twenties, I would be used to experiencing death as a combat soldier at war. I didn't know that four letters of the alphabet would turn my life upside down, leaving me to sort out the pieces.

I didn't know that I would watch my best friend die.

My friend Kevin and I took a Greyhound bus cross-country. I kept worrying that my timing would be off, and David might die before I could reach him. However, the bus was all that Kevin could afford, and I certainly wasn't complaining. Through the three-day trip, I couldn't help imagining the worst. I would arrive the moment he passed away, unable to hold him and tell him everything I needed to say. None of these things happened, luckily, but it was still a tense three days. I was very distant and withdrawn from Kevin, but he took it like a true friend. The thing I remember the most was a song that was popular at the time by Oleta Adams. It spoke of getting to someone at all costs. It mirrored everything I felt at the time. That song still makes me cry.

I silently spoke to David in my mind. I pleaded with him to hang on. After his death, his lover Gary told me that he believes the knowledge of my arrival kept David going. Riding on that bus, staring out at the dark farmlands, I thought of everything that David was to me.

For a few years, we were brothers. We both knew that our relationship was predestined. It wasn't anything obvious, we just knew it. Staring out that bus window, huddling down into my jacket, I remembered it all...

I went to Ventura, California with a lover in the summer of 1987. I was twenty-four years old, and I still thought I had the world on a leash. I had everything I ever wanted in life. I had a lover, a job, and I could now live in California where I always wanted to be. Life was really going well.

Well, within a year, my father died in Detroit, my lover walked out at Christmas, and I was severely gay-bashed on a beach. That's how life can be sometimes, and, come to think of it, probably will always be. The point is that it was a hell of a rude awakening to a spoiled, only child who had never depended on himself before. I guess I needed to grow up, and life was giving me one long crash course.

After all of the disasters settled, I moved from Ventura to L.A. with a newfound friend, Michael. We shared an apartment in West Hollywood, and so began my adventures in the great City of Angels.

The only angel in my life would soon exist in the form of a small, dark-haired Indian man, with an attitude that never stopped.

David might have looked more like a Hell's Angel in his leather, riding his Suzuki Savage motorcycle. The first time I met him, I was actually a little intimidated by him. That would soon change. Like in the first ten minutes.

Surprisingly enough, I stayed friends with my ex-lover Larry, even after I moved to L.A. I say this is surprising because of the extenuating circumstances associated with our breakup. Whatever the reason, I'm glad that I did. Larry's new boyfriend invited me to a party with them at his friend David's apartment. I almost didn't go, but I figured what the hell. I didn't have many friends in L.A. yet. I might as well be social.

When we arrived, I was introduced to David, and I know this sounds corny, but our eyes actually locked for a moment. We just looked at each other, knowing we were there because it was right. By the end of that first evening, David and I were at one end of the couch, with a lot of bored guests around us. We talked like we knew each other our entire lives. The bonding was natural. Everyone else kept commenting that they couldn't get a word into our conversation. It was something they would have to get used to in the next few years.

Los Angeles was a different creature to adjust to for a boy raised in small-town Florida, later small-town midwest. I had a difficult time getting used to everything, but David was a native, and he showed me the ropes.

This was a time when my self-esteem was smashed to bits. My problems had followed me around the country. L.A. is the type of place that feeds on instability, so it was great that David was there to be my boost.

He was the most confident man I ever met. His good looks and personality were astounding to me. I stood back and admired him at least once a day. This sometimes bothered David because he didn't like being put on a pedestal. I didn't realize that he was trying to help me find my own pedestal. David would hug me when I tried and failed, but he would turn away if I didn't try at all.

The first time I had to ride on the back of his motorcycle, I was terrified. I kept whining (a horrible habit left over from childhood), and David just sat down on the bike and started the engine. He told me that I had a choice. Either I could give in to my fear and sit at home, or I could ride around L.A. and see it like I had never thought possible. I tentatively climbed on. After that, I rode it hundreds of times. David showed me every spot of L.A. that was off the beaten path. David knew that I could do it, but he also knew that I had to know. Taking risks was one of the biggest lessons that David taught me.

Eventually, the bus pulled into L.A. The ride was hell, but I wanted to see David immediately. I went to his Section Eight apartment the first day we arrived. I didn't know what to expect when I went into his bedroom. When my father died, I arrived after he went into a coma. The sight of him lying on the hospital bed still haunted my thoughts. I was expecting to see the worst with David.

The person I found was a man whose strength and integrity were still intact. He was very weak physically, and he weighed no more than a feather, it seemed. However, the light in his eyes still existed. It was the same look as when our eyes first met. David's spirit was as strong as ever.

The next four weeks would be filled with visits to his bedside. My heart ached every time his body went into spasms of coughing. He insisted on smoking pot, even though his fragile lungs could barely handle it. I knew that the pot was easing the body pains and the mental stress that he tried so hard to hide.

We talked about our lives and all of the fun we had together. One of our favorite things to do was to visit different cemeteries and look at all of the ornate headstones. These particular memories were very somber for me, considering the circumstances. I could not bear the thought of visiting David's grave. I just couldn't believe that he was going to die. It's funny how a person can have death staring him in the face and still cling to the thought that the person will survive against all odds. I was, I suppose, experiencing a slight case of denial at that point.

The weeks went by too quickly. There is never enough time to spend with someone when he or she is dying. I feel lucky that I had at least four weeks to spend with him. Most people wouldn't get that opportunity. When it came time for me to leave and go back to Michigan, I visited David for what I knew would be the absolute last time. I cannot describe the feelings that swirled around inside of me that day. What would I say? How could I express all of the love that I felt for David? It seemed impossible to put all of it into words. I knew it was my last chance, but I didn't know how to start.

I expressed all of this to David. He told me to sit on the bed and put my arms around him. He felt so fragile underneath my hands. It was one of the first times that I felt like David's support. He had gotten me through so much, and now I needed to help him. We lay there for about an hour not speaking, just hugging each other. Finally I stumbled for the right words, but David said it wasn't necessary. He said we both knew all that we needed to know. I hugged him harder, and we both began to cry. I stroked his long, dark hair with my fingers. I put my face in the base of his neck. I wanted to remember how he felt and smelled that last day. I still do remember.

We had to say goodbye. I told him that I would call him after the bus ride back to Detroit. He told me to get his Batman watch from the dresser and take it with me. David was a Batman fanatic, and the watch rarely left his own arm the entire time I knew him. We had stood in line together for four hours for the premiere of the original movie at Mann's Chinese Theater. I treasure that watch. I still wear it today.

When I left his apartment in tears, I stood looking at his bedroom window from the street. It was as if my feet were unable to move. After standing there for a while, I knew I had to leave and walk away.

I knew the bus trip back to Detroit would be the longest trip of my life. My best friend, and ultimately, a main part of my Los Angeles life, would now be gone forever.

After returning to Detroit three days later, my friend Kevin and I had to go to a party at another friend's home the next evening. I didn't really want to go, but Kevin insisted that it might cheer me up.

During the party, I felt an overwhelming sense of despair, and I walked out to the back sundeck to sit and stare at the stars in the night sky. The party was not going well for me, but I had suspected that it wouldn't.

As I was sitting there, I suddenly felt David's presence. I could feel him all around me. I had heard of such experiences, but I never really believed them one way or the other. I heard David's voice whisper to me, "I'm gone now, Darrell. Everything is wonderful. There isn't any reason to be upset." As quickly as I felt him, I was suddenly left alone. I sat staring at the stars, crying uncontrollably. It was over, and David had chosen to say goodbye one last time.

When I returned to my mother's home that evening (I had moved in just before the trip), I asked Kevin to come inside. I knew that I would need his moral support. I knew that my mom would give me a phone message. When I entered the door, she said that Gary had called from L.A. and that David had died. I had hoped that I was wrong, but I knew that I wouldn't be. He was gone.

Looking back, I feel blessed that I had a relationship such as ours. Even in death, David and I were bound in spirit. People like that don't come along often enough in someone's life. I'm just glad that I had the experience. I miss him, but I know he went on to something wonderful. After all, he told me so himself.

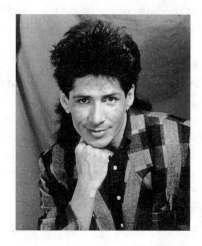

In memory of my soul mate:
David Trujillo
May 19, 1958–May 3, 1991

Going Home (A Nonfiction)
May 1990

Hernán Poza III

Tuesday, a.m., Nicholas' apartment

His "God's Love We Deliver" meal arrives as we are preparing to leave for his clinic appointment at the hospital. We're interrupted in our discussion about his deteriorating condition, the painful admission that very little about his body is holding together anymore, that he may likely be admitted into the hospital during or after the clinic checkup.

The delivery man, handsome, cheerful and gregarious, mentions that he heard that Nicholas has three birds looking for a good home. He says he has an aviary at home and would love to adopt them. It's quickly agreed that he can have them, he skillfully and gently catches them, places them into the carrier cage. As he leaves he promises to give us an update tomorrow on the birds' acclimation to their new home.

Suddenly the apartment is unnaturally quiet, "I've had those birds a lot of years," he says, tears running down his cheeks, "I'm glad they have a good home. How quickly that happened, he seems like a really nice guy. I guess it's a relief…" He pauses and begins to smile as he stares at the now empty aviary, "Too bad I probably won't be here to see what tomorrow's meal is. Wouldn't it be a little suspicious if it was miniature squabs?"

Tuesday, p.m., Infectious Disease Clinic/Memorial Sloan-Kettering

The doctor leaves the examining room, her face flushed, hair disheveled, eyes red and tearing. He is sitting up on the examining table trying to pull the gown around his emaciated, purple-scarred body. I step into the room, he looks up at me, his eyes catch mine, the terror jumps from his eyes and my heart leaps. I can't breathe, I can't take my eyes away from his. "I'm going to die. She told me I have maybe a few weeks, if I'm lucky maybe months. She says it's just gone too far, my body is shot. I thought I had more time. I'm thirty years old. I don't want to die, I don't know how to die. What do I do? How will I die? I don't want to die. Who will tell me what to do? Oh, God." We hug fiercely, my arms squeezing his frail body, his sobs and tears exploding into my neck and chest.

Thursday, p.m., room 409, Memorial Sloan-Kettering

I enter his hospital room, his eyes connect with mine and he says brightly, "When I go home we're going fishing together, my dad and me, he says he knows a perfect spot. He says he can bring the car right up to the shore and we'll just sit and fish in the sun. Now that we're both retired, we can go as much as we want."

His eyes look out, looking through the hospital wall, past the I.V. tubes, the oxygen tank, the "Warning/Fluid Caution" signs, past the dirty, crowded city. Looking out over the faraway lake of his childhood, the lake of his memories, over the icy clear waters, the clean blue Washington sky. His father sits next to the bed, also looking off, through the hospital walls, perhaps visiting the lake, holding his son's hand, tears running down his face.

Monday, p.m., birthday party, room 409, Memorial Sloan-Kettering

It's his thirty-first birthday and he lights up the hospital room from his bed, telling a story to the gathered friends about late-night TV, the addictive, seductive, thirty-minute "infomercials" for fantastic products and dramatic, sensational charities; his story is about watching too much TV and the resulting brain damage.

"...that cellulite show, with the fabulous, glamorous beauty queen, Erin Grey, interviewing the equally fabulous inventor of the diet plan. 'Tell me,' she asks, leaning across the glamorous coffee table, dripping jewelry and fashion towards her guest, `Is it true that you have no cellulite on your entire body, just between you and me, just between us girls, is it really true?'"

He then reflects on another marathon commercial for world hunger and saving the children.

"… I could just see it, the fabulous Erin Grey, sitting in her glamorous interview set, across from some starving third-world woman, Erin leaning across the coffee table saying, "Tell me, is it true, just between you and me, just between us girls, is it really true that you've had two (holding up two fabulously manicured, ringed fingers), two children die from malnutrition this year alone?' "

He is delighted with the selection of outrageous rhinestone costume jewelry I have given him. (His original rhinestone bracelet having 'disappeared' from his room the day before.)

He is very animated, laughing and putting on the earrings, the necklace, I have to help him fasten the bracelet, his arm is so thin that the bracelet slides easily up to his elbow. The rhinestones are bright, sparkling against the purple lesions.

A nurse comes into the room abruptly to adjust and check his I.V. tubes, seeing the mob of people, the balloons, the rhinestone jewelry, she is confused and loudly asks if this is some type of costume party. The crowd of friends is suddenly, awkwardly silenced. Shaking the fabulous bracelet away from the I.V., without batting an eye, without hesitation, Nicholas brightly tells her, "Oh no, it's my birthday today and I'm a fag, you know, and fags are allowed to give each other and wear tacky jewelry like this, *especially* on our birthdays!"

The room suddenly erupts into stunned laughter, the nurse's face evolves from shock to embarrassment, to a warm loving smile as she briskly says, "Well then, a Happy Birthday to you then, I hope you let me try on that bracelet some time!"

Tuesday, late a.m., hospital corridor, Memorial Sloan-Kettering

His mom is in the corridor alone, crying. I ask what has happened and she says, "I was doing just fine, just fine, and then he started talking about his funeral. About how he wants a simple ceremony like his grandma had. I was thinking, he was so young when she died, I just can't believe that he remembers. Then I realized that I can't do this, I can talk about my mother's funeral, I can talk about my funeral, his dad's funeral…But not his, he's my baby. I can't talk to my baby about his funeral. I just can't." She's crying, her tears running off her crumpled raincoat as she hugs me.

Tuesday, late p.m., room 409, Memorial Sloan-Kettering

I come into his room late after visiting hours; it's the night before he is to leave to go to the airport at 6:30 a.m. in an ambulance with his parents, going home, to his childhood home which he hasn't seen in many years, going home ("to die" he says repeatedly, brutally).

"My parents went shopping today at Macy's, to buy the makeup that the cosmetologist recommended to cover the lesions on my face, to make it easier for the trip. I wish you could've been here to hear my dad going on about the stuff. 'I'm telling you, Donna, we should've bought the complete set, came with a lot of other stuff, with powder, a brush and a nice little carrying case, real nice stuff, such a selection.' "

He laughs, "I think Dad just might have a new twist on his at-home retirement work. I can just see it now, back home in our neighborhood, the sign out front changed to "Wayne's Motorcycle & Car Repair/Mr. Wayne's Cosmetology Salon.""

Tuesday, later p.m., room 409, Memorial Sloan-Kettering

"I can feel the love from you," he says, holding my hand from across the bed. "I feel it in so many ways, the things you do, the things you always just know how to do without me asking, the way you look at me, I can feel the love in your eyes every time. It seems that I'm not here, that this isn't happening, when I'm with you. I don't understand why that is, why you should love me like this, why I deserve this, I don't understand. You know, you're my family, I'm so glad you're still here after all this, my family."

Starting to cry, I reach over the cold bars on the side of the bed, careful of the I.V. tubes, an awkward obstructed hug, growing tighter and more powerful, my tears unleashing in a torrent, overwhelming sobs burst forth as I hold his frail, pained body in my trembling arms.

"You know, it's about time," he says (about my tears). "I was worried that you were perfect, now I know, you are, it's okay, it's okay…"

Wednesday, very early a.m., Northwest Airline terminal— Kennedy Airport

I rush into the airline terminal, late, with the "babies," three cats, sitting, curiously peering out from their travel boxes. I pause and scan the floor. I see him, sitting at the check-in counter in his wheel-chair, holding his cane (the one with the ugly bulldog head). Looking closely, seeing him clearly, I'm paralyzed, unable to move or breathe. He's suddenly fine, healthy, a handsome, tired-looking young man waiting for his flight home, jet-lagged maybe. Wearing his favorite sweater and leather jacket, eyes staring off, his face lost in deep thought. His gaze drifts over in my direction, he sees me, the "babies," and a smile shines from his face, melting my paralysis. My heart pounding wildly, I stumble awkwardly forward, putting the boxes by his side. I reach down for him. In my hug I can feel his frag-ile body through the many sweaters he is wearing, I smell his hair, clean, fresh and sweet like a little boy's. His beard is soft against my face, his makeup mixes with my tears, rubbing off, onto my face and collar. His parents join the embrace. "It's time for us to go now," they say gently. "Early boarding." It's time for him to go home now, going home, going home to die.

Tuesday, September 12, Gay Community News, Obituaries

Nicholas Dana LaCasse, 31, died from complications related to AIDS at his childhood home in Bellingham, Washington, on Wednesday, August 1st.

Nicholas lived passionately and fiercely with HIV for over five years before returning to his parents' home in late May. Mr. and Mrs. LaCasse dedicated themselves to providing their son with compas-sionate, respectful care during his time with them. His hospice visit-ing nurse remarked that she had never seen anyone in such serious condition receiving such superb care from parents alone.

Nicholas was an active member of the Lavender Heights Neighborhood Association during his years in Washington Heights. Through his interest in holistic approaches to living with HIV, Nicholas was involved with and known to HEAL, Healing Circle, POWARS, Integral Yoga, Water-of-Life, ACT UP, PWA coalition and GMHC.

Nicholas will be remembered for his incredible strength, courage and bravery in the face of his illness, for his quick, biting wit and his sarcastic sense of humor, for his intense will to live and passion for life as well as a gift of charm and charisma that made him a person not to be forgotten by any who were blessed to know him.

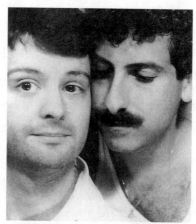

Nicholas, left

For Nicholas, in loving memory
Nicholas Dana LaCasse
May 14, 1959–Aug. 1, 1990

DEAREST RACHEL

MARCIA ROSE

Dearest Rachel,
It is eight months to the day since your death. How can it be? I used to count every day until you were born! I went down to the Dept. of Public Health to pick up a copy of your death certificate. It was a perfunctory process that I had put off for months. That building is old and cold and used. It reminds me of Duggan's funeral home, the last place we saw your body. At least there we had rainbow balloons, wild-flowers and Jacob's sweet, sad singing! I sat on a bench waiting and wondering if the woman at the counter thought very much about all of the names. I'm certain she does. There are so many young people who die. Did she notice what they died from, what kind of work they did, whatever became of their bodies?

Just one block down is your old apartment at 55 Polk, here in the heart of it all. There were lots of people lined up at the Tom Waddell clinic this morning. Anyway, we celebrated your twenty-sixth birthday at that apartment. You were sick that day. That year you went to the hospital so much. You always thought someone was going to bash out the windows. Lots of mornings on my way to work I look over at that building. It's weird but today I noticed that those street level windows had been busted out. Someone had tried to repair them with a piece of wood. That big mean guy with the diabetes is still the manager. I never liked that place either. It was so dark and so enclosed.

I'm still working at the same place. I don't take care of people with HIV anymore. I ache for you so much. I don't have adequate personal resources. I stopped when you came home to California. I think about you and Richard and Matthew. I think about and remember you every single day and night. Sometimes I go to demonstrations. I went to a funeral procession at the Capitol in Sacramento after the governor vetoed the needle exchange bill. You might like to know that we exchange needles anyway! I write to women in prison who have HIV. I picket and chant outside the prison for all of the women with HIV who are locked inside. You could have been there so easily. I'm making a dark, strong quilt piece for you. It's black and purple satin. I'm also putting together one for you and Matt. It's from the design you made. Jessica designed the rainbow. I have started a drawing for you, too. I want to write and talk. I hold on, Rachel. Sometimes I'm so angry! Some other days I'm feeling you are somewhere safe and beautiful. Then again, I could throw myself down in a heap from broken-heartedness.

I got out this poem I wrote to you when you were living in New York City. You were on the streets with Matt. Then I was taking care of lots of people with HIV. I was doing hospice work. I knew you were probably in deep trouble. I thought of you each time I cared for someone. I was looking for you. It never occurred to me to read you any of the things I had written, until now. I'm always working to make sense out of no sense.

Jessica is in rehab now. She ended there three months after you died. She ran away again the day of your funeral. She is sober now. You'd be "hella proud" as she'd say. Jacob is plugging along at White Hill. They don't want him there so he will go to Special Ed. He'll be thirteen in two weeks. I remember how you weren't so sure about treatment programs. It's a chance for change. Goddess knows we all could use that, don't you think?

I recall your childhood. It was so troubled, unsafe and lonely for you. I have a picture of you at eleven out in front of the garage. It's summer. The picture is a marker, a sharp memory of time slipping away, out of control. You have your arms folded defiantly in front of your chest. Your head is tilted to the side and your smile is mischievous, rebellious, tinged with the hint of adolescent anger. Your body is tiny. You were still a little girl.

You started using when you were so young. You did all those programs. It seems as if you just left one day with Matt. Then he was hostile, manipulative, handsome. Soon you had a heroin habit. Once during those years Nancy found you. She sent me stark, lonely pictures
in which you were thin and pale, heavily made up. Once in a while you
would call me. Calls would come from Bellevue. Endocarditis, kidney
failure, a slipped disc, detox. You'd end up in Miami, Atlanta. I have
the letter you sent when you told me you were HIV-positive. Your life
got harder and harder. Matt would hurt you and you'd want to come
home. You called yourself a junkie then. You and Matt were working
until he got too sick.

I was so relieved and scared when you and Matt came back to
California. He had barely made it through that episode of pneumonia. It was time to come home. Remember all those "famous" snapshots I took at the bottom of the front stairs of your new apartment?
Matt was kissing you on your rosy, round cheek. He was pale and thin.

Your new place was nice. You started using not soon after you
moved in. I'd not hear from you for a week or two and I'd start to worry.
You tended to isolate yourself when things got rough. It took me so
long to realize that you were protecting yourself, protecting us from the
despair of these episodes. I knew how ashamed you were. Finally, I'd
just get in the car and drive up to see you. Your place would be ruined,
your nicest things smashed and filthy. There'd be no food in the refrig-
erator. Sometimes your hands would be cut or burned from cigarettes.
Matt would be gone. One day I drove up and the house was silent,
shades drawn, no sign of you anywhere. The back windows were broken out and blood was spattered over the back porch floor and walls.
The smell of garbage was heavy and huge flies buzzed and crawled on
everything. My dread was so deep I decided to call the police. At that
moment I saw you coming down the street. You looked good and you
were smiling. Oh, Rachel, I was so glad to see you! I hated the pain.
There was always such predictable unpredictability to things.

At first I attempted to be with you when you were high. I got confused, sad and angry a lot. Back then it was hard figuring out what to
do. It still is. It put us all in a precarious, unsafe situation. I'd just want
to have time with you. Trying to control, trying to hold on. I returned
to twelve-step meetings and I agonized. Then I came to the decision
that I couldn't be around you when you were using. It was painful for
us both but it was a powerful decision. As you became sicker that

boundary changed somewhat. I just knew there would be consequences. I think we missed time but we also missed more crisis and confusion.

Matt's time got more and more fragile and precarious. He remained angry and withdrawn. He'd also flash that sweet smile now and again. He was proud and frightened. He certainly gave people a run for their money. He seemed to try and be tough sometimes. His respiratory distress could have been lessened by oxygen but he did not want nurses or anyone telling him what to do. He suffered. You cared for him. You suffered. I know you were afraid and that you were strong. People gave you shit for having HIV. You told us they threw eggs at your house and called you "the AIDS girl."

We sat at the table on Thanksgiving eve, myself, Jessica, Jacob and Judy. I was expecting your call. Matt had gone to the hospital the night before. I felt numb and in some heavily fogged place of denial and sorrow. "Mom, talk to Matt now." His voice was very distant and faint, a whisper, a strangling. "Marcia, take care of Rachel for me. I can't talk anymore. Goodbye." Then you left the hospital to feed your animals. When you came back, he had died. You tried to do CPR. You tried to save your man. They had to take you out of there. You staggered around in shock. You got high. You said he was free at last and over the rainbow.

A lonely funeral stuck out in Lodi. No peers, no friends, a few rehab counselors, a kind, cool-looking nurse. Someone had run off with all the donations from the people at the methadone program. Matt's mom had put up some pictures: a newborn, a cute third grader and a very serious, sullen, looking twelve year old. You got up and pinned a crumpled picture of you and Matt on a wreath. A strong, proud, sweet reminder. I was so moved by that act of yours. No one had asked you, Matt's partner, what you might want and need. Everything was just whisked away. There was no place for you to go, no ashes, no gravesite, no acknowledgment of the relationship you had. I know your grief was vast. You had to bear what is beyond description. I know that so well now.

I decided that I wanted you near us. It was time to come home. It was quite an undertaking to get you here. By then you had gotten close to Richard and he was going to come with you. The day of the move after we loaded up everything in the rented truck, we couldn't find you. We had found a great apartment on Taylor and had everything ready. We were just shifting into panic and there you were; high, unruly, pissed off. You were so sad to leave Stockton behind. You'd be returning to the streets where you met Matt, all the sights and smells and memories and grief to come rushing at you. You had so much courage to return to visit our house and to a town that did not welcome you home, a town that was fearful and ignorant about AIDS. This strange liberal suburban place where you spent your youth as an outcast, a misfit.

We were going to witness the unfolding of HIV, of love and of healing. No matter how unwelcome the visitation of this illness, it also, in a sad, profound, mysterious twist, brought you home. I feel a surge of agony and regret as I write this. It is a process of uncovering and it causes me turmoil and renewed grief. The time was so compressed! I sit here writing and, Rachel, the jolt, the stunning reality that you really did die hits me. Violent loss of you! It was so hard to watch the destruction of blood and bone, of tears and that laugh of yours. I watched as your world shrank down to medication schedules and obsession about your body. At twenty-six, the loss of youth. At first subtle changes, and then the eventual, inevitable horrible bloom of disease and debilitation.

I must have purchased a hundred flowers since you were in the hospital for the last time. I was obsessed. I have watched them slowly bloom, wild and fragrant, new and sweet. I'd try to understand the moments of change, of turning from fullness to death. I tried to hold onto you there. I thought I'd find you there again and again. I still do.

Some days I think a lot about the hard, complicated and desperate times of your life in San Francisco. I drive past all the places your memory haunts. You had toughness and wild rage. There was a place in you of hunger and need and restlessness that consumed you. As your mom, I will always try to understand this. I never will, but the pain of witnessing, of guilt, of anger, of love never changes. I sometimes hate a world in which a sick young woman, my child, could be standing on Ellis and Taylor in the night. Where is the mercy, the love, the accountability of men? I do not have words for this pain, Rachel. I know you did not either.

Because of your decisions about continued drug use, you returned to the streets, to living in a car, a hotel room in the Tenderloin. Even in this "conscious," model AIDS care city with all of its programs and resources, people were shocked by you. There were some kind ones and there were the cruel ones. The stares and the whispers, the absolute silences you often responded to with confrontational direct-ness. You'd tell anyone to fuck off. I admired your streetwise ways. As you became more frail and vulnerable you still wanted to look for your sister Jessica. I have that picture of you walking down Ellis Street, the last day you were able to walk outside. You are wearing your black leather jacket and your smile gives me light and soothes my pain. You have your cane and your cigarettes. You were happy that day. Jessica had gotten a pass from juvenile hall to visit with you. We went to the deli for cigarettes, coffee, fruit salad and ice cream. I did-n't dream that it was our last walk. I didn't dream that I'd carry you up the stairs to the hospital. Although I knew our time was limited, I thought we'd be forever. We had made different plans for your dying.

I remember how you looked when you had just died. My dear lost child, my dear lost girl. I still don't really accept your death. How could I? I see you with your head tilted back, turned partly toward the wall. You looked as if you were concentrating on something far beyond what we could grasp. You would look like that sometimes when you were very tired. It was almost as if you had a glimpse of something quieter, safer, much kinder. I touched your paleness, the smallness of your chest. The morphine was still pumping into your left foot, the oxygen hissing into your nose. I turned it off and removed the tubing. I looked at your beautiful feet, they appeared to be posed and tense. A gracious nurse came in and handed me a cup of coffee. She had a pained and panicked look. It was shift change and she had to leave. I thought she was so kind. What could she have pos-sibly said to me? I just stood there. A mother without a child. I did not know what to do.

I carried your cane, your old leather purse, your toothbrush and shoes, your package of five new cotton underpants out into the huge, dark blue silence of a June night. I struggled with the urge to run back and see you again, hear your voice. Eight hours later Elyse and I would be sitting at Manor School watching Jacob graduate, the same school you went to. No one said a word. No one mentioned our pain.

So, five months later Richard died. He died a few hours after Thanksgiving. The last time I saw him was a few days after your funeral. Elyse and I were wandering on Polk Street (I was looking for you). He had started using again, had locked himself up in the apart-ment, unplugging the phone as he had done when you went into the hospital, locked away to grieve in his own way and time. I saw him coming up the street pale and gaunt carrying some of your things. He was selling them. We saw each other. He crossed the street midblock and disappeared. Except for phone calls, I never saw him again.

I am still here doing much of the same. I'm trying to figure out what to do. I'm still Mom. I see you everywhere. The smells of an old hotel remind me of you. It's the rush of spring. Things are blooming with madness. They are opening and growing and you are not here. Your spirit haunts my days and nights. I pass women on the corners as they stand and talk to each other, turn to motion at the passing cars. I still look for you. I hear your voice and catch a split-second glimpse of you going slowly up the street, thin, persistent, resilient, and the pain goes on and on. I look into the eyes of pale, thin strangers in wheelchairs. My connections, my searches are deep.

> I love you, sweet child,
> Mom

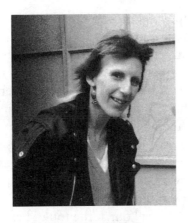

In memory of my second-born child,
Rachel Ellyn.
She was a fat, dark-haired baby angel.
She was born on Feb. 2, 1966,
and died on June 15, 1993.
She died a strong, defiant
and vulnerable angel.

AIDS WARS: D.C. JAIL

Susan Rosenberg

There are no happy endings in this skirmish. Sadness, loss, waste and neglect fill the encounter. In war there is supposed to be purpose and consequently meaning. But in the AIDS wars this story, like many, results from oppression and genocide, the product of the apartheid state of Black people's lives in the nineties in America. But there is a twist, a shining bright spot that illuminates this dark story and casts it in a different light. It is a love story. Love that is condemned and feared, love that is against the law, made illegal by the state, love that in its pure subversiveness intensifies suffering but eases the pain. A story of two Black women who loved and shared and made their way—together—if only for a short time.

I keep hearing Celia call out at the top of her voice, "Rider, Rider, where are you?" "Come here, Rider." And then Rider would answer, "Okay, baby, I'm coming, hang on." Rider would glide down the stairs to the bottom of the tier and slide into her cell and they would talk. Then she'd slide out and go on about her work on the unit. One day I was on the phone and I looked into the cell they shared, that Celia had fixed up. Rider was sitting on their trunk, back against the wall, leaning easy and looking at the bed where Celia was sitting, knees up, and the intensity and intimacy was clear as a day after rain.

Rider was one cool lady, and she has years and years of practice at showing nothing. She lives behind a mask of non-reaction. She's a pro at it. She never loses at poker or spades, never. She reveals nothing. But this feeling she had, this love for this lady, this lovely lady, her partner, she couldn't hide. The tug around her forty-five-year-old eyes right at the outer corner began to turn upward, and the squint lines slowly became laugh lines. Their love affair affected anyone who wanted to be let in. They navigated through the jailhouse rules and prohibitions with practiced grace and ease. The police knew the deal and let them cell together.

One night Rider came to my cell and said, "Celia is sick. She is really sick. Do you understand?"

"Yes, Rider, I think I understand."

For five months Celia hid herself, hoping it would undo her sickness. She wasted in silence. She hid against the rumors, the cruelty of other people's speculation, and the pain of her mental and physical suffering. She never was counseled, the medical care was inadequate and the social neglect criminal. Celia lied to keep it secret, to deny reality, her reality. But Rider knew, I knew. And then she was too sick to stay in the cell block.

Celia was dying in the prison ward of D.C. General Hospital. That her death was inevitable there was no doubt; that it had to be the way it was is left to health officials and prison officials to debate and analyze and then they will factor it into their statistical data. For Rider, nothing could take the stricken look of anguish out from behind her eyes. Rider was powerless to stop Celia from dying. Rider, like Celia, was a prisoner. She didn't count. The fact that Rider and Celia were lesbian lovers for nine years, in and out of prison, together and separately, didn't count. Their love went unrecognized. A lesbian lover is not next of kin. That Rider loved Celia more than anything or anyone, that she took care of her in sickness, that she wanted to spend her life with her, or lie down and die with her, does not count.

Nine days after Celia left the cell block, four days after her thirty-third birthday, Celia died of heart failure from complications from pneumocystis pneumonia associated with the final stages of AIDS. She was a prisoner treated in the intensive care unit at D.C. General. She was initially admitted to the ICU in a code blue state. Her heart had stopped. She was revived and placed on a respirator. During the course of those nine days she went into code blue again, almost died, was revived, and finally failed to respond to drug therapy. She thought Rider was there at the end and said, "Rider, I love you, my baby." A guard who was there told this to another prisoner.

Celia had been serving a nine-month bit on a parole violation. She had been scheduled for release in two months. She died while shackled to the bed. There is no compassion release in the District of Columbia.

The day after Celia died, Rider was at my door telling me that the funeral was Friday. She asked me, should she try to go, could she go, would it be possible for her to go as her husband, or her wife, or anything? After all, she said, I was real family. If I had been free, I'd have been at the hospital.

In general if you're in prison and a family member dies, you don't go to the funeral. It's a question of security, not humanity. But if a "grief furlough" is approved you go in chains accompanied by armed marshals to the funeral home where you are allowed merely a few moments to view the body alone.

Rider decided not to fight it out, not to go. Then she held out a plastic bag filled with jail-issued medications. Cream, pills, and suppositories. She said, "Can you explain all this stuff to me?" The hurt, the search as to what was this thing that took her beautiful girl, snatched her away, will never be answered. But now she had to know. The pills and cream with their specific instructions made it clear. AZT, acyclovir and steroid cream are the only approved medications for prisoners with AIDS. They had been dispensed irregularly and with no monitoring. I explained each medication and its use. And she stood at my door with tears streaming down her face. "I knew she was sick, but I didn't know she'd die. Why didn't she tell me?" And the pitch in her voice dropped to a whisper and she said, "You know, I am a very open-minded person, I would never have left someone that is sick, not ever, and never her. She was, well, you know, I love her."

If Celia had lived a little longer, Rider would have tried for a hospital visit, to take her in her arms one more time, tell her it was all okay and say goodbye. Instead she sent roses with a note to the funeral. The card read "To Celia, my love always, Rider." We heard that Celia's pimp wasn't happy.

To Teresa Paige—
one beautiful sister—age 29

ONCE IN A LIFETIME

SUZANNE SABLAN

I sit here writing this article about my husband Joseph as I recover from MAI tuberculosis. AIDS has changed my life dramatically, but this story is not about me. It is about a man named Joseph Sablan—my husband, lover, and best friend—who knew more about enjoying life than any other person I have ever met. AIDS changed his life, but it did not take away his pride or dignity. I hope this story will provide some inspiration to others suffering from this disease.

Joe was only nineteen when I met him: we worked at an Orlando area hotel together. What attracted me most about him was his bubbly personality: he trained me to do my job with exuberance and a smile. While we did not date for several months, I always enjoyed his company. He had a throaty, full laugh that others found contagious. And although many young women flocked around him, he seemed very shy about dating. So I was surprised when he agreed to go out on a date with me.

The rest is history. After a brief courtship Joe and I eloped. My parents fell in love with Joe, too. He had a passion for cooking that he shared with my mother, and he always knew exactly what to say to endear himself to my siblings. While Joe's family did not welcome me with open arms, they did begrudgingly accept our union. Joe's family was from Guam, and they preferred a traditionally patriarchal union. Our marriage was nothing like that. Joe and I made all decisions—

monetary and otherwise—together. He cooked dinner and cleaned the house more often than I did. In fact, Joe worked two and sometimes three jobs so I could afford to finish my degree at a local private college. Joe loved to shop for clothes for me, and he'd sooner buy me something than buy something that he'd been yearning for. Joe was the most generous man I knew: he was always thinking of others' needs and desires before his own.

We had been happily married for six years when Joe became very ill. At first, he was diagnosed with walking pneumonia. As his condition worsened and he had to be hospitalized, one of the doctors asked permission to run an HIV test. I said sure, because Joe did not fall into any of the high risk groups. He never did drugs, was not bisexual, and had not had blood transfusions. We were both shocked when the test came back positive. I was sure that I had given the virus to Joe, because I had been sexually active before I met him (he had not been). But there was another factor here that we had to consider: both of us had been raped while in our teens, and we could only deduce that one of those attacks had exposed him to the virus. Thus we were not surprised when my HIV test came back positive as well, although my CD4 cells were still in the normal range. The good news was that, once Joe was accurately diagnosed, the doctors were able to treat him effectively.

The period immediately after Joe's diagnosis was a difficult transition for him. His doctor told him he could not work more than one job unless he planned on an early grave. At the time, Joe's main job was as a department store manager, which required him to be at work sixty hours a week. After a lengthy discussion with his manager, Joe moved to a commission position where he would make close to the same salary without the stress of managerial responsibilities. He had to learn to listen to his body and rest when he needed to. Joe never gave up his zest for life, however. We spent a lot of time with our friends and their children. Joe loved kids, and since we now seemed destined never to have our own, he cherished the time he spent playing with our surrogate children.

One wonderful thing happened because of Joe's battle with AIDS: we spent more quality time together as a couple. I had completed my degree by now and was teaching high school English, so I enjoyed the extra time off that teachers get at Christmas and in the summer. We took trips to Nashville and Honolulu—trips we surely would have postponed indefinitely under other circumstances. In fact, one of my most cherished possessions is a videotape of a friend's wedding in Hawaii on which Joe narrated the events. The sound of his cheery voice comforts me. We also made time for dates to go to the movies or the mall. If we had relatives in town visiting, Joe still played tour guide to Disney World or Sea World. Joe did not let the disease control and destroy his life.

I would be remiss if I also did not mention that we began counseling immediately after his diagnosis to help us deal with the crisis. I had been seeing a counselor about dealing with my mother's death in June of 1988, so the counseling just naturally led to the discussion of Joe's illness. Joe began attending sessions with me, and it helped greatly. More than anything, the counseling helped Joe to learn to set limits with those around him. Joe always wanted to be everything to everybody, which meant sometimes that he got burned out when people used him. For example, his father was always asking us for money, or to borrow the lawn mower, and Joe generously helped him out. Well, inevitably, the money was never repaid, and the lawn mower was returned to us in disrepair. I had a tougher resolve about such matters, but Joe's optimistic attitude always caused him to hope for the best. In addition, our counselor helped both of us come to terms with Joe's inevitable death. I still see her, eighteen months after Joe's death, because she not only helps me with my grief, but with my own battle with the disease. Counseling helped us enjoy our time together and appreciate the life around us. This was especially important for Joe, as he became weaker and had to slow down his pace of activities.

Joe did have a few setbacks. He developed MAI tuberculosis in January of 1990. At that point, he had to leave his job and go on permanent disability. That was a very difficult time for him, because he was so used to being busy. Joe did not just sit and vegetate, however; he found a job off the books for about twenty hours a week just to keep busy. He baked banana bread for me to bring to school. He visited friends during their lunch hours and took them out to eat. He took a book to the park and sat in the sun to relax. For someone who was so ill, Joe was busier than some healthy people I knew!

It was obvious by the summer of 1992 that Joe's health was failing. He was not as peppy as usual, and he lost more weight. I watched helplessly as he physically faded before my eyes. But he had a goal to strive for: we were throwing ourselves a big tenth year anniversary party at my father's house. Joe pumped all of his energy into the preparations for that party. My cousin, aunt, brother, and sister all attended, even though they lived in New York, because they knew how important this party was for Joe. My father cooked all of Joe's Italian favorites, and we enjoyed a wonderful party with fifty or sixty of our closest friends and family members in attendance. The day after the party, my aunt and her friend even took Joe to Epcot, where he still played tour guide from his wheelchair.

Joe's death six days later did not completely surprise me because of something he did the night before he died. We had not slept snuggled together in months because Joe was so bony from his weight loss. The night before he died, he slept wrapped around me: I had to slide out of his grip the next morning to go to work. He knew he was dying, and he wanted to be as close to me as possible. Joe showed me right at the end how much he loved me and valued our relationship. Eighteen months after Joe's death, I still get a suffocating ache for him. We loved each other completely and passionately for ten years. I get frustrated with people who ask me if I am angry with Joe for possibly exposing me to this virus. Who infected whom was never an issue for us.

Would I have forfeited my life with Joe because of AIDS? Not on your life. Although his death has left a large void in my life, what I stress to people is not that Joe died of AIDS, but that he lived with AIDS for four years during a time that AIDS patients were expected to live only a year and a half after becoming ill. He did not waste one precious moment feeling sorry for himself or blaming God for his predicament. He treasured the gift of life and shared that enthusiasm with all those around him.

Now I have to deal with the ravages of AIDS. I pray every day for the fortitude and optimism Joe exhibited during his battle with the disease. I will be out of work for the rest of this school year because of complications from the MAI, but my doctors have told me I can return to teach in the fall. I spend my time now seeking outlets for me to share my experiences with others, so they can see that AIDS can affect anyone, of any race, creed, or economic background. I want to share his strength and resolve with others who are faced with AIDS. This is my tribute to my husband: I will continued to fight the battle in his absence. Joe, this is for you.

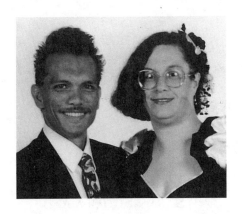

*To my husband of ten years, Joe Sablan,
who died Oct. 9, 1992, after a four year
battle with AIDS.*
*Born Oct. 23, 1961, he was only thirty
years old at the time of his death.*

In the Hall

Susan Schulman

The windows in the small room
are hung with daily print curtains.
Fields of yellow and purple wildflowers
decorate the ivory colored walls.
All the cold medical instruments
are tucked out of sight
in small wooden drawers and cabinets.

But we know where we are—
the black examining table, its paper cover
crinkling under your weight,
the cool metal sink,
clanking medical scale.

The KS is spreading.
Jagged spots populate your body,
colonize your throat and lungs.
You sit on the table,
head bowed,
shoulders drooping,
legs dangling over the edge.
My fingers touch your shoulder
but cannot reach you.

I slip outside
to the noisy hallway,
my back jammed to the unyielding wall.
Others wait their turn, shifting restlessly
in chairs that line the corridor.
A stranger moves before me, blur
of beard and open arms, his body
like a giant pillow where I
sob and sob, my arms hugging
his wide middle, his slow hands
stroking my back.

He asks no questions,
only holds me in his careful embrace.
And when my grief is exhausted,
our bodies no longer touching,
we exchange pleasantries
like former lovers at a chance meeting.
Then I go to wash my face
and he to take his seat
waiting next to his young son.

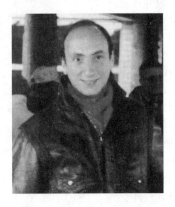

*For Steve Grossman. He was a singer of
poetry, a writer of songs and my friend
for 20 years.
His music and memory remain.
Sept. 1, 1952–June 22, 1991*

FOR STEVEN

SUSAN SCHULMAN

After we scattered your ashes
over jagged rocks
between broad summer leaves
and the hard brown earth,
and sorted through
your green dresser drawers
with their mismatched socks,
half-finished musical scores,
prized collection of pink triangles;
after we finished packing your possessions
into neatly labeled boxes
and the out-of-town mourners had departed
leaving me alone to breathe the air
that no longer carried your scent;
when all the wearing tasks of death
had been completed,
    grief took over
pierced my body cutting through layers of muscle and skin,
exposing tender nerves   forcing my eyes and mouth wide open

One long cry that stopped only after endless months
to take an awkward breath and begin again.

MIKEL

DIANE SEUSS-BRAKEMAN

I

Little did we know back in high school that sex could kill you. You told me when I was fourteen that I had the most beautiful eyes in high school. In spite of the fact that I had the reputation of a whore, that everyone on the football team knew the pattern of my underpants, you treated me like a virgin. And I treated you like a man in the running for my company even though you were called a faggot and a queer. We sat in art class coating the big table with rubber cement and, after it dried, rolling it into big translucent nightcrawlers. The art teacher sat at her desk knitting long gray scarves, clicking her needles, glaring at us now and then but keeping a respectful distance, as a Schnauzer will look at a chained German Shepherd. Knowing you wouldn't want to touch me made you more alluring, deepened my eyes, gave my lower lip more fullness and color. You, the thin-lipped one, the one with the pale, white hands more sensitive than photographic paper. You, who lived in the leaning yellow house on a dirt alley behind the fruit stand. With your words you gave me back my silly little cherry. *You are pretty*, you said. *You wear pretty clothes. Your eyes are number one in this school, better even than Robin Starr's. Someone will love you, girl. Someone will love you.*

II

We discussed everything over hard pieces of coconut pie at the Swordfish Café right over the state line. We both craved sweets and knew even then that they were a substitute for love. Hot Fudge Cake at Big Boy, Pecan Pie at Denny's, fat, rose-colored cupcakes at the downtown bakery. Like all people from our town our teeth began to go bad, our eyes took on a sugary glaze and looked dull and unfocused. When you won the township tennis tournament and leaped over the net, tripped and cracked your head open, you called me from the hospital. With your FM radio voice, which you used when you were trying to be superficial, you told me how your father was ashamed to go to work the next day. Your mother cried her big tears all over your sheets and I knew I was losing you to your history and to your pain, that you would head out to California to find a cure and never come home again.

III

You would go to California but not for two years, two years in which you were a saint, you later said, a walking, talking, feeling saint. You worked in a leather shop—during those years everyone tooled and stained it, leather decorated with scallops and hearts and deer heads and cattails, leather made into billfolds and belts and boxes and boots. You later blamed your deep feelings on the chemicals used to stain the leather. You sat on your wooden stool and watched poor people and drunks stagger by, tooling your leather, tears rolling down your cheeks. You noticed everything. The colors in mud puddles, bird shit in the shape of Abraham Lincoln, the beauty of donuts and good coffee. Later, you said you fell in love with me during those years and found being in love just what it was supposed to be. I remember you as very still and graceful in those years, somewhat Buddhist, always looking balanced and perfect in the way you wore your soft cotton shirts and baggy pants. Your love was just sitting there waiting for me. Later, you would describe this as my Wildwoman Phase, before the Bitch-Goddess Phase which preceded the Victim Phase and was a decade before the Sweet Little Wife and Mother Phase. Wild, I came to your junky yellow door smelling like coconut, drenched in rain, missing a shoe, drugged and drunk and sick from too many Camels and sad screwing and bad speed and weak coffee. I'd end up on your mattress with you toweling me off, chattering silly words and freaking out over a ladybug on the pillowcase. I made you sob, my sweetheart. It took towels and towels to mop up all the tears. You thought I was killing myself. Then the night calmed down and I threw the alarm clock out the window. It hit the alley and shattered, holding us to whatever we were feeling and saying at 2:53 a.m. We followed it downstairs and slept on your porch listening to the all-night news on the TV next door and keeping a cigarette's width of distance between us. We looked at each other in the blue light with the casualty numbers from Vietnam like bad jazz in the background and I could see in your eyes you'd had it with me, right when I was getting ready to fall in love with you, you were free of your sainthood, done with me and ready for San Francisco.

IV

But before you left, you were in your Existential Cowboy Phase and visited me in my basement apartment with red carpet and black walls. The darkness of the room had the texture of velvet. On my huge mattress we drank schnapps and beer and got so loaded we forgot not to touch. We rolled toward each other like the two ends of a scroll and that's when you named the middle of my upper lip *Cupid's Cusp* and involved yourself in my round body on those old pink sheets. Oh, those pipes hissed, those ghosts talked. We slept close as sled dogs all night long, never getting to sex, touching for the first and last time.

V

Ten years later you call to tell me you have AIDS, you are dying. You went out to San Francisco looking for a man like a baked potato, you said, one you could cut through and find only mealy white meat. Instead you found your death, saintlier and bitchier than either you or I could ever have imagined. My tears fall over my five-month-old baby boy. You have always been out there, way at the farthest coast of my broad black mind, still preserving my virginity, cloaking my nakedness with your white bath towels. We have talked and talked for all these ten years but haven't seen each other. You paint my portrait from an old photograph and I chip away at poems about you, none of them right, none of them lasting. Then you call asking me to take your ashes. *Don't spread them in Indiana, you say, don't cry over them, don't put them in ice, in France, don't be a slave to them, Di. They will be*

*feathery and gray. They will puff and float. They belong to you and I trust
your decision about them to be tender. It is not a crucial decision. They are
what I can give you.*

VI

My brother is an Elvis impersonator, you say, *my sister makes satellite
dishes and I am dying. Sometimes I can see it that clearly. Other times I sob
and shake, terrified, humiliated by the lesions on my face and feet. Limping
and in pain, I wonder if I should kill myself.*

I am embarrassed by all the excesses of my childhood. If only we
had known how important it was to be alive. How precious that pie,
the snow, the rubber cement nightcrawlers.

Art is everything, you say. *If my fingers weren't numb I'd paint myself
into the grave.*

Right now my stomach is shaking. Writing this breaks my heart.
I think about the day we went to take pictures of the haunted house
and just as you clicked the shutter the door swung open. *Hello,* you
said. *Goodbye.* And it swung shut. I dream of holding you around your
skinny waist with my face in your neck and hair. I dream of standing
with you on the banks of the old river, the dirty one running through
our hometown. We're eating apples, the fruit of the surrounding
fields, and we are not ashamed.

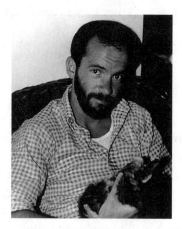

*For Mikel Allen Lindzy,
with all kinds of love
Sept. 14, 1954–Sept. 28, 1987*

Conquering Fear

John R. Sharkey

I used to be afraid of electricity.
Once I cleaned a bathroom wall heater with a wet sponge. Smart,
huh? The shock sent me sailing into the tub.
Years ago I installed a dimmer switch. As I proudly turned it on
sparks flew, smoke rose and fuses blew.
Since then the thought of changing bulbs or, God forbid, rewiring
anything makes me shudder.
One day our visiting nurse taught us how to use my lover's catheter.

Create a sterile field.
Sterile gloves.
Sterile needles.
Sterile gauze.
Sterile everything.
Cleanse the infusion site.
Pour antiseptic skin cleanser on a sterile swab stick.
Wash the chest—always clockwise in ever-widening circles.
Swab likewise with alcohol to remove the cleanser.
Insert the needle.
Flush with 5ccs of saline solution.
Stretch the skin tightly over the catheter.
Insert the needle in a straight line.
No! No! No! Never on an angle.

Flush the line.
   Don't use too big a needle.
   Don't use too large a syringe.
   Don't flush too quickly.
   Don't flush too slowly.
Begin the infusion.
   Connect the drug to the line.
   Connect the line to the catheter.
   Program the pump hanging on the I.V. pole.
   Infuse for exactly one hour—no more, no less.
End the infusion.
   Flush with 5ccs of saline solution and 5ccs of heparin.
   Remove the needle from his chest.
   Discard all appropriate waste into the chemo container.
   Check the infusion site for bleeding, redness or swelling.

Always remember that the line connected to this catheter goes directly into a major coronary artery. If you screw up, if you cause an infection, you could kill your lover.

This was our morning ritual every day for months. Evenings too, depending on how his body was responding to the drug, ganciclovir.

Last night a bulb burned out in my bedroom. Without so much as a second thought I replaced it with a new one.

Electricity doesn't scare me anymore.

To Frank Metcalf, my best friend and
lover for twenty-one years
Frank H. Metcalf, Jr.
June 19, 1944–May 25, 1993

ONE IF BY LAND...

JOHN R. SHARKEY

Most Americans are familiar with the story of Paul Revere and his famous midnight ride. On the evening of April 18th, 1775, Revere rode through the streets of Boston proclaiming, "The British are coming." Following prior arrangements, the steeple of the Old North Church which sat on a hilltop was the site chosen to warn people across the Charles River that the British were marching to Lexington and Concord. Two lanterns were placed in the steeple. If the enemy approach was by land, one lantern was to be lit. If the British arrived by sea, both lanterns were to be displayed. I am by no means an avid American history buff. This particular piece of Americana came to mind while I was remembering an event that occurred almost five years ago.

My lover Frank and I had two very close friends, Russ and Andre. In June of 1988, Frank and I began attending HIV support groups. We met Andre at the very first meeting. Several weeks later we began attending another group. It was there that we met Russ.

Andre's lover Donald died in 1987. Russ' lover Dan was suffering from advanced stages of Kaposi's Sarcoma when we met. A few months later he died. Not long after Frank and I met Andre and Russ, they met each other one Wednesday evening at the Living Well group. There was a mutual attraction from the start, and in time they became lovers. Andre had recently purchased a house and Russ was unhappy living alone in the house he had lived in with Dan, so the inevitable occurred. While I can't remember the exact date, sometime shortly before Christmas they began living together at Andre's.

Since becoming HIV-positive, both Andre and Russ had remained asymptomatic. Aside from the usual minor afflictions brought on by HIV, both were healthy and happy. Suddenly, almost in unison, both developed cryptosporidiosis. This is one of the major opportunistic infections brought on by HIV. It is a diarrheal infection caused by a protozoan which attaches itself to the lining of the small and large intestines and prevents absorption of nutrients. The diarrhea is severe and frequent with intense abdominal cramping.

After several weeks of hell there was a glimmer of hope. The University of California at San Diego (UCSD) Medical Center was accepting patients with "crypto" to test a promising new treatment. Both Andre and Russ were accepted. One of the requirements of the study was that they both be hospitalized at UCSD Medical Center so that the treatment program could be closely monitored.

On a sunny day in April of 1989, Frank and I drove to UCSD to visit Russ and Andre. We rode the elevator to the tenth floor (the AIDS floor) and walked the corridor to the last room on the east side. After duly noting the warnings posted on the outside of their closed door, we went in.

The room was surprisingly large—as hospital rooms go. There were two beds which faced each other from opposite sides of the room. Andre was lying in the bed nearest the door and Russ was sitting up in his bed next to the two large windows. When we walked in, it was immediately apparent that they were both very glad to see us. After exchanging some awkward hellos and rather meaningless chitchat we hugged and gave them the gift and card we brought for them. They both enjoyed the playful poster of a child's birthday party in full swing. The card, which I remember vividly, was somewhat more serious. The front showed an elephant with his trunk wrapped around the neck of a giraffe—both strolling silently through the jungle. The message inside read: "Friendship needs no words."

They began telling us all about the study: what the regimen was, how they felt, what the side effects had been like so far. Rather quickly they began to ask us about mutual friends and what we had been up to. It was obvious that they had changed the subject deliberately and preferred talking about anything but the reason they were hospitalized. That's right about the time I looked out the window and made "the discovery."

To begin with, the view was spectacular. It was an extremely clear day and we were looking south. Not only could we see downtown San Diego, the bay, the harbor and the ocean, but also the hills of Tijuana. The "discovery" lay between downtown and the hospital. We could see our building! Frank and I lived on the fifth floor of a twelve-story building which stood out from the shorter buildings surrounding it. For some peculiar reason being able to see our building became a really big deal. The four of us spent some time talking about it. The observation was eventually made that if we could see our building this clearly from their windows, then surely we could see the hospital just as clearly from our building.

As we continued to talk we became more and more like the little children in the poster we had given Russ and Andre. What would little kids do in a situation like this? How could we take this revelation and turn it into something fun? It didn't take us long to decide.

That evening, at approximately ten minutes to eight, Frank and I rode the elevator to the top floor of our building. There is a large rooftop patio which faces the ocean, but which also affords views to the north and south. We were armed with a pair of binoculars, two flashlights and a great deal of juvenile anticipation.

At precisely eight o'clock we watched as the far right corner of the tenth floor of UCSD Medical Center became dark. Then the lights came back on and the two huge windows were again lit. Then dark. Then lit. Frank and I each took a flashlight and began to alternately turn them on and off. As we blinked our prearranged code toward the hospital some two miles away, the top floor would acknowledge our message and blink their reply. This was great. We blinked back and forth for about a half an hour and then rode the elevator back down to our floor.

We called the hospital at once and two very excited little boys were trying to talk into the phone at the same time. "We saw your lights as clear as a bell. Could you see the lights go on and off in our room okay? Did you understand the code? We got yours."

That night will remain in my memory forever. For just a brief time the four of us were able to forget about AIDS. We took a rather insignificant observation and transformed it into an unforgettable experience.

It wasn't until years later that Andre's mom told me that the bed arrangement in the hospital room was quite deliberate. Andre's former lover Donald had died in one of the beds in 1987 and Andre insisted on sleeping in it.

Russ passed away in September of 1990, followed by Andre the next March. After almost twenty-one years of loving each other, my beloved Frank died in May of 1993.

I often close my eyes and picture Frank, Russ and Andre (along with some other devil-may-care angels) inventing and playing the silly little games that bring out the childlike innocence in all of us.

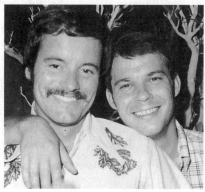

Frank, left

To Frank Metcalf, my best friend and
lover for twenty-one years
Frank H. Metcalf, Jr.
June 19, 1944–May 25, 1993

GLOVES

MARCY SHEINER

White gloves in spring.
Leather gloves in fall.
Woolen mittens in winter.

Keep hands soft
Keep hands warm

Rubber gloves for washing dishes.
Cotton gloves for dyeing hair.
Oven mitts for hot pots.

Keep hands safe
Keep hands clean

Glove rhymes with love:
Rub down with a velvet glove/
you're not sick, you're just in love.

The cops wear
big yellow gloves
and dentists wear plastic gloves
and doctors
and people who kiss in the night.

We are sheathing hands and cocks.
Our cunts are dammed.
But the heart:
how
to protect
the heart?

Your gloved hand enters me.
My gloved hand moves clumsily around your cock.
Protected fingers speak an ancient language.

The rubber
the latex
the avoidance of tongues
cannot stem the flow of passion.

I need a glove for my heart:
it breaks the same when you leave
as if we'd touched skin to skin
my heart
unprotected
still breaks.

CHARISMA

MARCY SHEINER

On what should have been
your fifty-second birthday
I buried your ashes
in the Rose Garden
at Golden Gate Park
beneath a flaming orange flower
called "Charisma."

They were only some of your ashes—
most having been strewn in the Atlantic—
and I wondered exactly what I had buried.
Your cock?
Your kneecap?
A piece of your skull?
There was no way of knowing
what my secret stash contained
shards of bones
sequestered from the others.

But I had resolved
not to scatter them to sea,
to give you in death

what you refused from me in life:
the rootedness you craved
towards the end.

Nearby bloomed a bush of pink Duets
and another of yellow Simplicity.
I replaced the damp earth around Charisma.
The name of the rose was my only concession.

TESTED

MARCY SHEINER

Three years later I am still getting tested.
Six months, say the clinicians.
Eighteen years, a counselor friend told me.

At first I felt paranoid
sitting among legions of gay men
at the health center
but now more women are getting tested.

When I tested negative
a month after you died
I was dismayed.
The next time they took my blood
I was terrified, then relieved.
Now the whole thing has become routine
if not ritualistic.
When the needle pierces my skin
I remember telling you:
I regret nothing. Even if I get AIDS
I will regret nothing.
Perhaps you thought me mad:
I wasn't sure.

By then you were hooked to a respirator
and never spoke again.

Except with your eyes.
They crinkled at the corners
when I reminded you
of the morning we'd clung to one another on Broadway
and cabs rolled by until I missed my flight.

The faint bruise on my arm is oddly reassuring.
Until I get the results
I repeat like a mantra my resolve of no regrets.
So far
this has not been tested.

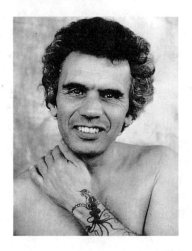

For Marco Vassi
Nov. 3, 1937–Jan. 14, 1989

DIVIDED AGAINST ITSELF

SIMON SHEPPARD

Ash's ashes! Your mama named you Ashley;
Black as she was, she'd loved *Gone With the Wind*.
You never told your mama the truth about yourself:
how you sought out other men to hold you in their arms.
Nor how you railed against the church that she held dear.
She never saw that anger that split apart your soul.
And suddenly, all that was left of you
could be held in two large hands.

We opened the box and found you there, white ashes.
A sneeze or breeze could launch you into space. So
we took you to a hill in a park you used to cruise
and sent you skyward with the birds:
squawking Steller's jay in blue,
serene gray mourning dove.

Were you there, floating, gone on a gentle breeze,
looking down at us like that crane shot looks down
at the rows of wounded rebels
on the railway station platform?
Did you drift on up to the God you always doubted?
Did you find only emptiness?
Were you there anymore at all?

Later, over juleps, we remembered your black fists
seeming to turn pale against your mint-green hospital robe.
The way you wheedled promises from us,
so willful you were you should have been named Scarlett:
"Swear you'll scatter my damn ashes on the State House lawn.
Send them in a bucket to the Goddamn President.
Spread my remains on the consecrated host and shove it down
the Holy Father's throat." We figured
that you'd become lucid one last time,
just before your body was defeated from within

And now we're left fighting this war that you fought
with one fewer soldier who wouldn't give up,
this war fought against us on such uncivil terms.
　　(When I pass by a church, there's a rock in my hands.
　　In my mind I make Jesus explode into space,
　　shards of stained glass become airborne like birds.)
(All fall down.) We go to demonstrations.
(All fall down.) We go to funerals.
And often we miss you and rarely we pray.
And sometimes I can almost believe
that tomorrow is another day.

For those who are lost to us,
and for those who fight on.

IN THE ROOM THE WOMEN
COME AND GO

DEBORAH SHOUSE

Al lies sick, his hand across his head, his dog covering his feet, a bowl of pitted cherries on his bedside, the telephone on his stomach, in case Jay should call. The women come and go, most of them volunteers assigned to him from the Good Samaritan Project.

Laura is a sales rep who just wants to make a difference. Eve is an artist, who buzzes his house into cleanness and blends his carrots just the way he likes them. Mary, his day person, is a wet rag of a woman, dim in the head. She can't tear the lettuce right for his salads, won't vacuum when he is awake and accidentally bruises his arm when she helps him into the tub. Still, he senses, she is a good woman.

The good women come and go, forming a family among themselves, leaving notes for each other about him downstairs in the kitchen, where he is almost too weak to go. The women are making new friends, having fun, being socially responsible, while he is dying.

Before his illness, his friend Rachel was the only woman he let hug him. He spent his life avoiding women, and now they cluster around him, hover over him. He is a fifty-year-old-man with forty-year-old mothers.

His head feels like an overripe cantaloupe. He hears Mary downstairs talking to soap opera characters. Rachel comes in, sits on his bed, moves the phone from his stomach to his bedside. She knows he's waiting for Jay to call and she knows he can barely lift the receiver. She'll answer for him on the first ring.

"I have a fever again," Al tells Rachel, in case she doesn't want to hug him.

"I'm sorry," she says and leans down, resting her head on his chest like Peter used to. For a moment, Al lets the fever take him back to bed with Peter; the sacred warmth of that spent man lying across him, the hallowed rhythm of two breathing as one.

The phone jars Al out of the sun-soft spot with Peter. Rachel answers. "Just a minute, I'll check and see." Rachel is the only one who has not stolen his voice, who does not talk about him as if he were a feeble dog.

She puts her hand over the receiver and mouths, "The social worker."

Al shakes his head. He'll save the social worker for later when Rachel's gone. The women, there's always one of them around. The men have disappeared.

Jay moved back in with his mother two days after promising he would love and take care of Al forever. Jay shouted grand words like "always" and "forever," then melted into nothing like a wet witch. And he wouldn't even call.

"I brought you some fresh carrot juice," Rachel says. The bottle is cool. Rachel's face looks inviting, like an unread page. She understands that Mary makes him feel crazy. Mary never reads, never talks about anything but her dog and her gas pains. Mary won't follow his directions and believes it's okay to use yesterday's carrot juice.

Rachel pours and Al tastes the sweet gritty juice. Mary walks in wiping her hands with a washcloth.

"I'm leaving," she says. "Eve's here, when you need something." Eve stands behind her and waves.

Mary leaves, Eve goes downstairs. Rachel sits holding his hand, reading to him, until she too will be pulled into her other life.

And so that is the way of it, these last days, only women left to care for him and possibly about him. He feels their presence and yet when he wakes from his fevered sleep, his room is empty. Nothing is certain. Even the women come and go.

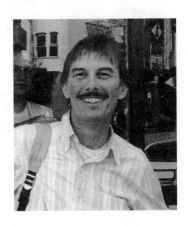

To my beloved friend, Al Bright,
writer, dreamer, soulmate
July 4, 1939–July 30, 1989

FOR ROBERT:
A GIFT OF COMMUNITY

CHARLES SPAETH

I recently watched a friend die of AIDS. He was not the first to die of the disease, nor will he be the last. In that his death was not noteworthy. What was noteworthy was that twenty people volunteered to nurse him through the last weeks of his life. They were not afraid to make time in their busy lives to do something they thought was important. They were not afraid to confront the emotional messiness of death and their fear of it. I felt someone should tell the story of the gift of community which grew from Robert's life and death.

Robert Auric, thirty-seven, was gay, a Vietnam veteran and a professional gourmet chef. Witty, with a slashing sense of humor, his large eyes were as practiced at making you squirm as making you feel warm and accepted. He had come from a large family in Ohio and lived several years in New York City before migrating to Seattle. In the summer of 1984 he bought a house with a heterosexual couple named Grace and Charlie who were friends of mine. That fall, after developing pneumonia, Robert learned he was HIV-positive. The following spring, once more in the hospital with pneumonia, he was diagnosed with AIDS.

Though I saw Robert frequently, I never knew him well. He was the first of my contemporaries I have known who knew he was dying. I often wondered how he was coping with the idea of his death and how I would have coped had I had been in his place. How were his priorities shifting? What envy or resentment might he feel for someone like me, healthy, with the prospect of living another forty years? Perhaps the time I spent thinking of Robert made me feel I knew him better than I did.

Though he had medical insurance and was in and out of the hospital several times, he decided early on that when the time came, he wanted to die at home. Grace and Charlie supported his decision. By mid-August, 1986, the disease was beginning its final stages. Robert slept eighteen hours a day and had lost forty pounds. He was weak, his feet were swollen and walking was painful. He had to be driven to see the doctor. To avoid dehydration his fluid intake and outgo had to be measured. His room slowly filled with bedpans, gauze cartons, intravenous tubes and clamps, hypodermic needles, disinfectants, emoluments and prescription bottles, as well as the normal accretion of a person confined to bed.

Grace, Charlie and Tom, Robert's lover, were overwhelmed by the physical and emotional demands of Robert's deteriorating health. All had full-time jobs, yet Robert required full time care.

Pat and Dan, friends of Grace and Charlie, called my wife Becky and me to ask if we would come to their house one Friday for a potluck dinner to discuss Robert's illness.

It was a warm summer evening. People stood in the kitchen sampling hor d'oeuvres and sipping wine, making small talk, laughing. After an hour the party came to order. Grace and Tom reported on Robert's condition and explained where help was needed. They were explicit in all details: what he would eat and how to coax him to take it; where his medications were stored and how and when to administer them; what kinds of magazines he liked; how his medical chart was to be kept; when to talk to him and when to leave him alone; how to guard against taking personally what he might say or not say. The whole thing reminded me of an old war movie where the wing commander briefs a roomful of pilots about a mission so dangerous that it's voluntary. And of course, everybody volunteers.

Pat took out a calendar divided into four-hour segments from eight in the morning to eight at night. People consulted their daytimers and signed up for shifts. Alternates were designated in case conflicts arose. Names, addresses and phone numbers were collected for typing and distribution. Phone trees were organized so news could be communicated quickly. The gathering broke up soon after business was concluded.

As I drove home it was difficult to believe that the reason for this pleasant party had been to lay a schedule grid over a man's dying. For a year we had all known it would happen. In the same way I put off thinking about my tax return I had avoided thinking about Robert's death. Now there was no avoiding it.

I had not signed up for shifts but offered myself as an alternate. Within several days someone asked me to take his shift. I said I would.

When I arrived at the house a man I had never met quickly briefed me on what I should know and left. The chart showed Robert had eaten a small piece of fruit for lunch, needed medication in an hour and had urinated four-hundred cc's since eight that morning. I hadn't seen him for two months. I knew he'd lost weight but I wasn't prepared for the hollow cheeks, sunken eyes, and arms little more than bones. He breathed heavily as he slept in an unnatural position with a forearm cocked against a pillow and the hand hanging limp. I left the room quietly, afraid he would wake while I watched and nervous about how I would handle myself if he did, as though impending death lent him some terrible authority over me. I hoped my shift would end while he still slept and I wouldn't have to face my fear of dying.

But he did wake, was only slightly surprised to see me, asked for nothing and went back to sleep. Later I brought him a protein milk shake. We talked while I leaned against the door jamb. It wasn't hard after that.

Many people brought meat loaf, quiches and casseroles so Grace, Charlie and Tom (who by now had set up a cot in the basement) wouldn't have to add shopping and cooking to their responsibilities. While Robert slept, there were floors to mop, dishes and clothes to wash. "I don't do housework anymore," Grace laughed. "I leave that for the help."

I never heard a complaint about anyone being late for a shift. It wasn't uncommon for three or four people to be at the house at a time. Conversation about Robert was common, but there was laughter too, ringing phones, dogs to be let in and out, reimbursements for supplies bought, doctor and therapist visits and the working out of ad copy to sell Robert's Volvo. The house became a place to leave and pick up messages, linger over a glass of wine and get to know people. In the face of Robert's death it was also a place to find someone to share sadness, someone who could read in the lines of your forehead, "How much longer will this go on?"

Robert was sleeping when I arrived the next time, on a Thursday afternoon. I sat down to read, fell asleep, and awoke to find him watching me from his wheelchair. He'd once confided to Grace that if ever I had doubts about my sexuality he'd be pleased to offer counseling. The vacant stare was gone. He greeted me with darting eyes, a smile, and chided me that my incompetent nursing had been noted.

We chatted. I said, "You know, what is going on here is unusual. All these people, coming to this house...A lot of us don't even know each other. You've been to AIDS support meetings. Do you know of anywhere else this has happened?"

He shook his head. "Most people are alone."

"Somebody ought to say something about how no one here is afraid of the disease."

He agreed.

"If I could get someone up here from one of the local TV stations to do a story would you be willing to be a part of that?"

"Of course." He was pleased there might still be something useful he could do.

That evening we watched the news together. A five-minute spot was devoted to a promising new drug for treating AIDS patients. I was wondering if he still harbored hope, or was he beyond that now? His face was blank. Grace later told me he asked the doctor if he could get the drug. The doctor told him none was available and taking Grace aside, said it wouldn't matter anyway.

That weekend Tom said Robert had felt well and spent several hours a day in his wheelchair. When I came on Tuesday things had changed. Robert called me to his bedroom. His eyes were glassy, his face rigid with fear. In a breathy, raspy voice he asked if I would prop up his legs; they wouldn't move anymore, he said, and he couldn't lift them with his arms. I bent his swollen knees, larger by far than his thighs, and braced them against each other so they wouldn't fall over. He said it hurt less that way. Later, he asked for the urine bottle that sat on a shelf on the opposite side of his double bed. He was too weak to roll over and reach for it, and, I soon discovered, too incoherent to use it. When Grace came home we rolled him from one side of the bed to the other and changed the sheets. She was cheerful and joked as we worked. Robert could only lie helplessly and watch. The next day he told Tom the worst indignity of dying was having no privacy.

Grace called to ask if I would pick up morphine on my way over on Thursday. At the doctor's office the nurses were sad and asked me to tell Robert they were thinking of him. Back at the house I crushed morphine into a spoonful of yogurt, and holding Robert's head with my left arm, fed it to him slowly. When he deliriously complained of pain I tried to explain the morphine would take a while to work. He didn't understand but fell into fitful sleep.

A friend of Robert's came to see him an hour later. I discouraged a visit. Though he was too weak and disoriented for conversation, with hindsight I admit I had become protective. Then Grace came home from work and cried. "Things are getting real bad now," she sobbed, "I'm real scared." We held each other.

Robert got worse for three more days and he died on Sunday. Monday he was cremated.

Word went out that the party was on Wednesday. "Wake?" I asked. "No, a paaarty," Grace corrected. "A bring-your-own-champagne party, Dom Perignon or better. Robert said nobody was going to drink cheap shit at his 'gone away' party." The people who had nursed him were all there and many more. The August gathering had only been six weeks before. It seemed longer. We were relieved that the suffering and the waiting and the tension were over.

Dozens of snapshots of Robert were spread out on a table. People told stories about him and laughed, even if later they cried quietly in dark corners. Someone who might have been tagging along with a friend and hadn't known the purpose of the gathering, at first might have thought it reminiscent of an earlier era, maybe a 1969 smoke-pot-in-the-kitchen party, maybe a little unusual for a Wednesday, but otherwise a fun time.

I thought it was more like the last act of a ballet where the townspeople come out after the terrible storm to dance a mazurka for the hero who has died to rid the land of the evil sorcerer. The applause, of course, was missing; other than that we accepted from ourselves or what a friend conveyed with a touch or glance.

The people who cared for Robert ran the gamut of age, sex and sexual preference. They included teachers, attorneys, social workers, architects, homemakers, academics, and commercial real estate brokers. Far from being a source of discord, our differences knit us together without homophobia, heterophobia, or resentment over income or education. From Robert's death I learned that compassion is learned by doing; that death is real; that lives are shaped within the unknown parameters of mortality and that there's no time to waste in shaping the lives we want—valuable in-kind payment for a few of my afternoons.

I can only guess what all this meant to Robert. That so many people would reaffirm my value as a human being by volunteering to keep watch over my unglamorous death would have been significant to me. He didn't talk much, though.

The TV spot never materialized. He died too quickly. There was, however, still time to write of those few weeks before memories were lost behind the screen of more recent events. Not to let that moment slip away, as I have let so many slip away, was something I thought I owed Robert.

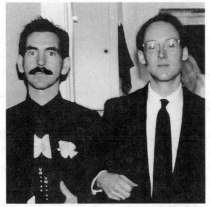

Robert, left

Dedicated to Robert Auric,
died Oct. 1986 at age 37,
and to the family of his friends.

LETTING GO

SU STOUT

The first time I met Ron Markle was early in 1977. I was on the Pastor Parish Committee at Christ United Methodist Church, and we had the task of hiring a new pastor. Ron walked in, regal in his black cleric, exquisite parchment-white skin and aquamarine eyes that seemed to see through me. I watched him walk across the room and knew he was gay. It would be a long time before he would acknowledge this to me although I was out to him and everyone else who would listen. Funny, but based on his interview that January night, I voted not to hire him. Not because he was gay, but because I believed he wasn't a very good minister. I was the only NO vote. Ron came to Christ Church in Jersey City that June.

From the beginning, Ron and I disagreed in church. He loved formal high worship style, with candles and choral responses and acolytes and a crucifer and wafers for communion and genuflecting. I asked why he hadn't sought an Episcopal or Catholic pastorate, rather than the informal, freethinking Methodist church. None of what he said or did fell into my twenty-year-old concept of the tradition I had grown up in and loved. As I listened to his sermons each Sunday, I was struck by the way I heard Ron describe the God he knew. It was an angry, sad, disappointing relationship as he told the story. We debated his theories until he said, in words that chill me even in retrospect, "I'm gay. I'll never be good enough for God."

From that moment, I began to look for all the good in Ron and to affirm it. Ron had a haunting tenor voice and loved to sing with the church choir. He loved to listen to Bach's sacred works and Mahalia Jackson. He had stereo speakers wired all over his house so he wouldn't miss a note. An antique collector, Ron loved odd pieces. He had a leather barber's chair in his kitchen, and on the sun porch was a collection of antique chamberpots. Ron was one of a kind!

In the six years he was at Christ Church, we became good friends, even if we seldom agreed on church doctrine, theory or practice. I house-sat, dog-sat and plant-sat when he was away. He cared for my critically ill puppy so I didn't have to leave him alone while I worked. I met his mom, helped nurse him through hepatitis, and let him cry on my shoulder more times than I can count. I met his new lover and celebrated their new love with them.

Yet in church we would bicker. I would never accept my homosexuality as a separation from God, and Ron could not accept the love that encompassed, even celebrated his sexuality.

By the time his term at Christ Church was up in 1983, I was so disgusted by his sermons of self-flagellation that I had left the church. For the first six months after he left, we had no contact. When my youngest nephew needed baptism, Ron officiated at the service. He looked gaunt under his cassock and surplice during the service, but Ron had sort of a Dresden quality. Lose an hour's sleep and he had dark circles under his eyes and was digging out some coverup. When he removed his robes, I gasped. I wrapped my arms around him in our familiar hug and he was skin and bones. I held him tightly, feeling him relax into me and return my hug. I wanted to ask, but how does one say, "Do you have IT?" when nearly all my gay male friends do or did? I settled for hugging him longer and tighter. I settled for looking him directly in the eyes when we spoke, for cupping his cheeks in my hands to tell him I loved him as we parted. I settled for calling him more often and listening to his gripes about the new church without my usual witty repartee about his impatience. One night, I awoke screaming from a dream. Ron was dead and came back to tell me so. The next night, I awoke in a cold sweat. Ron was dead. I just knew it. I called him that day after the second dream. No answer. I had the dream for five nights in a row. Each day I called him and got no answer. On the sixth day I got a call from Ron's ex-lover. Ron was in St. Vincent's Hospital with severe bleeding from the AZT. He refused a transfusion. He refused medication. He refused to eat. Ron had chosen death. He said if I wanted to see Ron alive, now was the time.

Before work the next day, I went to St. Vincent's. When he saw me, he cried. He was very weak. I sat on the side of his bed, gently holding his hand. I kissed his fingertips. I leaned down and pressed my lips to his hollow cheek. He touched the tears on my cheeks and said, "Nobody touches me anymore. Thanks."

I came back after work and Ron had lapsed into a coma. There was little I recognized of my old friend except his caramel-colored beard. I smiled, remembering how much he loved his beard, and how it distinguished him. I touched his cheek just about the beard line. He wasn't conscious, but his head moved slightly so that his cheek rested heavily against my hand. "It's me, Rev. I'm gonna visit for a while," I whispered in his ear.

The lesions on his arms and chest were an angry purple. He was skin stretched across bones except for his big belly where the blood was seeping. There were tubes everywhere. His face was serene, but I couldn't believe it wasn't painful for his body to be invaded like that. Tears slid warmly down my cheeks.

Letting go was hard. Ten years ago, my close circle of friends included seventeen gay men. Ron was the fifteenth to be dying. My sense of loss smothered me. I sat holding his hand, feeling his long, slender fingers and hoping he knew it was me.

In fifteen minutes the nurse came to the doorway to tell me my time was up. I reluctantly stood to leave.

The numbers flashing over his head had been in a downward spiral since right after I got there. As I stood to go, the beeping from the gray machine in the corner got louder. I touched his cheek again and realized the noise was louder when I was touching him. Holding my hand still, I watched the bright green numbers get smaller and smaller. My eyes moved from his face to the numbers and back to his face. A hand on my shoulder told me the nurse had returned. Together we stood—her hand on my shoulder—my hand cradling his cheek until all the sounds stopped.

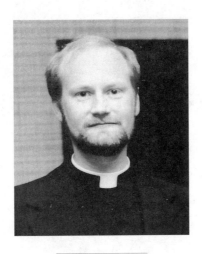

For Ron...you are loved.
Rev. Ronald R. Markle
Sept. 27, 1941–March 3, 1989

PRAYING FOR DREAMS

JEAN E. SWALLOW

Last night I dreamt I finally cried for Nicholas my friend,
the man I loved who died on Friday. Do you think we could
rest here for just a moment? I'm so tired I can't
move; it's been like trying to run underwater—could we
sit a moment? I'd like to lie down I'm so tired;
I could just lie down in the middle of this room but
I wouldn't sleep of course; I think I must sleep
but I lie awake, drift, toss and turn, get up, lie down.
Nicholas died on Friday. I wish there was something left
to do but there isn't. All that's left
are dreams and prayers.

I haven't been able to cry since he died, well, those times
in the middle of the night, and yesterday after I finished
cooking supper, I stood at the end of the table, and saw
the number of plates, the amount of food I had set out—
I cried then, dishtowel stuffed in my mouth, I cried then,
but not too loud; I didn't want him to hear me—he
mustn't hear me—he has to go. I have to let him go,
open my hand, open my heart to him, one more time.

I wanted him to go; I knew it was time; so much pain,
his endless racking cough tearing his heart out and

mine too—I couldn't ask him to stay; I didn't want
him to stay, didn't want anything to stop him, didn't want
him to see how I laid my head down at work and wept when
everyone was at lunch, how I held the checkstand
at the grocery store to keep from collapsing before I
could get out of the store; there was that incident
by the bread, on the sidewalk, driving the car, reading
the paper, and every night wrapped, weeping, around Betsy,
but I haven't really cried, because if I did, my body
would have split apart, the world would split open, the center
of my self cleaved, between my breasts, my heart exposed:
see how it still beats, see how blood seeps out everywhere;
there is nothing I can use to stop, it just keeps coming.
I cannot see anymore; I'm tired, so tired, I must lie down
and rest, just a moment, I must lie down. Nicholas is gone.
There is nothing I can do, nothing left to do, nothing
here but my oozing heart, quietly trying to pray.

I am praying for dreams, no more, no less. Last night
I dreamt I went up to the ridge, and night became day.
I began to weep then, to moan, fell to my knees; I could
not stop. The buzzards came at the sound of carrion, five
riding thermals as they do each day, circling as I rocked,
looking for the dead. They recognized mourning's
awful daybreak; I heard someone screaming; the birds waited,
kept vigil, and a russet-winged hawk who appeared when Nick
died came too, in my dream, soundlessly circled. There
were no other sounds, even crickets ceased singing. There
was no other sound but the unhinged howl of my keening:
Listen, Nicholas is gone; hurry, I must tell God, hurry,
the valley is filled with sound, the world is one long
shriek; hurry, something terrible has happened here, hurry
oh hurry; we must hurry, for only in dreams is there enough
room to receive my grief, only in the silence of dreams.

There had been other silent nights, those nights at the end
when he couldn't speak and I grew self-conscious at the
sound of my own voice, trying to be cheerful, times when I
could think of nothing to say except, go to sleep, darling,

go to sleep. I sang him lullabies and stroked his hands,
his face, his feet, whatever I could still touch; there
were times in the end when I couldn't speak any longer and
I laid my head down on his shoulder, listening to his machine
breathe for him, wheezing. I listened for oxygen bubbling
hastily through tubes into his mask; I listened to him moan,
struggling to breathe and I tried to reassure myself he was
not in pain, that he was only panting for the uphill journey
he was on, groaning the way he did when he could still lift
weights, as long as he breathed the force of his will kept
him with us, so long the force of his will, pumping iron
after two bad bouts of pneumonia, rebuilding his forty-inch
chest, finishing his novel, falling in love one more time,
the force of his will illuminating the sky, pushing night
back like a full moon, so bright he made it seem like
daytime, but it was night after all.
I am waiting for his return, please understand, this is
all I can do. I am praying for dreams.

Before he was gone I dreamt he had come back—an angel
dream. I couldn't ask him to stay, not even with my tears,
but I could ask him to come back and I did. He smiled his
slow smile, his lips thickened and parched, but he said yes.
That night I dreamt he came to me as an angel, filled
out again, his taut skin tanned, without lesions anywhere,
hair cropped like last summer, bleached blonde trashy roots
showing; he had grown wings taller than either of us and we
walked down Market Street to get some dinner, and the boys
stopped and started just like they used to; he smiled at me
just like he used to, and he was with me again, and we were
laughing just like we used to when we were delighted with
all God had given us to cherish—you understand now why
I am praying for dreams. This is where he will come,
resurrection in the present moment. The love I carry in me
has a past but also a present and a future, has an always.
I have been loved by Nicholas Carter, and I will be, I will
continue to be, if now only in dreams; someday those dreams
will fall from my heart and enter into my blood, and I will

have him: an angel on the street or flying as he danced
a hawk's grace or laughing, his hand in mine, as always,
all my life. This is resurrection, this love stronger
than death, you understand now why I am praying for dreams.

For his memorial service
Nicholas Carter
Sept. 20, 1948–July 9, 1993

WALKING IN A BLIZZARD: THE
WHITE DRESS

DIANA TOKAJI

W*hen you die, Andy, will you hiss hard at the change, or put on the white dress, pirouette and leap—offstage.*

In my dreams I do not fight change. It is only awake that I am a snake hissing at every intruder. It is only when I am awake and a snake that I whip back and glare, head raised high off my neck: Get back, you. It is only when I am awake that I am compelled, by habit, to attack any change such as death.

Though I go to dreams involuntarily, I want to be made to go there. There I speak freely, like my friend Andy, whose brain has been attacked by the AIDS virus, leaving his mind, away, like mine when I dream.

I ask him about his visit with our friend, Marcia. He says, I was hanging off the top of the chariot a little. I say, Sometimes it's like that, isn't it: hanging off the top of the chariot. Yeah, he says, and we laugh. But sometimes it isn't, he says. I mean, I did see her, and we talked. I mean, I did SEE her.

He tells me later, she turned into a lollipop. I say, yeah, people'll do that. We talk about our past, dancing together, and he recalls names and places I've forgotten. He recites the poem his brother wrote, which we danced to twenty-three years ago—all of which I've forgotten. For half an hour he strokes my head, MY head, as I sit on the floor beside his chair. You look like a musician, I tell him. It's the uncut hair, wavy down the neck, brushed back off the forehead. Someone fabulous, I say, whose hair dances while he waves a baton. Leonard Bernstein, I say, as he runs his hands through his hair. Leonard Bernstein.

Sun pours through the bay windows, a balm to my body, but bright for Andy's eyes which are going blind. He puts on a pair of sunglasses with round, dark green lenses. John Lennon, I say. In his lap he is kneading yellow Play-Doh.

We talk about how he broke up with me when we were teenagers. I say, I'll forgive you, Andy. Eventually. Maybe. If you're lucky.

We talk about his career. When I ask him if he has enjoyed dancing all his life, he says, enjoy? Enjoy is not the word; and I smile. He is picky about my language these days, and I like it. The day before, talking about dances we choreographed at age fifteen, I'd said, We were advanced for our age, weren't we? And Andy had corrected my word choice. I'm not sure that *advanced* is the word I'd choose, he'd said. I would've said, *accomplished.*

But today he cannot come up with a word to replace enjoy. Maybe there isn't one, I say. During his career, Andy hated the backstage politics in ballet, but he did what his body was carved for—with Stuttgart, Frankfurt, and the Joffrey. Now, he is quiet and his eyeballs vibrate swiftly as he searches for a way to describe his life. I had a lot of great times, he says, and looks straight at me. I had a lot of fun.

Aside from your technique, Andy, I say, you always had that timing, that musicality. You always had that, didn't you? Yeah, he says, I understood music. It was a gift.

And that body didn't exactly hurt your career either, did it? No, he says. It was good to have a beautiful body, actually. Aesthetics help. I mean, aesthetics matter, don't they?

I always knew you were bright, Andy. I say, but I never saw it so clearly. Until now, (I think to myself), your genius was channeled through those thick, high-arched feet, that flexible back, the flick of your head—a signature of yours—and the lyrical extension of your long, beautiful legs.

Now, I see your genius while you're still. Sitting here. Emaciated. Now, I hear it in your words.

When I leave Andy's house crying, my son, who has been running up and down the street with Grandma in tow, greets me with wet overalls and a blow-out diaper. I change his diaper cautiously inside my mother's car, taking care to avoid the upholstery.

But before this, I have had to say good-by to Andy. I have told him, I will miss you. I am going back to D.C. where I live. Oh you've moved, he says. Yes, I did move about seven years ago, I say, and I haven't been able to see you too often. I will miss you, I say, nodding my head.

We'll see each other again, he says. And you know you're always with me. I whisper, I'll keep you right here, Andy, and press my palm above my heart.

I go into the kitchen to say good-by to his parents. We hug and they are still talking to me as I walk back to Andy's chair and he says, Thanks for all the things you brought. I assume he means the cake and fruit—watermelon, kiwi, pineapple, blueberries, bananas. The clothes, he says, speaking of something I have not, I have never, brought him. They are fabulous.

One week later I am walking in a blizzard, and I remember this conversation as if it were all a dream.

Especially the white dress, he had said. I can't wait to dance in it.

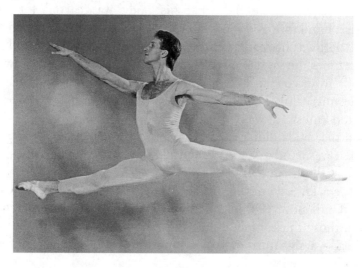

To the family of Andrew Levinson who
held him at birth and at death
July 23, 1954–March 19, 1993

SITTING WITH GUS

JACK VEASEY

I didn't mind watching you hook yourself
to the I.V. There was no need
for your apology. It was another way
of being close to you—
after we'd rehearsed
your song, one of your many songs
that are not written down yet, though AIDS
makes the issue pressing.
The concert we rehearsed for
would be cancelled, but we didn't know that
yet.

Your hands had moved so skillfully
beneath my voice, which you'd let soar
beyond uncertainty—effortlessly
changing keys, to comfort me,
to suit me as so few have.
No, we haven't known each other long,
but time means more to men like us
in these cold days, these too-clear days,
these racing days.

And so I sit beside your bed
and watch the liquid
flowing into you—the liquid that will save you
from this latest scare, the one
which might have led to blindness.
And I am grateful
for your eyes, bright, deep
as ever. And I'm conscious
of the ticking
of the timer
that you've set, so you can stop
the moment that the bag is empty—so
your heart will not start
pumping out your blood, the blood
with which you are at war, but which is still
source of your life.

I sit with you, and want
to take your hand, and
do not let myself—though I am not afraid
and have embraced you, and will
when we say goodbye. And
I watch your face, pale, fragile
and so haunting.

And I love you, very suddenly,
as I have loved few things:
as I loved the light in the sky
on the day I left home.
I'd wished that light
could be a solid thing.
I would have grasped it
firmly in my hands.
I would have never let it go.

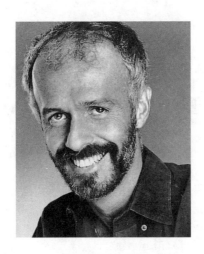

In loving memory of my friend
Gustavio Motta
June 20, 1944–Feb. 6, 1993

THOM'S DREAM

MEGAN WELLS

We weren't particularly close in college, Thom Miller and I. We paid our tuition as graduate assistants working in the theater box office. Our desks were right next to each other; our social lives, worlds apart. Our acquaintance revolved mostly around food. We shared a weakness for cheesecake, and commiserated about the extra pounds neither of us could shed. Thom's wrapped around his middle, too early for his thirty-one years. Mine padded my thighs and hips. Thom and I traded diet tips, not confidences.

I graduated in 1985 and returned to my home town, Chicago, MFA degree in hand to launch my theater ambitions on the sea of the city, opening yet another off-off-loop theater company. In 1986, Thom moved to Chicago and joined our venture. We managed crisis to crisis, show to show, for three years. Finally, we ran out of money, energy, and hope. Thom moved to Seattle to try his luck there. I found a corporate job. We promised to write, you know how it goes...

I thought about Thom every time I went to the theater, which wasn't often—it hurt too much to get too close to my lost dream. I'd ease the sting with my imaginings. What would Thom think about this? God, how he would have hated that!

One night, I was seeing a play at Victory Gardens theater. I stopped to grab a gulp of water before the second act. I saw this skinny guy hogging the fountain. Something about his hand on the silver push bar jarred me. He turned. "Thom Miller? What the hell are you doing here!" We laughed right into a hug. That's how I knew before he told me. I could feel his ribs through his shirt.

We skipped the second act. Over coffee and chocolate chip cheesecake, we told each other our stories. He'd done fairly well in Seattle, but his debt finally brought him down. He'd accepted a job at Barat College in Lake Forest working the theater box office. "I meant to call you so many times." "Yeah, me too." Then walking out the door of the coffee shop, "Megan?" "Yeah, Thom?" "I've got ..." "I know."

When I drove him home, he lingered in the car, his hand on the car door handle. "You wouldn't happen to know anybody with a room to rent, would you?" I'd been thinking about getting a roommate. I lived in this huge two-bedroom apartment and needed a break in the rent. "Why?" I asked. "Well, my lease is up and...I was going to stay with a friend for a couple of weeks, just until I could find a place..." I waited. "She backed out..." I could hear his feet shuffling on the floor mats. "She's afraid she'll catch it." One week later Thom moved in with me.

My parents worried. I never knew what to say to quiet their fears. He was so careful to protect me, bleaching the tub and basin every morning after his shower and shave.

The bathroom...seems like it all happened in the bathroom.

It was a Wednesday morning, 7:45 a.m. I was getting ready for work, Maybelline coverstick in hand. Thom's alarm went off. I wondered how he slept. We'd had a particularly tough week. His cough was getting worse, keeping him up at night—keeping us both up.

He came in. He was wearing his lime green pajamas, thin cotton with a drawstring waist, his hair unruly, sculpted by his pillow. He put down the toilet seat, sat down and said, "I had a dream..." I watched him through the mirror. He leaned his elbows on his knees to continue.

"I was on the beach, an ocean beach. My sister and her husband and...yes, the kids were with us, too. We were all standing on an embankment, overlooking the ocean. Then I saw other people, in the water...playing in the waves. And then I was in the water. They were...tremendous...the waves. Not violent but powerful. They were..." He closes his eyes for a moment searching for a word. I hold my breath. "...tremendous.

"Suddenly, the sands shifted and I lost my balance. I was being buffeted about. I started scrambling in the water, fighting to get my balance, but the more I fought the more I seemed to lose control.

"And then someone... I didn't know who, just a someone... appeared and said, 'Lean into it... the wave... just lean into the wave.' So, I did. And then, I was flying. It was... I kept leaning, and each time I leaned further and further until I was almost...flying." He's gesturing now. His arms spread wide.

"Then there was this huge wave. Grand...bigger than anything...and it wrapped me up and I was pinned on the beach, up against the embankment. My arms pinned against the rocks and the wave just holding me, pressing me, pressing my chest so that I couldn't breathe. It didn't hurt, no, but it frightened me. Really, really frightened me. I felt helpless, scared...alone. I remember knowing my sister was there but she couldn't help, she wasn't meant to help. I started to panic. Then I remembered...I leaned."

He falls silent. I watch his eyes moving slowly back and forth behind closed lids. He straightens his upper body, a deep breath presses the outline of his ribs against pink white flesh. He sighs, "It's hollow, but not empty, no...it's full...peaceful. I'm just hanging here, floating, leaning, and all around me is..." He starts to cry. I watch mesmerized as a tear curls slowly, gently, over a long blonde lash and stops. Hanging on his lash as he hangs in his wave. A crystal ball reflecting all the light we feel at this moment.

Then it's over, just that quick. He stands up, runs his fingers through his sandy hair and starts to go. At the door, "I guess it was more a vision than a dream, don't you think?" "Yes. Yes, Thom, I think it was more of a vision than a dream." I tell him he should write it down. "Oh, no need, I'll always remember." As he leaves the bathroom, his bare feet echo my heartbeat on the floor boards.

After that dream, Thom and I practiced "leaning into" everything. We spent hours with crayons and poster paper drawing pictures of our dreams and fears. We gorged on books about mysticism and soul and death and love. We went to all the movies we'd ever wanted to see and always got popcorn. I pulled out my theater dream, polished it up with my résumé and launched my hopes again.

Two months later, Thom made a decision. He moved back to Seattle and regathered his group of artist friends. They put together a production of a play Thom had always wanted to direct, Samuel

Beckett's *Endgame*, then toured the production around the West Coast. At the end of a year, when Thom was too weak to tour, he moved in with his sister, her husband and children who live in a big house on an embankment overlooking the ocean. I often imagined him at night, lying in bed, listening to the waves.

Toward the end, when he was in the hospital, Thom wouldn't let me come see him. He said he needed me to remember him as he was. One night we were on the phone, he was in terrible pain and I tried to soothe him. "Thom, Thom, remember your dream? Your vision of the waves?" "No, Megan, what dream?" I couldn't sleep that night. I wrote down everything I could remember about our morning in the bathroom and mailed it to him. When he got it, he called me, "I'm leaning now." A few days later, Thom Miller died.

My life did not change miraculously after that. The truth is, Thom changes me a little bit at a time—when I'm questioning my life, when the waves of fear threaten to overwhelm me, when I'm running low on money and energy and hope—I remember Thom's dream...and *I* lean.

Hi Thom. Thomas Edward Miller,
Dec. 23, 1958–Dec. 28, 1990

PRISON HEARTS

LAURA WHITEHORN

Like a lot of other people I know, I've taken to reading the obituaries every day. I scan the page looking for ages—anything under sixty, I stop and read. Sometimes the cause of death is cloaked in code—"cancer," "respiratory disease," "pneumonia,"—and then I have to search for other clues in career or survivors. When it's plain—"He had AIDS"—I stop and read every word. It's only very seldom that I actually know or have heard of the person. I'm just paying my respects. I hope that when my friends Eliot Espana and Mike Riegle died, someone paid them the respect of poring over their obituaries, committing to heart the scant facts of another life lost to the epidemic.

But most of my friends who have died of AIDS never made it into the pages of any newspaper. No obituary; rarely even a death notice. Women. Some of them died of AIDS before it was even acknowledged that women *get* HIV. Joyce Cooper, for example.

I met her in the D.C. Jail in 1988. I was on lock-down status. She defied the guards in order to bring me a hot cup of coffee in the morning. In jail, you tend to get close to people pretty fast, because things are so intense, you spend so much time together, and your survival depends on one another in a lot of ways. It was like that with Joyce and me.

Joyce had a clear, uncynical smile, and the strength to fight to be a human being in a situation geared to prevent that. Late in the winter of 1988, she caught a bad cold. The next thing she knew she was waking up in D.C. General Hospital's prison ward, chained to the bed, breathing through a mask. When a doctor finally visited her he told her, "What's the matter with you, don't you know you have AIDS and you're dying?" By the time I saw her again, back on the cold, damp unit at the Jail, her smile had collapsed into a haunted, terrified look.

One Monday morning, following a long, icy weekend during which we'd been locked in our cells for most of every day, Joyce sent someone to get me. I ran downstairs to her cell and found her soaking in sweat, moaning with the pain of a high fever. The guards locked themselves in the bubble (their command post) and locked down the whole unit. Joyce and I refused to go into our cells. We sat in the metal-benched dayroom, where I cradled her in my arms, demanding to see a P.A. I asked the guard to come out from behind the glass to look at Joyce, to feel her skin to see how hot she was, so that there could be no doubt that this was an emergency, and immediate medical assistance was needed. The guard wouldn't even answer me—too scared to open her mouth or look me in the eye.

Finally a P.A. came to the unit for the regular sick call. I was able to convince her to look at Joyce, whom I'd carried back to her cell, too weak to walk or sit or lie on the metal bench. The last time I saw Joyce she was being wheeled out of the unit on a gurney. Knowing the loneliness awaiting her, I had no means of managing the heartbreak. I've never learned to do it any better in the five years since.

Joyce died a few months later. She'd been released not long after that crisis in the Jail, because her sentence was up. I can only imagine the bleakness she encountered outside. Her family, who tried to protect her, was utterly unable to find resources for a woman—especially an African American woman—with AIDS.

The virus blind-sided Joyce. She didn't have a chance to choose resistance, she didn't have enough time and backup to exhibit her nobility in the face of AIDS, because she never saw it coming and hardly knew what it was when it hit. This was before the important option of *living with AIDS* was available to poor people, to women, to Black people, and certainly to a Black woman in prison.

Like many people on the outside, the only way I could begin to deal with my grief over Joyce—and Theresa, and Eliot, both of whom died around the same time as Joyce—was to throw myself with a vengeance into AIDS education, support, and (to the extent it's possible in prison) activism. In doing so, I've met some strong, courageous, at times heroic women; some frightened and inconsolable women; some new forms of inspiration, and new forms of heartbreak.

I knew Dawn Copeland at D.C. Jail, but I didn't know her well until we were both at FCI Lexington in 1991. By then she had full-blown AIDS and had been moved to the hospital unit. She was in her mid-twenties, but was wide-eyed and childlike enough to seem much younger. She didn't care who knew that she was HIV-positive, as long as people would respond by caring for her. She craved attention and support and loved to be babied. That was fine with some of us—we poured our anguish into attentiveness.

Dawn's impishness did an end-run around the bigotry and prejudice. Once when I accompanied her to a Saturday night movie, she got a gleam in her eye. She turned to another prisoner and asked her for a red-hot out of the woman's bag of candy. The woman thrust out her hand, said, "Here, take the whole bag," and eased off into the crowd outside the auditorium. Dawn said, "The stupider they are, the harder they fall. She thinks she'll catch AIDS from me if she shares her candy with me."

"Work it, sister," I said.

And she did, feeding her sweet tooth and her affectionate nature. She didn't want to deal with her medical problems—not that she could have done much in the way of controlling her own health care in those conditions—preferring to trust the doctors and be taken care of by others. Dawn finally went home to D.C., her sentence completed. She lived only a short time after her release. By letting a group of us take care of her, shower her with attention, she left a wake of sentiment on which we could begin to build our AIDS work at Lex. That was quite a contribution. Lex had about 1,800 women then, and most of the HIV-positive women in the federal prison system were held there. At the time I arrived at Lex, AIDS education at orientation consisted of a white male guard saying, "I can't tell you much about AIDS, but I'll tell you two things: you and I might not like it, but it's the law that people with AIDS can work in Food Service; and don't share an apple with someone with AIDS, because the skin can cut your gums, and if they bleed on the apple and then you bite it, you'll get AIDS." So AIDS education was drastically needed at Lex. By accepting support, Dawn helped us start to work together to initiate AIDS education and support. I don't think she realized that. I wish she had, because it might have been a comfort to her.

Geri Norwood spent time in D.C. Jail, too. She was transferred to Lex at the same time I was, in January of 1991. Unlike Dawn, she never got to go home. She died in the hospital at Lex, a few months after our arrival.

Geri chose to fight aggressively, with a lot less hugging and cuddling than Dawn. Geri would tell you what she wanted; then if you didn't give it she'd say "fuck you." She knew that ultimately she was in a very lonely situation. Picture yourself as an African American woman prisoner with AIDS, suffering from "mysterious" gynecological problems that were dismissed by the prison doctors, who ignored both the excruciating pain and the fact that these were opportunistic infections, part of AIDS. There was no AIDS support group at Lex yet, and Geri's main support came from a terrific lifelong friend, also a prisoner there, and from a prison chaplain. Her friend, Niecie, had to sneak to see her (at that time, the hospital unit was out-of-bounds to the rest of us; that changed as we began the AIDS work). The medical staff treated Geri as a hostile, uncooperative prisoner/patient, because she didn't meekly accept their diagnoses, judgments, and their pressure to let them operate. She died as she lived, deciding for herself, fighting for herself. The fact that she'd had to wage so much of that fight all alone was part of what compelled a few people to join in the formation of the "A Team," an AIDS education and support group at Lex, late in 1991.

Much of the spirit and strength to make the A Team work came from two prisoners with AIDS at Lex, Rosalind Simpson-Bey and her dear friend Doloris Hatcher-El. For a long time, Roz and Doloris were the only two women at Lex who talked openly about having AIDS, insisting on being respected, making it clear that they were in the process of living, not dying, and that the problem wasn't with them for being HIV-positive, but with those too ignorant to deal with that. This was at a time (still befor the Center for Disease Control did not recognize gynecological diseases as opportunistic infections) when "she's got AIDS" was a behind-the-back curse at Lex, as at most prisons. Doloris and Roz together provided a daily example of faith in life and the strength of women overcoming fear and prejudice. After Doloris left Lex to be released from prison in D.C., Roz provided the political and spiritual heart of our AIDS work, standing in the Chapel addressing an audience of four-hundred women, saying, "I am living with AIDS, and so can you. We have to conquer deathly ignorance with the spirit of life."

Doloris went out of prison and, until she died last year, she spread that strength, doing HIV/AIDS education and support through a D.C. organization, The Positive Woman, Inc. That organization has played an important role in bringing resources, information and support to the African American community in the fight against AIDS. Happily, Roz is alive and active still, recently freed in D.C. on "compassionate release."

Shortly before I was transferred from Lex to the Shawnee Unit, FCI Marianna, I was asked to write out a dying woman prisoner's Last Will and Testament to her small son. I hadn't known Yvonne well, and I only spent a few hours with her in her hospital cell. When I returned to show her the completed document, she was asleep. I sat down and waited until she woke up—ashen, sunken, emaciated, confused. I sat with her and held her as long as I could, until she fell back asleep. In the overheated stuffy stillness of that cell, I thought about the times when, as a child, I would awaken in a fever of measles or some other childhood disease, hurting and miserable, to see my mother sitting reading across the room...just sitting there, having taken the day off to be with me. And I thought, that's such a simple thing, but what a difference to awaken in a prison cell all alone, with only death watching over you.

I have known and loved all these women, along with others who have died, about whom I can't write because they kept their HIV hidden to the end, and many others who are still fighting. It's funny how enormously thankful you can be every day for your friends' lives when those lives are threatened The high point of my days now is the moment when I can call Roz and hear the vibrant strength of her voice, laugh together, and tell her how much I love her. It has been on these women's lives and deaths that prisoner peer advocacy AIDS programs have grown in Lexington and other federal women's prisons. This work has enabled other HIV-positive women prisoners to take a little more control over their health, to live a little better and to be more at peace. But we are so limited by prison conditions and the oxymoron "prison health care" that the demand for release of all prisoners with HIV and AIDS is the only humane and reasonable resolution to the problem of AIDS in prison.

To all who read this, in memory of Joyce, and Dawn, and Geri, and Doloris, and Yvonne, and too many others: fight for the release of all prisoners with HIV and AIDS.

To all those fighting to live with AIDS in prison and in memory of those who have died there

MY RICE QUEEN
BASED ON AN INTERVIEW OF M
SEPTEMBER, 1992

MARTI ZUCKROWV

He was in the main lounge fucking some guy, when I first saw him. Back then, everyone went to the baths. For ten bucks you could spend a few hours there, and for a little extra, get a private stall. I always paid the extra, but then again, I'm shy. Allen, he had absolutely no modesty whatsoever, just walked around the place completely naked. Most guys covered up a little, just to keep you guessing, but not Allen.

Funny, that's something I admired about him from the very beginning, how easy he was with himself. I don't think that he saw me while he was fucking the guy, but I could almost swear that immediately after they were done, he looked straight up at me, probably looking for more. I hung around the lounge for a while. Allen and the guy left. Then I decided to go back to my stall.

No sooner did I get there when the guy Allen was fucking appeared and asked me if I wanted to do a threesome. He seemed very fucked up on something, I think it was alcohol, but I'm not sure. I figured, why not, I was there for some action also, so I followed the guy out into the hallway while he tried to hustle another man into completing our trio. Somewhere along the line he got too loaded to do much of anything and left. In the meantime there was Allen, parading around the halls, stark naked. The ease with which he did this really turned me on. It also left me feeling very envious. You know, in Japan, sex is much more discreet, nothing is done in public.

I was coy and played hard to get. Allen went for it. I never knew if he was really a Rice Queen or not, but I know that he liked Asian boys. We were back in my stall pretty quick, having sex. It's funny, but I remember the exact date, don't ask me why. It wasn't much after I first got to this country, July 9th, 1981. Hard to believe, I was thirty-one and Allen was thirty-three.

Well, out of the blue, Allen asked if he could come home with me. I was totally surprised, but I agreed. He had his bicycle, and I liked that. I remember how he put a rubber band around his ankle to pull his pants leg away from what do you call that, oh yes, the spokes. He was athletic, and I liked that too. Especially, because up until the time I was in Kindergarten, I thought I was a girl.

We went back to my place, I was living close to the baths. He took an apple and some cheese out of his backpack and offered me half. I liked that, too. He seemed natural, wholesome. We took our shoes off and started to play footsies. Somewhere around that time, between the apple and cheese and footsies, I decided to trust him. It's not easy for me to trust people, but usually my intuition is right. He stayed the night. Well, I figured it was a one-night stand, which was okay with me, although I have to say, I liked him.

He called a few days later, though, to tell me that he had gonor-rhea, and he offered to take me to the clinic with him. I didn't know much about the clinics, because I was so new to the country. We met at the Sutter Street Clinic, he gave me directions to get there, and we both got treated.

That was the first time I saw how Allen could take charge of a sit-uation. The receptionist wanted us to come back the next day, instead of treating us that afternoon, but Allen insisted on talking to one of the doctors, and he did get us in right away. It wasn't a big deal to treat, not like today. One shot and you were cured. I was impressed at how he spoke up, I don't like to do that—speak up.

In my country, when someone you love gets sick, you don't ques-tion what to do. You just do it. Here, it's different, more selfish, I think. I started to take charge, because I had to. I always tried to be there for him. Even with his art work, I always talked to him about his art work. Something was missing in his work, a nuance or something. Allen didn't allow himself to follow his intuition, maybe his feminine side. I always tried to tell him that, because I admired his work, and I thought he could do better work, I really wanted him to listen to me, not so that he would do it my way, but so that he could find a better, a fuller way to work, but I don't think he listened to me. I don't think that Allen really respected me.

Sometimes I miss him, sometimes I'm relieved that he died, sometimes all I want to do is get on with my life, for however long that is. If I wasn't sick too, I could take all the time I need to heal, but I don't know how much time I have left. I want some good times before I die, I can't wait. Sometimes all I want are some big strong hands to hold me, some comfort, some relief. The last two years were hell, and now this. Life isn't fair.

The first time Allen got sick, we were in Japan. It was his first trip there with me. He got sick from eating sushi, he thought, but now I don't think that was it. We were in Tokyo then, and he thought that it was food poisoning. I didn't and I still remember how delicious that sushi was. Funny. Well, that's when his diarrhea started, after the sushi.

Next he got these weird red spots on his feet. We joked about it, said it must be AIDS. We both knew about AIDS, but it seemed like AIDS had nothing to do with us. The red spots went away, but then Allen got a terrible toothache and his gums started to hurt him all the time. He went to see a dentist he'd met at the school where he taught English as a Second Language. The dentist did a root canal, and gave him antibiotics for his gums. Allen said that the guy prescribed too much medicine, and that it caused his Candida, which he never got rid of.

I remember a conversation we once had, after we moved to the countryside, in Makioto. Allen said that if he ever got AIDS, he would read the newspapers for updates on information and take lots of vitamin C. That makes me laugh, how little we understood back then.

Soon after we got to Makioto, Allen was starting to feel pretty sick and on top of that he got the news that his father had died. That's when he left Japan and went back to Maine. I didn't know yet, but I was worried. I got sick once myself, with shingles, but it was easy to treat and I got over it fast. I didn't hear from Allen for quite some time, then, after he'd gone back to Maine. I was getting very worried, so when he called me up to tell me, I wasn't really surprised. But I didn't know how to respond. I was cheerful. I wanted him to be okay. He asked me to come back to the States with him, and I agreed right away.

Maybe I believe in fate. I'm not sure, but I did feel that he was my mate. In Japan, there is a myth which says that the right person for you exists somewhere in the universe. And that person will have a thin ribbon tied around their pinkie finger. You have to find the string, but it might be tied up in knots with someone else's string, so you may never get to be with this person, but this person is still your true mate. So I guess I knew, I had found my mate and it was Allen. So it was easy to come back with him.

He came back to Japan first for a few weeks to help me pack up and move. Then we returned together. I'm not sure exactly when it was, but I know that we were living on Eddy Street in 1987, so it must have been a little before then.

When we were at Eddy Street, that's when things began to really change, after he got PCP. Our roles started to shift, a little at first, not like how it got to be when he couldn't do anything for himself, but enough that I saw it happening. He probably did too. And that's when AIDS started to be what Allen's life was about. Doctors, medicines, night sweats every night. Everything started then. But it was the last year when it got really bad.

I was glad to take care of him. Only thing is, I wish he'd thanked me for it. He got so angry and bitchy at me all the time. I think he hated to have to ask me for help. I think he hated not being the Captain. I didn't like having to become the Captain, not at first. Not ever really, but it felt good to see that I could do it. I didn't know that about myself, he always did everything before.

A few of our closest friends couldn't touch him. When he was in the hospice, they got too scared. It wasn't like that for me, but once I felt his body dying, I couldn't have sex with him anymore. Having sex, being so physical together, that scared me, because he was becoming a death presence, not Allen anymore. But by the time he got to the hospice, it was all okay. I just tried to help him feel more comfortable. I couldn't stand the pain he was in. That was the worst, just watching him suffer, feeling so helpless. But you know, I think he knew that I was there, an hour before he died, because he squeezed my hand. His face was so beautiful at that moment, I took a picture of it. I carry it around in my backpack, actually it's Allen's backpack, but I use it now. I never did understand why he always used a backpack, but now, now I'm coming to understand.

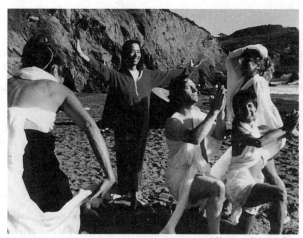
Mikeo, standing, in robe

To Mikeo and Allen
Mikeo: Dec. 10, 1949-June 1993
Allen: April 2, 1947-June 1992

Epilogue

Lunch on Sixth Ave.

Lesléa Newman

Keith and I can hardly breathe
let alone order, with you
suddenly at our table
pen and pad posed,
beautifully balanced between
male and female
black and white
adult and child.
You wait puzzled, then dazzle
us further with your smile
which so unnerves Keith
he spills his water
into my lap. You rush off
and return with napkins
that look like flowers
in your strong, delicate hands.
Finally we order and you leave
us to our stunned selves.
Neither of us will say it:
you look just like Gerard
a decade ago when he was
my roommate and Keith's lover
and none of us could imagine

ourselves middle-aged
or dead. Suddenly it is hard
to eat but we order more food
another drink, dessert, anything
to bring you back
to our table one last time.
You bring the check
which we argue over
then tactfully walk away
so we can leave you an obscene
tip neither of us can afford
along with both our business cards.
Keith wonders who you'll call
first. I imagine you adding
our cards to a mile-high stack
teetering in your apartment
or pasting them in place
among the hordes you've fashioned
into adoring wallpaper. But who cares?
Knowing beauty such as yours
still exists in the world
is enough to make Keith and me mad
with joy as we rush out
into the razzle-dazzle street
forgetting just for a moment
how mad we are with grief.

For Gerard Rizza, 1959–1992
"most ordinary boy"

THE CALLING OF THE NAMES

"I'll be somewhere, listening for my name"

—Melvin Dixon
Keynote Speech OutWrite, 1992

So many people sent their stories to *A Loving Testimony*, I wasn't able to include them all. However, I do call the names of everyone who was written about, as a way to honor them and to remember them:

Aaron Cohen: died October, 1989
Al'zeen
Al Bright: July 4, 1939–July 30, 1989
Al Parker
Alan
Alan D. Hutchins
Alex Smith
Allan
Allan Bednarski: May 3, 1952–Aug. 10, 1993
Allan Eric Grams: Feb. 14, 1952–Sept. 10, 1986
Allen: born April 2, 1947, died in June 1992, age 45
Allen Lucian: April 24, 1964–Dec. 19, 1990, forever young
Allen Sperl: died June 11, 1992, age 45
Andre, died March, 1991
Andres Herendez, alias Picasso
Andrew Levinson: July 28, 1954–March 19, 1993
Angela
Angelo
Anonymous
Anthony Calloway
Arthur
Arthur Ashe: 1943–Feb. 6, 1993
Arthur Robbins, Ph.D., died Jan. 1989, age 39
Ashley

Barbara C.: died Sept. 28, 1993, age 37
Barry Godfrey
Bart: June 26, 1961–Aug. 31, 1990
Ben
Ben Collins: Dec. 22, 1953– Feb. 28, 1991

Bill
Bill Harren: died Oct. 1989
Bill Quinn: Dec. 19, 1957–Dec. 20, 1992
Bill Rossiter, Ph.D.: died Jan. 26, 1988, age 38
Bill Upton
Bill W.: 1936–1989
Billy
Billy Pollard: died in 1992
Blande E. Cornell ("Buddy"): Oct. 17, 1955–Jan. 4, 1988
Blane F. Feulner: April 12, 1954–July 12, 1992
Bob
Bob: Jan. 4, 1957–May 2, 1993
Bob Colagrande
Bob Hart: died Feb. 1989
Bob Mony: 1940–1990
Bob Sappenfield
Bobby Lawlor
Branch
Branch Hastings: died in 1992
Brian Pocar
Brian Pomerleau
Bruce Hoffman

Calvan Vail
Cap Moran
Charles Jones: died Aug. 1990, age 46
Charlie
Charlie Halloran: died Feb. 7, 1993
Charlie Kurtz
Chester
Chris Angeles: died April 6, 1992, age 27
(Miss) Chris Steve: March 14, 1957–July 22, 1993
Christopher Colt: Oct. 15, 1953–Dec. 17, 1992
Christopher ("Kippy") Conway: 1960–1994
Chuck Macintyre: died Aug. 1990
Chuck Solomon: March 10, 1946–1987
Cirby: died in 1992
Dr. Clark A. Thompson: March 22, 1935–Jan. 14, 1990
Colin: died in 1993
Conrad Reny: June 29, 1954–Sept. 11, 1991
Cookie Mueller
Craig Anderson: Jan. 19, 1952–Spring 1987
Craig J. Philip: July 27, 1954–June 6, 1993

Craiger Black
Curtis Walter Schmeider: July 9, 1946–Dec. 8, 1985

D.D.
Dale
Dan
Dan: 1947–1992
Dan S.: June 10, 1951–July 25, 1993
Dan Turner: died June 1984
Daniel
Danny Bova
Danny Thompson: Aug. 23, 1960–March 16, 1991
Daniel Haight
Daniel Lynn Stimmerman: Aug. 10, 1947–Aug. 17, 1992
Darrell Cole: died Sept. 11, 1992
Daryl E. Fredrick: Feb. 4, 1949–June 20, 1992
Dave Williams: 1952–1990
David
David Cobbett
David Lemieux
David A. Loebl: Feb. 19, 1956–May 24, 1993
David Riel: Nov. 11, 1962–Nov. 22, 1990, 11:03 a.m.
David Trujillo: May 19, 1958–May 3, 1991
David Ward: Aug. 30, 1948–Aug. 29, 1989
David Wojnarowicz
Dawn Copeland: died 1992
Dene Ralph Greenough: 1960–1992
Dennis
Dennis Janis: Dec. 18, 1954–Dec. 19, 1993
Dick Carey
Doloris Hatcher: died Aug. 23, 1993
Don Meuse: Aug. 1950–June 1992
Donald
Doug Fraser
Duane Kearns Puryear: Dec. 20, 1964–Oct. 8, 1991

Ed
Ed McCoy: July 19, 1939–July 22, 1992
Ed Parente
Ed Weissenborn
Edward Hunter: 1945–1991
Eliot España: died Fall, 1990
Eric

Eric Lerner
Ernie Acosta: died Summer, 1991

F.B.: March 19, 1939–Oct. 30, 1991
Francis Paul Pedornock: March 27, 1945–March 16, 1992
Frank
Frank Cream: Aug. 2, 1944–March 19, 1991
Frank Dost
Frank H. Metcalf, Jr.: June 19, 1944–May 25, 1993
Fraser MacBeth
Fred Shepler: July 10, 1940–March 5, 1984
Freddie Mercury
Frederick Mandel: born April 28, 1948, died at age 42

Gabe Kruks: 1950–1992
Gary
Gary Prutsman
Gary Reynolds
Gary Roberts: June 18, 1949–March 7, 1993
Gary Vavrinek: April 17, 1958–March 14, 1990
Gene
George Ash
George DeSipio
Gerard Anthony Rizza: Oct. 20, 1959–April 4, 1992
Geri Norwood: died March, 1991
Gerry
Glen
Glen Holt: died in 1987
Glen Spiegelhalden: died 1990
Gordon A. Juel: died at age 39
Gordon Young
Goyo
Gregory Kolovakos: 1952–1990
Gustavo Motta: June 20, 1944–Feb. 6, 1993
Guy

Harry
Harry Earls
Harry Varjean
Henri
Henry R. Weitzer: 1929–1987
Hugh: died July, 1985

Ira

J.F.
(Dr.) James Finkelstein: Feb. 14, 1930–July 22, 1989
James Marshall: died 1992
(Rev.) James Sandmire: died May, 1991
James Turcotte: Nov. 30, 1945–May 11, 1993
James Gray Vaughan: Aug. 9, 1949–March 8, 1993
Jan Sutter
Jay: June 1, 1950–Feb. 27, 1989
Jeff
Jeff: April 14, 1950–May 25, 1991
Jeff: died Nov. 4, 1990
Jeff Cowles: Nov. 12, 1957–Oct. 16, 1992
Jeff Dames: April 14, 1950–May 25, 1991
Jeff Gold: died Oct. 1991, age 30
Jeffrey D. Byers: July 13, 1953–Jan. 17, 1989
Jeffrey Keith Cowles: Nov. 12, 1959–Oct. 1992
Jerry Rogers: 1959–1990
Jerry White: Nov. 7, 1943–March 17, 1989
Jim
Jim: Feb. 14, 1930–July 22, 1989
Jim Hely: 1957 or 1958–March 4, 1986
Jim Hickman: April 20, 1941–June 15, 1993
Jim Perry: Jan. 1950–Oct. 1990
Jim Thanos: 1951–1992
Jimmy
Jo: died 1981
Joe
Joe Campo: June 14, 1961–Nov. 7, 1990
John and James
John Brewer: Dec. 27, 1953–1992
John A. Bubb: 1950–1993
John David: May 15, 1966–June 9, 1993
John A. Davidson, Jr. 1959–Nov. 12, 1989
John Lewis: Dec. 23, 1953–Dec. 31, 1989
John Carl O'Brien: Sept. 27, 1953–Sept. 3, 1989
(Dr.) John George Sampson: April 1, 1959–Dec. 17, 1992
John Williams: died 1982
John Willig
Johnny
Jojo Gillan
Jon

Joseph
Joseph McAllaster: Feb. 3, 1955–June 18, 1993
Joseph C. Patton: July 14, 1950–Oct. 25, 1991
Joseph Andrew Sablan: Oct. 23, 1961–Oct. 9, 1992
Joseph Wickline
Joyce Cooper: died Spring, 1989
Judith McDonnell: 1952–1993
Jurgen Tilsner: died July 9,1988

K.M.: June 14, 1951–Jan. 3, 1994
Keith Gann
Ken Hamilton
Ken Johnston: July 9, 1957–July 16, 1989
Kenneth Roger Alsleben, Jr.: April 15, 1950–July 9, 1987
Kenneth L. Dawson: Oct. 9, 1946–April 9, 1992
Kenny: Sept. 29, 1959– Sept. 25, 1990
Kenny B.
Kevin: died Jan. 1987
Kevin O. Gessler: 1959–1992
Kevin Patterson: May 23, 1955–March 18, 1988

L.N.
Larry
Larry: died April 1990
Larry Fodrocy: Sept. 2, 1949–March 30, 1992
Laurence
Lenny Malone
Leon McKusick
Lew, died at age 50
Lionel Cuffie
Louis F. Homyak
Louis Smith Weingarden: 1943–1989
Luis Felipe Pereira: Jan. 4, 1955–June 28, 1992
Luis Armando Valdes: 1952–1986

Marco Vassi: Nov. 3, 1937–Jan. 14, 1989
Mark
Mark: died Nov. 1986
Mark Hardwick
Mark David Horowitz: May 3, 1948–Sept. 27, 1993
Mark P. Prantner: June 3, 1957–Feb. 28, 1989
Mark T. Rifkin: died 1984
Marty B.: Sept. 12, 1954–Sept. 20, 1991

Marty Selim: Nov. 8, 1951–Jan. 7, 1992
Matt
Melvin Boozer: June 21, 1945–March 6, 1987
Michael
Michael Arnsmeier
Michael Callen
Michael Carson: Aug. 29, 1954–Aug. 8, 1992
Michael Johnson (aka Mijo): 1953–1988
Michael Robert Kindred: Feb. 23, 1952–Oct. 20, 1992
Michael Maletta
Michael McKinnon
Michael Rubin: 1935–1989
Michael Schaefer: July 31, 1950–Nov. 5, 1990
Michael Watterlond: Nov. 4, 1946–May 17, 1988
Michael Young: Oct. 8, 1963–Dec. 19, 1991
Mike Clark: 1948–1993
Mike Riegle: died Jan. 10, 1991
Mikel Allen Lindzy: Sept. 14, 1954–Sept. 28, 1987
Mikeo Kondo: died June 2, 1993, age 46
Mitch
Mommy, died Nov. 21, 1991
Morgan Fine
Myreon Taylor: 1947–1992

N. Craig Geist: died Nov. 30, 1990, age 38
Neil Sandstad: died 1990
Nicholas Carter: Sept. 20, 1948–July 9, 1993
Nicholas Dana LaCasse: May 14, 1959–Aug. 1, 1990
Nicholas Reigh: died Dec. 26, 1988
Nick: Dec. 9, 1931–June 28, 1985
Norman Armentrout: died 1988

Oren K. Clark, Jr.: Oct. 16, 1949–April 3, 1993

P.T.M.
Pat
Patrick: died in 1992
Patrick Sweeney: 1956–1993
Patrick Toner
Paul
Paul: July 2, 1954–Jan. 14, 1993
Paul Abels: Aug. 4, 1938–March 12, 1992
Paul Binkley

Paul Fini: died Oct. 15, 1985
Paul George Hornyak: Aug. 2, 1955–Oct. 27, 1993
Perry: died March 1984
Peter
Philip Harmon Porter: Dec. 8, 1957–July 15, 1992
Philip Sciaroni: 1957–1992

R.H.: Aug. 20, 1953–Sept. 5, 1987
R.J.
R.W.
Rachel Ellyn Hertzberg–Thurman: Feb. 2, 1966–June 15, 1993
Raeburn Miller: died Sept. 6, 1990
Ralph
Rana
Randal Alan Myers: Nov. 30, 1956–Feb. 25, 1991
Randall Harrison Lowe: July 11, 1941–Feb. 9, 1988
Randy Brown
Randy Gillenwater
Ray
Ray Cork: died in 1991
Raymond Jacobs
Raymond Navarro: Oct. 6, 1964–Nov. 9, 1990
Richard: Nov. 18, 1938–March 25, 1993
Richard Davidoff: died Aug. 3, 1990
Richard Bruce Fried: Feb. 19, 1952–Aug. 17, 1986
Richard Gibson: July 10, 1952–May 21, 1991
Richard Hall: 1926–1992
Richard Benjamin Kaplan: June 24, 1943–Nov. 14, 1993
Rick: died at age 35
Riley Patrick Liming: 1961–1991
Rob McCall
Robb Caramico: Feb. 17, 1964–Nov. 30, 1992
Robert
Robert Bruce Arganbright: Oct. 22, 1938–Oct. 22, 1992
Robert Auric: died Oct. 1986, age 37
Robert F. Bucci: Feb. 9, 1949–April 29, 1991
Robert Scott Chase: July 26, 1954–Oct. 16, 1991
Robert Cooper: died in 1983
Robert Scott Ford: Feb. 2, 1960–May 23, 1991
Robert Hancock: 1948–1993
Robert Haule: April 13, 1948–Aug. 8, 1993
Roberto Galindo: Sept. 14, 1950–Sept. 8, 1993
Roddy Soma

Roger
Roger Childs
Rolando Reyes: Nov. 29, 1959–May or June, 1989
Ron: died in 1990
Ron Duda: died Dec. 1992
(Rev.) Ronald R. Markle: Sept. 27, 1941–March 3, 1989
Ross Johnson: May 3, 1966–March 13, 1993
Roy Raoul Gonsalves: Oct. 5, 1959–July 10, 1993
Roy Mark Harrison: Dec. 20, 1951–March 3, 1993
Rudolph Nureyev: 1938–1993
Ruffin Cooper, Jr.: Jan. 4, 1942–May 31, 1992
Russ, died Sept. 1990

Scott Caldwell: died in 1984
Scott Ford: Feb. 9, 1960–May 23, 1991
Scott Griffith
Scott Shipe: Nov. 10, 1957–May 29, 1993
Sean
Sean Heggarty
Seth Kimmelman: died Dec. 5, 1991
Sidney Burstein
Skip
Stephan: died July 1, 1992
Stephen: died April, 1987
Stephen John Risch: Jan. 10, 1950–Sept. 17, 1990
Steve: Jan. 10, 1950–Sept. 17, 1990
Steve Cee: died Fall, 1989
Steven
Steven Grossman: Sept. 1, 1952–June 23, 1991
Stormy: died Jan 12, 1990, at age 33
Stuart Teitler
Swami Danesh (aka Jerry Phieffer)
Sylvester

T.W. McKinsey: 1920–1990
Ted
Ted Schoen: Sept. 15, 1946–Aug. 18, 1993
Tede Matthews: July 29, 1951–July 19, 1993
Terry Vander Heyden: Aug. 19, 1950–Aug. 18, 1992
Terryl Joseph "TJ" Myers: Feb. 7, 1960–Aug. 28, 1990
Theodore T. Urban: Aug. 7, 1950–Nov. 14, 1991
Teresa Paige: died in 1990, age 29
Thomas Edward Miller: Dec. 23, 1958–Dec. 28, 1990

Thomas John Knobblock: June 10, 1958–Nov. 29, 1991
Tim
Tim Salvner: died 1992
Tim: March 29, 1956–April 4, 1994
Timothy Harold Foster: March 29, 1960–Jan. 30, 1986
Timothy McDonnell
Todd De Meza
Todd Lawson: 1941–1987
Tom
Tom C.
Tom Black: April 27, 1958–Oct. 2, 1990
Tom Brown: June 11, 1958–July 24, 1992
Tom Cunningham: Jan. 5, 1960–Dec. 9, 1992
Tom Perry: June 20, 1952–June 26, 1988
Tom Ratzin
Tom Rosinsky: died in 1987
Tom S.
Tonio Gonzalez: April 21, 1949–July 20, 1993
Tony
Tony Beam: July 1949–Sept. 11, 1990

Uncle Bobby: May 25, 1940–Oct. 8, 1985

Victor Petersen
Vincent Cage

W.M.: July 23, 1957–Aug. 18, 1981
W. Paul Bingo: April 18, 1854–July 1991
Ware Smith
Warren Hadler: died Aug. 1986
Wayne
Wayne Friedman
Wayne Marcy: May 4, 1954–April 8, 1992
Wayne Slusher
Wendal: died in 1989 or 1990
Wesley Jackson
William "Skip" Alfredson: died in 1990
William Paul Bates
William Hague: 1956–1985
William Albert Walson: Dec. 22, 1956–Dec. 31, 1993

Yvonne: died in 1992

RESOURCES

ORGANIZATIONS

AIDS Hotlines
1–800–342–AIDS

Spanish AIDS Hotlines
1–800–344–7432

National AIDS Information
Clearing House
1–800–458–5231

Mothers of AIDS Patients
P.O. Box 1763
Lometa, CA 90717
(213)542–3019

PFlag (Parents and Friends of
Lesbians and Gays)
PO Box 27605
Washington, DC 20038
(202)638–4200

The NAMES Project
310 Townsend Street
Suite 310
San Francisco, CA 94107
(415)882–5500

Lambda Legal Defense and
Educational Fund
666 Broadway
12th Floor
New York, NY 10012
(212)995–8585

National AIDS Network
2033 M Street NW
Suite 800
Washington, DC 20036
(202)293–2437

Positive Women United
P.O. Box 34372
Washington, DC 20043
(202)898–0372

National Association of People
with AIDS
2025 I Street
Suite 1118
Washington, DC 20006
(202)429–2856

Compassionate Friends
National Office
P.O. Box 3696
Oak Brook, IL 60522
(312)990–0010

Gay Men's Health Crisis
129 W. 20th Street
New York, NY 10011
(212)337–3694

PWA Coalition
31 W. 26th Street
5th Floor
New York, NY 10010
(212)532–0568
outside New York City:
1–800–828–3280

Senior Action in a Gay
Environment (SAGE)
208 W. 13th Street
New York, NY 10011
(212)741–2247

PUBLICATIONS

Periodicals

Art & Understanding:
The International Magazine of
Literature and Art About AIDS
25 Monroe Street
Suite 205
Albany, NY 12210

POZ
Box 1279
Old Chelsea Station
New York, NY 10113–1279

Books for Children

Girard, Linda Walvoord. *Alex, The Kid With AIDS.* Morton Grove, IL: Albert Whitman & Co., 1991.

Jordan, MaryKate. *Losing Uncle Tim.* Morton Grove, IL: Albert Whitman & Co., 1989.

Merrifield, Margaret. *Come Sit By Me.* Toronto: Women's Press, 1990.

Moutoussanmy-Ashe, Jeanne. *Daddy and Me.* New York: Knopf, 1993.

Newman, Lesléa. *Too Far Away To Touch.* New York: Clarion Books, 1995.

Quinlan, Patricia. *Tiger Flowers.* New York: Dial Books for Young Readers, 1994.

Wiener, Lori S., Best, Aprille, Pizzo, Philip. *Be a Friend: Children Who Live With HIV Speak.* Morton Grove, IL: Albert Whitman & Co., 1994.

Books for Teenagers

Durant, Peggy. *When Heroes Die.* New York: Atheneum, 1992.

Gleitzman, Morris. *Two Weeks With The Queen.* New York: Putnam, 1991.

Hein, Karen and Digeronimo, Theresa Foy. *AIDS: Trading Fear for Facts: A Guide for Young People.* Yonkers, NY: Consumers Union of the United States. 1989, 1991, 1993.

Humphreys, Martha. *Until Whatever.* New York: Scholastic, Inc., 1991.

Kittredge, Mary. *Teenagers with AIDS Speak Out.* Englewood Cliffs, NJ: Julian Messner, 1991.

Landau, R. *We Have AIDS.* NY: Franklin Watts, 1990.

Nelson, Theresa. *Earthshine.* New York: Orchard Books, 1994

Porte, Barbara Ann. *Something Terrible Happened.* New York: Orchard Books, 1994.

White, Ryan and Cunningham, Ann Marie. *Ryan White: My Own Story.* New York: Dial Books, 1991.

Books for Adults

Alyson, Sasha. *You Can Do Something about AIDS*. Boston: Stop AIDS Project, 1988, 1990.

Brown, Joe. *A Promise To Remember: The NAMES Project Book of Letters*. NY: Avon, 1992.

Brown, Rebecca. *The Gifts of the Body*. New York: Harper Collins, 1994.

Currier, Jameson. *Dancing on the Moon: Short Stories about AIDS*. NY: Penguin, 1993.

Donnelly, Katherine Fair. *Recovering From The Loss of a Loved One to AIDS*. NY: St. Martins, 1994.

Eidson, Ted. *The AIDS Caregivers Handbook*. NY: St. Martin's, 1988, 1993.

Feinberg, David B. *Queer and Loathing: Rants and Raves of a Raging AIDS Clone*. New York: Viking, 1994.

Fries, Kenny. *The Healing Notebooks*. Berkeley, CA: Open Books, 1990.

Froman, Paul. *After You Say Goodbye: When Someone You Love Dies of AIDS*. San Francisco: Chronicle Books, 1992.

Hitchens, Neal. *Voices That Care: Stories and Encouragement for People with AIDS/HIV and Those Who Love Them*. NY: Simon & Shuster, 1992.

Hubley, J. *AIDS Handbook: A Guide to the Understanding of AIDS & HIV*. New York: MacMillan, 1990.

Jones, Carolyn. *Living Proof: Courage in the Face of AIDS*. NY: Abbeville Press Publishers, 1994.

Klein, Michael. *Poets For Life: Seventy-six Poets Respond to AIDS*. NY: Persea Books, 1989.

Mars-Jones, Adam. *Monopolies of Loss*. New York: Knopf, 1992.

Martelli, Leonard J., Peltz, Fran D., Messina, William and Petrow, Steven. *When Someone You Know Has AIDS*. NY: Crown, 1993.

Monette, Paul. *Borrowed Time: An AIDS Memoir*. NY: Harcourt Brace Jovanovich, 1988.

Monette, Paul. *Love Alone: Eighteen Eulogies for Rog*. NY: St. Martins,1988.

Reiner, Ines and Ruppelt, Patricia. *AIDS: The Women*. San Francisco: Cleis Press, 1988.

Rudd, A., Taylor, D. *Positive Women: Voices of Women Living with AIDS*. Toronto: Second Story Press, 1992.

Shelby, R.D. *If a Partner Has AIDS: A Guide to Clinical Intervention for Relationships in Crisis*. NY: Haworth Press, 1992.

Shiltz, Randy. *And The Band Played On*. NY: St. Martin's, 1987.

Verghese, Abraham. *My Own Country: A Doctor's Story of a Town and its People in the Age of AIDS*. NY: Simon & Shuster, 1994.

CONTRIBUTORS' BIOS

Daniel J. Barone is a social worker and a church musician working as an HIV counselor and a church organist in Hartford, Connecticut. His mom, brother, and gay family are his biggest supporters. Beauchamp and Sappho, the two "kids," are a constant source of affection and amusement for him.

Judith Black struggles to live, love and come to terms with regrets in San Francisco, California. At twenty–nine, her survival is dependent on making art, writing, sewing, kite–flying, the kindness and love of friends, and high hopes for better days.

Maureen Brady's novels, *Give Me Your Good Ear* and *Folly*, were reprinted by Spinster's Ink and The Feminist Press, 1994. Her meditations for women in midlife are forthcoming, Harper San Francisco, 1995, and her new novel, *Ginger's Fire*, will follow soon after. "Lovers" was a finalist for the Katherine Anne Porter Fiction Prize.

James Breeden was raised in the quiet, uneventful suburbs of Grand Blanc, Michigan. Currently he is editor of "Books To Watch Out For," newsletter for A Different Light Bookstore in San Francisco, and has resumed a quiet life in the Inner Sunset neighborhood of that city.

Marisa Brown has been a marketing/public relations professional in the arts for more than ten years. She is now changing careers, finishing a Masters of Social Work degree. She resides in western Massachusetts with husband, Peter Ludwig, where she volunteers as an AIDS buddy, and studies yoga and meditation.

Jill Cagan is a writer of fiction, nonfiction and poetry. She is a graduate student at San Francisco State University in Counseling. She has worked as an actress on stage and television. Raised in New England, Jill now lives on a houseboat in Sausalito, California, with her husband and son.

C.A. Carmel grew up in Cincinnati but for the past thirty years has lived in a one-hundred-year-old house in New Jersey. She is married and has two grown children. Her stories have appeared in *The Quarterly* and in *Christopher Street*. She is currently working on a novel.

Kim Christensen has been active in the feminist, antiracist, disability and bisexual liberation movements for many years. Since 1988, she has worked with ACT UP/NY and is coauthor of *Women, AIDS and Activism*. She currently teaches Economics and Women's Studies at SUNY Purchase. She misses her dear friend, Ray Navarro.

Cynthia Lee Clark is currently committed to one of the most optimistic acts of her life: writing a novel. *Luck of the Draw* tells the story of four family members, one a PWA, on a trip to Las Vegas. Cynthia lives in Arizona with her husband and two young daughters.

Louie Crew has published 518 items including the poetry volumes, *Sunspots* (Lotus Press, 1976), *Midnight Lessons* (Samizdat, 1987) and *Lutibelle's Pew* (Dragon Disks, 1990). The University of Michigan collects his papers. He has read at more than threescore venues in Britain, Canada, China, Hong Kong and the USA. He teaches English at Rutgers University.

Donna Decker is an assistant professor of English at the University of Wisconsin–Stevens Point. She is very interested in choreopoetry and recently performed an extended work, "Dear Riz," merging poetry, music, dance and visual arts, about her soul friend Gerard Rizza's life and subsequent death from AIDS.

Helen Decker is a teacher of English and Poetry at Susan E. Wagner High School. She shares her time and her words between New York City and Woodstock, NY.

Denise Duhamel is the author of *Girl Soldier* (Garden Street Press, 1995), *The Woman With Two Vaginas* (Salmon Run Publishers, 1994), and *Smile!* (Warm Spring Press, 1993). Her poems have been included in literary magazines such as *American Poetry Review*, *Mudfish*, *Ontario Review*, *Poet Lore* and *Hanging Loose*.

Ms. Dutkowsky lives comfortably in beautiful Ithaca, N.Y.

Alice E. was born in Madison County, Illinois, in 1923, and was the third of four children. In 1939, she moved with her family to the same village where she currently resides. She is the mother of three children: Mike was the youngest. She is a founding member of the Vermillion County (Illinois) AIDS Task Force.

Jenna A. Felice is a part–time editorial assistant at TOR Books, as well as a student at Sarah Lawrence College. She has had criticism published in *The New York Review of Science Fiction*, of which she is a staff member. Ms. Felice lives in New York City with three roommates, one spousal, two quadrupedal.

Miriam Finkelstein's *Domestic Affairs* was published by Houghton Mifflin in 1982. Her stories have appeared in magazines such as *Ascent*, *Arizona Quarterly*, *Kayak* and *Kalliope*. She began writing poetry in 1990, shortly after the death of her husband. Her poems have appeared in *Commonweal* and *Women and Death*.

Carie Ford–Broecker works in Monterey, California, counseling people with HIV, and has spoken to numerous audiences about her experience living with HIV/AIDS. She has received several awards in recognition of her contribution to the fight against AIDS. She is dedicated to spreading a message of hope to HIV-positive people.

William H. Foster III has been a writer since age eight and was first published at age twelve. Poet, essayist, playwright and short story writer, Mr. Foster is a regularly invited author at the Celebration of Black Writing. He is presently a Professor of English at a Connecticut community college.

Suzanne Fried is a published writer, licensed psychotherapist and a public speaker on transforming our lives after loss. She facilitates grief groups entitled "Healing for Broken Hearts." "Frozen in Time" is excerpted from an unpublished book entitled *Loving Richie*.

Jane Futcher teaches English in Marin County, California, whre lives with her lover, Erin. She is a founder and editor of *The Slant*, a gay/lesbian/bisexual newspaper, and has published two novels, *Crush* and *Promise Not to Tell*, as well as *Marin: The Place and the People*.

Joyce Gallegos, born in Swanton, Ohio, married H.E. Brooks in 1955. Had two sons, Timothy, born 1956, and Steven, born 1959. Married Joe Gallegos in 1986 and now resides in Warren, Michigan. Joyce spent the last few months in New York, caring for Tim who died peacefully in his own apartment on April 4th, 1993.

David Garnes was born and grew up in Springfield, Massachusetts. He lived in New York from 1963 to 1981 and is now a reference librarian at the University of Connecticut, Storrs. He has several writing projects in progress and is still studying Spanish.

Kimberly Gerould coordinates a bilingual education program for teen mothers and their children in Holyoke, Massachusetts. She is also a writer, friend, wife, and mother of Yamila and Diego.

Harry Gipson was born in Shreveport, Louisiana, on February 4th, 1939. He is a teacher in Los Angeles, California, where he met Gary Roberts, his deceased life partner. He believes that the journey through AIDS with a loved one can be one of the most profoundly transforming experiences one can have.

Jewelle Gomez is the author of a novel, *The Gilda Stories*, and a collection of essays, *Forty–Three Septembers* (Firebrand Books). Originally from Boston, she lived in New York City for twenty–two years. She currently lives and teaches in San Francisco.

Norman C. Greenough married Beverly in 1954, and just tried to be a good husband/father and provider over the last forty years to his wife and four children: Dorene, Jody, Dene, and Meg. A silent majority citizen, he pretty much minded his own business, until AIDS became a part of his life. Nothing has been the same since.

Robert H. Gross was born and raised in New York City. A technical writer by trade and an AIDS activist by circumstance, he currently lives in San Francisco with his partner of fifteen years, Tony Mariano, and their cat Chester.

Marny Hall, San Francisco Bay area psychotherapist and author of *The Lavender Couch*, is the sister of the noted author and critic, Richard Hall.

Nels P. Highberg grew up in South Texas before moving to Houston to earn a B.A. in English from the University of Houston. He currently studies in Columbus, Ohio, at the Ohio State University where he will earn an M.A. in Women's Studies in 1995.

Paul E. Hoffman is a Human Resource professional living and working in Providence, Rhode Island. Currently dating again, he is looking forward to building a new life and perhaps relocating.

Evelyn Horowitz is a poet and publisher of *The Bad Henry Review*. Married to the poet Michael Malinowitz, she is currently writing a memoir about her brother Mark Horowitz, from which the piece "Our Lives Expire As A Sigh" is taken.

Kathryn Udetiz Hulings of Fort Collins, Colorado, is married, and the mother of five young children. She is studying to become a registered nurse, and hopes to work in a hospice setting. She enjoys creative writing in her spare time. Most of all, Kathryn cherishes every moment shared with family and friends.

Terence K. Huwe was born in Hermosa Beach, California, and grew up in Ka'u on the island of Hawai'i. He has lived in Berkeley, California, for seventeen years, where he works as the director of a research library at the University of California at Berkeley.

David Israels has worked as a freelance journalist since 1978. His column, "Gay Matters," was probably the first gay column in a nongay newspaper. It appeared in the *San Francisco Bay Guardian* from 1988 through 1990. He currently writes about computer entertainment and lives in San Francisco with his cat, Renee.

Donna Jenson, midwest born and raised, lived and worked as an activist in Brooklyn, New York, for twenty-five years. Months after Ken died, she moved to the Pioneer Valley of western Massachusetts. She now resides in the hilltop home her husband Chug built for them, and runs a consulting practice.

Robert Kaplan is a radical Jewish fag who is trying to turn poetry into political action. He currently lives in San Francisco. Other recent publications include *Modern Words: A Thoroughly Queer International Literary Journal,* and *Beyond Definition: New Gay and Lesbian Writing from San Francisco.*

Sylvia Kimmelman taught high school English for twenty–six years in Brooklyn, New York. Her remaining son Burt is a poet who teaches literature in a New Jersey College. He is the father of Jane, age four, a very good artist.

Gabe Kruks (1950–1992). For many years Gabe Kruks worked in the film industry, but since 1984 he had worked at the Gay and Lesbian Community Services Center in L.A. where he was Chief Operating Officer at the time of his death from AIDS in 1992. Gabe's lover Jurgen Tilsner also worked at the Center, and since 1992 the Center's shelter for homeless youth has been renamed in their double memory.

Stephen Kyle has written for *Bay Windows* and the *Boston Phoenix*. "Words" is part of a collection titled *Fine Lines* which he aims to publish. He's also writing a novel about growing up gay and Catholic called *Going To Hell in My Sleep*.

Jay Ladin's poems have appeared in many magazines. He lived in San Francisco from 1982 to 1992, before returning to the east coast.

Laura Rivero Marcy resides at the South Jersey seashore with her three children, three dogs and four cats. She majored in photography at the School of Visual Arts in New York City. Her work has been shown in Boston and Manhattan. Besides numerous speaking engagements, Laura devotes time to her writing and being director of the Daddy Wayne Pediatric AIDS fund.

William L. McBride is a writer and consultant for educational materials. Other publications include AIDS study guides for schools and a chapter in *You Can Do Something About AIDS*. Bill also helped create *Specialties of the House,* a Chicago restaurant cookbook which raised money for PWAs. He now lives in San Francisco.

John McFarland is the author of the prize–winning *The Exploding Frog and Other Fables from Aesop* (Little Brown). His short stories have appeared in *Ararat, Caliban, Cricket* and *stet*. He is also represented in *The Next Pariah Over: A Collection of Irish–American Writing* (New Rivers Press).

Stephen W. McInnis began writing six years ago after working as an advertising copywriter. He has written a number of short stories and has just finished his first novel. McInnis currently resides in San Francisco, where he is starting his second novel.

Martin McKinsey now lives in Richmond, Virginia. His translations from modern Greek include Andreas Fraghias' novel, *The Courtyard* (Kedros, 1994), and *Late into the Night: The Last Poems of Yannis Ritsos* (Field Translation Series, 1995).

Margaret McMullan's first novel, *When Warhol Was Still Alive* (The Crossing Press), which explores a young woman's friendship with a transvestite who dies of AIDS, is partially dedicated to Ken. She recently received a grant from the Indiana Arts Commission and the National Endowment for the Arts to work on her second novel.

Dorothy Merton is the pseudonym of a National Endowment for the Arts Fellow living in a small Midwestern town where Jay's death is discussed in hushed voices. This voice is hushed only by an alias.

Victor Mingovits was born in New York City. He now lives in Missoula, Montana, where he is a production manager at a weekly newspaper. His collection of poetry, *A Satan Worshiper's Guide to the American Northeast*, was published in 1991 by Watershed Press. He is currently working on a novel.

Beverly Mire is the editorial director of GAVIN, a music industry trade magazine, and an instructor at Youth Radio, a nonprofit program that teaches teenagers all aspects of radio. Ms. Mire was encouraged to write by her late father, Joseph Mire. She lives in Berkeley, California.

Michael Kiesow Moore has won awards for his writing and has been published nationally with articles and short stories appearing in *Equal Time, The James White Review* and *The Evergreen Chronicles*. He is currently working on a Masters of Fine Arts in Writing at Hamline University.

J. Fraser Nelson is the HIV services coordinator for the Minnesota Department of Health. Her next project, "Not Waiting for a Cure," is an oral history of the personal impact of living in the age of AIDS.

Lesléa Newman's poems have appeared in publications ranging from *Common Lives/Lesbian Lives* to *Seventeen* magazine. She has published two collections of poetry: *Love Me Like You Mean It* (Clothespin Fever Press, 1993) and *Sweet Dark Places* (Her Books, 1991). In 1989 she was awarded a Massachusetts Artists Fellowship in Poetry.

Allison J. Nichol is a member of Chicago's Pink Key Writers, and publisher of the *Queer Planet Review*. She has been published in a wide variety of literary magazines and anthologies. Some of her work can be heard on Chicago's Dial–A–Poem.

Nina lives in New York City and works as a copy manager for a direct mail company. She credits her husband Dennis for instilling in her a respect for life and showing her how to live hers to the fullest.

David O'Steinberg grew up in Niantic, Connecticut and now lives in San Francisco. He has published poems and stories in *Cups, James White Review*, and *Processed World*, and in the anthologies, *Bad Attitude* and *The Gay Nineties*. His first book, *Buttoned Up*, is forthcoming from All Is Vanity Press, San Francsico.

Felice Picano is a novelist, dramatist, essayist, poet, small–press publisher, troublemaker, and member of the Violet Quill Club. New books are a gay novel, *Like People in History*; a Sci–Fi novel, *Dryland's End*; and with Jenifer Levin, a book of Lesbian and Gay biographies for children.

Darrell A. Pittman has been involved in a number of AIDS–related projects including college speaking engagements. His poetry has appeared in a variety of gay periodicals in L.A. and Detroit, and also in AIDS organization newsletters. He is currently working on his first novel.

Hernán Poza III has been a social worker in New York City for over fifteen years, working with abused children, runaways, and gay and lesbian youth, as well as HIV counseling and testing. He is currently working as a clinician with severely emotionally disturbed children, and facilitates a support group for men and women with AIDS.

Marcia Rose is a forty-nine-year-old lesbian, mother of six, grandmother-to-be. Currently she has moved from deep mourning, isolation and chaos to a more hopeful survival in San Francisco. Loss, middle age and rage have returned her to activism through writing and making art.

Susan Rosenberg is a longtime political activist. She is in her tenth year of a fifty–eight year prison sentence for politically motivated activities against the government. She is an AIDS educator and peer advocate, as well as a struggling writer.

Suzanne Sablan is a writer and teacher who resides in Orlando, Florida. Her work has appeared in the *West Orange Times* and *Southwest Orlando Bulletin*. Suzanne's most recent work appeared in an anthology entitled *Cupid's Wild*

Arrows: Intercultural Romance and its Consequences. She, too, struggles with the ravages of HIV.

Susan Schulman is a forty-eight-year-old Jewish lesbian living in Oakland, California. She is originally from New York City. She loves creating things— poems, buildings, relationships, origami, films, quilts, animation, programs— and being quiet in the countryside.

Diane Seuss-Brakeman was raised in Niles, Michigan. She currently teaches creative writing at Kalamazoo College in Kalamazoo, Michigan, and has a clinical social work practice above a women's bookstore. She's had poems published in a variety of literary magazines and has recently completed a book-length manuscript of poetry.

John R. Sharkey, a native Chicagoan possessing an M.A. in Communications, moved to Los Angeles in 1972 where he met his lover-to-be, Frank Metcalf. In 1987 they relocated to San Diego and began AIDS volunteer work and activism. Frank died in 1993, leaving John twenty-two years of beautiful memories.

Marcy Sheiner is a freelance writer living in San Francisco. Her work has been published in *Mother Jones, San Francisco Bay Guardian,* and many anthologies and journals. She is currently editing *Herotica 4,* a collection of women's erotica.

Simon Sheppard's work has appeared in a number of magazines including *The James White Review, Five Fingers Review,* and *Art & Understanding,* and in the anthology *Beyond Definition.* He has been a member of ACT UP and is now a volunteer at the San Francisco AIDS Foundation.

Deborah Shouse often feels a restless dissatisfaction with reality. So she creates fiction. Sometimes Deborah feels a quirky fondness for certain versions of reality. So she creates essays. She has a petite book of fiction, *White Bread Love,* and is coauthor of *Working Woman's Communications Survival Guide* (Prentice Hall).

Charles Spaeth lives with his wife and two children in the Methow Valley. He is currently writing a novel.

Su Stout is a writer of fiction, a recent graduate of Fordham University and a copyreader at *Wall Street Journal.* She writes mostly fiction and personal essays, sometimes reporting on gay life in New York. She and her partner Sharon share their lives with four dogs and a cat.

Jean E. Swallow's books include *Leave A Light On For Me, Out From Under,* and *The Next Step.* As he lay dying, her writing partner, Nicholas Carter, asked her to read one of her AIDS poems at his memorial. The poem published here was written to honor that request. Jean Swallow died in 1995.

Diana Tokaji, originally from San Francisco, is a published essayist and a dancer in Washington, DC. Her contributed essay describes a dancer whose artistry prevailed even when chair–bound, and whose dementia invited the two into lyrical dialogue like a last dance. He died the night this work was finished.

Jack Veasey is the author of six published books of poetry. His "Sitting With Gus" was featured with an accompanying photo by Glynis Berger in the national AIDS-themed art exhibit, "A Need To Respond" (Watchung Art Center, Watchung, NJ, 1993).

Megan Wells is a storyteller, actress, and writer. She performs for children and adults, writing and telling original stories from her life including this story, "Thom's Dream." Megan still lives in her hometown, Chicago, with her husband, Gary Shunk, and two wonderful cats, Shakti and Gratitude.

Laura Whitehorn is an anti-imperialist political prisoner, a lesbian, and an HIV/AIDS peer educator/advocate. An antiracist activist since the Civil Rights Movement, she has participated in community organizing, political art, militant demonstrations, and the acts for which she is imprisoned: symbolic bombings directed against U.S. government property, including the Capitol.

Brooke Wiese lives in New York City where she works with young adult volunteers in a service program which might best be described as an "Urban Peace Corps." Her work has appeared in or is forthcoming in *Brooklyn Review, Hawaii Review, The Laurel Review, Plains Poetry Journal,* and elsewhere.

Marti Zuckrowv lives in Oakland, California, where she works as a fitness instructor. Originally a dancer/choreographer, she discovered writing and shifted her focus although not her intent: to create honest, powerful, raw art which is generally (in her own words) not very pretty stuff.